Treatment and Prevention of Malaria

Treatment and Prevention of Malaria

Edited by Kyler Hall

STATES
ACADEMIC PRESS
www.statesacademicpress.com

States Academic Press,
109 South 5th Street,
Brooklyn, NY 11249, USA

Visit us on the World Wide Web at:
www.statesacademicpress.com

ISBN: 978-1-63989-531-1

Cataloging-in-Publication Data

Treatment and prevention of malaria / edited by Kyler Hall.
p. cm.
Includes bibliographical references and index.
ISBN 978-1-63989-531-1
1. Malaria. 2. Malaria--Treatment. 3. Malaria--Prevention. 4. Fever. 5. Protozoan diseases. I. Hall, Kyler.
RC156 .T74 2022
616.936 2--dc23

Table of Contents

Preface

The world is advancing at a fast pace like never before. Therefore, the need is to keep up with the latest developments. This book was an idea that came to fruition when the specialists in the area realized the need to coordinate together and document essential themes in the subject. That's when I was requested to be the editor. Editing this book has been an honour as it brings together diverse authors researching on different streams of the field. The book collates essential materials contributed by veterans in the area which can be utilized by students and researchers alike.

Malaria is one of the diseases which spreads to humans through mosquitoes. It can also spread through blood transfusion or from an infected needle. It is caused by a parasite. Some of the common symptoms of malaria are chills, high fever, diarrhea, cough, vomiting and headache. If not treated timely, malaria can cause severe health complications such as organ failure, cerebral malaria, breathing difficulties and anemia. The most common method to avoid malaria is to take precautions in order to not get bitten by infected mosquitoes. Preventive medicine can also be given if there is a risk of catching infection. The diagnosis of malaria can be done through a physical exam or through a blood test. This book contains some path-breaking studies on the treatment and prevention of malaria. It discusses the fundamentals as well as modern approaches of research within this field. This book will provide comprehensive knowledge to the readers.

Each chapter is a sole-standing publication that reflects each author´s interpretation. Thus, the book displays a multi-facetted picture of our current understanding of application, resources and aspects of the field. I would like to thank the contributors of this book and my family for their endless support.

Editor

1

Severe and Complicated Malaria due to *Plasmodium vivax*

Wilmer E. Villamil-Gómez,
Melisa Eyes-Escalante and Carlos Franco-Paredes

Abstract

Contrary to the widespread belief that severe malaria is mainly caused by *Plasmodium falciparum*, malaria caused by *Plasmodium vivax* infection may also lead to severe clinical manifestations including a plethora of renal, pulmonary, hematologic, neurologic, and multiorgan dysfunction. Anemia and thrombocytopenia are considered as two major important markers of severity during the clinical course of severe *P. vivax* malaria. In highly endemic areas of *P. vivax* transmission, early diagnosis is crucial in preventing uncomplicated episodes progressing into severe and complicated clinical forms. In fact, given the wide geographic distribution of *P. vivax*, there is a large burden of disease, often not adequately acknowledged, and resulting from the combined effect of the large numbers of uncomplicated clinical episodes and the increasingly recognized severe and complicated clinical presentations.

Keywords: *Plasmodium vivax*, clinical manifestations, diagnosis, treatment, severe, complicated

1. Introduction

Globally, malaria remains one of the most important infectious diseases affecting humankind in terms of morbidity and mortality [1, 2]. *Plasmodium vivax* infection and *Plasmodium falciparum* represent the two most frequent and severe forms of human malaria. Individuals acquire the infection by the bite of the female *Anopheles* mosquitoes inoculating microscopic sporozoites that subsequently reach the liver via the bloodstream. Once in the liver, the sporozoites evolve into a schizont that produces merozoites and then releases them into the bloodstream coinciding with the onset of the clinical syndrome of malaria [3]. Most importantly, most deaths associated with malaria occur in children living in highly endemic settings [3]. The large social and economic burden attributable to *P. vivax* in highly endemic settings results from the elevated number of cases that require medical care in an already impoverished economy diverting cash and family members from work to attend the sick [2, 3]. Uncomplicated *P. vivax* malaria refers to a febrile illness where there are no hemodynamic instability, no evidence of major hemolysis, no absence of severe anemia, no evidence of pulmonary edema or ARDS, and no evidence of severe metabolic acidosis, renal failure, hepatic dysfunction, focal neurological deficits or seizures, or multi-organ failure [4, 5]. Historically, severe malaria is often considered exclusively within the clinical spectrum of disease caused by infection due to *P. falciparum*. However, albeit less recognized, infection due to *P. vivax* can also lead to clinically severe manifestations and complications including (a) fatal bleeding due to traumatic or spontaneous rupture of an enlarged spleen, (b) seizures, (c) shock, (d) hepatitis with cholestasis, (e) renal failure, (f) severe anemia and thrombocytopenia, (g) respiratory distress and acute lung injury (ALI), (h) miscarriage and preterm delivery, and (h) multi-organ failure [6]. Of all these complications, the most significant source of morbidity is by far the occurrence of severe anemia and its consequences. Furthermore, in many geographic settings, coinfection of *P. vivax* and *P. falciparum* may occur in the same host, and this can be associated with severe clinical manifestations. Therefore, identifying coinfection in settings where there is co-circulation of both *Plasmodium* spp., the peripheral blood smear is of utmost clinical importance in the early course of a febrile illness in which malaria is a consideration [7]. *P. vivax* malaria was originally described clinically as "benign tertian malaria"; however, this is a misleading concept because *P. vivax* is not a benign disease. In fact, it is increasingly recognized as a major cause of morbidity and mortality in highly endemic settings.

The clinical spectrum of disease associated with *P. vivax* infection ranges from asymptomatic parasitemia and uncomplicated febrile illness to severe and fatal malaria. In this regard, the host response influences the clinical expression of the disease. Fever may occur with low parasite densities and may be identified 2–3 days before the parasites are detected in blood, underscoring the need for serial peripheral blood smear examinations [8]; *P. vivax* has a lower pyrogenic threshold (parasitic density required to evoke a fever) compared with *P. falciparum*. Globally, it is estimated that there are more than 80 million episodes of *P. vivax* malaria every year resulting in a considerable amount of morbidity and mortality. The prevailing neglect of the substantial public health impact of *P. vivax* that occurs in many settings in comparison with that of *P. falciparum* relies on its low incidence in Sub-Saharan Africa as a result of the evolutionary trait of the Duffy antigen negativity selected among many African populations [9].

P. vivax causes almost half of all of the 70–390 million clinical cases of malaria each year. In countries endemic for both major *Plasmodium* species, *P. vivax* infection may account for up to 38% of patients hospitalized with malaria. In Indonesian Papua, *P. vivax* accounted for 24% of malaria admissions in all age groups, of whom 47% (415/887) are infants [6]. The need for hospitalization among these cases indicates significant morbidity, and at least moderately severe disease. Thus, clinicians should be aware of the spectrum of severe disease and of potential multi-organ affection among patients presenting with *P. vivax* malaria [10–37].

2. Parasitology and epidemiology

Infection due to *P. vivax* challenges human health in many settings, particularly in Southeast Asia, in some areas of the Pacific Islands, and in many areas in Latin America, particularly in Venezuela and Brazil [38, 39]. This type of malaria infection affects approximately 100–400 million people each year within a population living at risk of 2.5 billion. Interestingly, *P. vivax* occurs with an extremely low prevalence throughout much of Africa likely as selective pressure led to the emergence of the Duffy antigen negativity or red blood cells across African populations, particularly in West Africa. However, *P. vivax* produces substantial morbidity in some settings at subtropical and temperate latitudes in Asia [11].

P. vivax is responsible for approximately 3.3–30.3% of complications of malaria. In Colombia, *P. vivax* is responsible for almost 75% of cases of malaria. In the country, mortality from 130 to 150 cases per year is recorded, because this situation has been considered the disease as a public health concern with a growing number of complications [10, 11]. *P. vivax* accounted for 24% of malaria admissions in all age groups, including 47% of them among infants. In a recent autopsy-based report from Brazil, at least four of 17 (23.5%) *P. vivax*-associated deaths in Brazil were attributable to alternative causes at the time of death, including meningitis and yellow fever, underscoring the ability of this infection to manifest with severe disease often mimicking other conditions traditionally considered to produce severe clinical manifestations. Mortality rates in those hospitalized in Indonesian Papua with microscopy-confirmed *P. vivax* were reported as 0.8–1.6%, similar to that of *P. falciparum* infection (1.6–2.2%)). The adjusted odds ratio of death from severe anemia in Papua, Indonesia, was 5.9 for those with *P. falciparum* and 4.4 for those with *P. vivax* infection [12, 13]. Differences in intensity of transmission might contribute to the variation in the spectrum of disease severity, as it occurs with falciparum malaria. Prospective studies from Papua New Guinea conducted to address mortality associated with *P. vivax* infection have shown a mortality rate of 1.6% among hospitalized patients with *P. vivax* and of 2.2% among those infected with *P. falciparum*. These facts illustrate the similarities in terms of clinical outcomes between both types of human malaria. Further studies are needed to define *P. vivax* attributable mortality in endemic areas along with clinical studies to elucidate the precise pathophysiological and clinical spectrum of disease and from a public health perspective, the overall magnitude of morbidity and mortality associated with *P. vivax* malaria [14].

3. Pathogenesis and disease transmission

The clinical spectrum of disease of *P. vivax* infection in humans is influenced by many factors: the parasite, parasite-host interactions, host factors, and socioeconomic environment in which these infections occur [3–5]. For example, low socioeconomic status is associated with higher risk of developing severe anemia [3]. Studies of specific organs have also shown that the inflammatory response during infection with *P. vivax* is of greater magnitude compared with that seen in *P. falciparum* infection and also with a parasite biomass similar or greater. Moreover, cytokine production in *P. vivax* infections is quantitatively more robust than in *P. falciparum* infections with a similar parasite biomass.

P. vivax infections relapse at intervals of 3–4 weeks, and progressive anemia is associated with recurrent episodes of hemolysis and dyserythropoiesis. In areas with chloroquine resistance, this is further aggravated by the elimination of delayed parasite infection and risk of reactivation. The low number of *P. vivax* parasites indicates that severe anemia may not be produced by the destruction of infected erythrocytes. This is further evident from the fact that it has been shown that during *P. vivax* malaria therapy studies have shown that for each infected erythrocyte destroyed, 32 uninfected erythrocytes are cleared from the bloodstream. This contrasts with the loss of only a few infected red blood cells during *P. falciparum* malaria. The mechanisms underlying this difference are not known; the proportion of uninfected erythrocytes destroyed compared to the proportion of extravascular subject (e.g., splenic) pooling is also not known. Recent studies show an increased fragility microfluidics of infected erythrocytes [14–16]. Pathogenic mechanisms leading to severe symptoms not known exactly, but it have suggested that a failure of the immune system to control parasite replication or immunopathological response resulting from excessive inflammation; they are considered as contributing factors in this response malaria parasites and parasite-infected red blood cells that activate dendritic cells activate dendritic. Parasite antigen presenting T helper (Th) 1 cells triggers a pro-inflammatory response. The inflammatory response required to eliminate parasites may produce tissue damage and activation of phagocytes with production of a cytokine cascade [17].

4. Clinical manifestations

When evaluating patients presenting with a clinical syndrome compatible with malaria, there are no specific signs or symptoms to assist clinicians in distinguishing infection due to Plasmodium vivax or plasmodium falciparum; or when there is coinfection by the two species. Fever in young children may produce seizures. Some individuals progress rapidly to respiratory failure caused by either pulmonary edema or even acute respiratory distress syndrome (ARDS). Among those with rapid clinical deterioration, we should always consider the concomitant risk of gram-negative bacteremias among individuals with either *P. vivax* or *P. falciparum* infection [6, 7]. The main serious manifestation in most series of vivax malaria in children is severe anemia, defined as hemoglobin < 5 g/dl in children and < 7 g/dl in adults [18]. The pathogenesis of severe malaria is caused by erythrocyte destruction after the invasion of the parasite by its multiplication and also by morphological deformity of the infected red blood cell with opsonization and antibody-dependent lysis of erythrocytes. Indeed, *P. vivax*-infected red blood cells are minimally tacky and are more deformable than *P. falciparum* erythrocytes resulting in relatively low red cell sequestration in microvasculature and bone sinuses and the passage of a greater proportion of erythrocytes through the reticuloendothelial spleen and other organs infected [19]. Recurrent episodes of *P. vivax* infection in highly endemic settings contribute to a higher risk of severe anemia [20, 21]. Acute respiratory distress syndrome (ARDS) occurs often in patients with severe *P. vivax* [22, 23]. Among patients with Plasmodium vivax infection and presenting with severe clinical manifestating it is important to identify splenic rupture early. In fact, the incidence of splenic rupture is as high as 24%. Factors leading to Splenic rupyure include: rapid hyperplasia and parenchymal splenic capsule, forming small infarcts bleeding, loss connective tissue fibrosis and alterations of primary immunity [6, 10].

Acute kidney injury may occur in both children and adults, and it may result for oliguric renal failure or even from acute tubular necrosis [24, 25]. Many patients present with multi-organ failure and hemodynamic instability requiring vasopressor support and often mechanical ventilation. Others may develop acute kidney injury from hypovolemic shock secondary to splenic rupture. All of these potential clinical scenarios should be considered among those with severe *P. vivax* infection and particularly among those with rapid clinical deterioration often requiring intensive care support. In some settings, *P. vivax* may present with concomitant bacterial infection including non-typhoidal salmonellosis or even with enteric fever [26–29]. Finally, patients may also develop seizure disorder or focal neurologic deficits during the clinical course of *P. vivax* mono-infection or when coinfected with *P. falciparum* [30–32]. Early recognition and institution of appropriate interventions are crucial to improve overall clinical outcomes.

5. Diagnosis of severe vivax malaria

Appropriate management of individuals with *P. vivax* requires confirmation of the diagnosis by peripheral smear examination. Coinfection with *P. falciparum* should be entertained in settings where there are co-circulations of both *Plasmodium* species [30]. Early institution of anti-parasitic therapy is instrumental. Additionally, ruling out coinfection with bacterial diseases such as non-typhoidal salmonellosis or by other enteric-gram-negative bacteria is of utmost clinical relevance. Supportive management in intensive care units should be early instituted among those with rapid progression to multi-organ failure and among those with persistent hypotension despite volume resuscitation or requiring vasopressors due to persistent hemodynamic instability. Search for potential splenic rupture needs to be considered at the time of initial presentation, or during the course of illness, among those with rapid clinical deterioration or those developing severe anemia.

6. Treatment of severe vivax malaria

A summary of core concepts in the management of severe malaria due to *P. vivax* is depicted in **Table 1**. Clinical trials to assess optimal treatment regimens of *P. vivax* malaria are limited. At this point in time, in many settings, treatment of vivax malaria consists of chloroquine or an artemisinin-based combination therapy. In those settings where chloroquine resistance remains low, chloroquine may be used as monotherapy with continuous clinical monitoring. However, in most settings, an artemisinin-based combination therapy has become the standard of care due to the growing recognition of vivax malaria causing severe disease, also due to the risk of coinfection with *P. falciparum* (in settings with co-circulation of both species), and finally due to the increasing rates of resistance to chloroquine. Some areas consider a universal policy of treatment with an artemisinin-based combination therapy (artemether-lumefantrine) that is considered the treatment of choice since this drug combination is well tolerated and safe to pregnant women and children [34]. Additionally, there is an increasing recognition of treatment failure when using chloroquine or the combination of chloroquine/sulfadoxine-pyrimethamine [35–37].

Clinical category	Core concepts
Respiratory failure	Protect airway Provide supplemental oxygen Rule out other causes of concomitant respiratory failure (i.e., bacterial pneumonia, pulmonary embolism, or others)
Acute pulmonary edema	Oxygen supplementation BIPAP or mechanical ventilation via endotracheal intubation if needed. Patient often requires PEEP given the possibility of ARDS
Shock	Potentially caused by either hypovolemia due to bleeding or septic shock from gram-negative bacteremia Obtain blood cultures; administer broad spectrum antibiotics; correct hemodynamic disturbances Rule out splenic rupture with abdominal ultrasound or computed tomography Surgical consultation
Acute renal failure	Exclude prerenal causes Fluid replacement Hemodialysis or hemofiltration if indicated (i.e., worsening acute kidney injury, acute tubular necrosis, concomitant severe acidosis, and/or hyperkalemia)
Seizures	Protect airway Benzodiazepines Other antiseizure medications: Dilantin
Acidosis	Exclude or treat hypoglycemia, hypovolemia, and sepsis If severe, performing hemofiltration or hemodialysis is indicated
Severe anemia	Blood transfusion
Antiparasitic treatment	First-line treatment Second-line treatment of complicated malaria Quinine dihydrochloride combined with either clindamycin (300 mg) or doxycycline (100 mg) tablets Presumptive anti-relapse therapy with primaquine is required to eradicate the liver stage of *P. vivax* (hypnozoite), similar to *P. ovale* in both low-transmission and high-transmission settings

Table 1. Clinical spectrum and management of severe/complicated *P. vivax* malaria.

The spread of drug-resistant *P. vivax* to parts of Indonesia, other parts of Southeast Asia, and South America highlights the urgent need to revisit the spectrum of disease and of the burden of vivax malaria in order to implement control measures and allocate adequate resources against this neglected infectious disease [1, 37].

7. Conclusion

Malaria infection remains as a leading infectious diseases affecting humankind due to its associated large burden of disease. There is a growing recognition that *P. vivax* contributes to a large proportion of this burden. In particular, coinfection of *P. vivax* and *P. falciparum* seems to be synergistic in terms of leading to severe disease, complications, and death among the most vulnerable populations. The spectrum of disease severity associated with *P. vivax* infection ranges from respiratory failure to renal failure. However, the most important marker of disease severity across borders is produced by hematological abnormalities including severe anemia and thrombocytopenia. Further research is warranted to address the large epidemiologic burden of disease associated with *P. vivax* and to identify preventive strategies. From a clinical perspective, there is a need for further clinical studies to identify strategies to optimize the clinical management of vivax malaria.

Author details

Wilmer E. Villamil-Gómez[1,2,3,4*], Melisa Eyes-Escalante[3,4] and Carlos Franco-Paredes[5]

*Address all correspondence to: wvillamil07@gmail.com

1 Committee on Zoonoses and Haemorrhagic Fevers, Colombian Association of Infectious Diseases, Bogotá, DC, Colombia

2 Infectious Diseases and Infection Control Research Group, Sincelejo University Hospital, Sincelejo, Sucre, Colombia

3 Doctoral Program of Tropical Medicine, SUE – Caribe, University of Atlántico, Barranquilla, Colombia

4 Biodiversity Research Group of the Colombian Caribbean, Faculty of Basic Sciences, University of Atlántico, Barranquilla, Colombia

5 Children's Hospital of Mexico, Federico Gomez and Infectious Diseases Department and Phoebe Putney Memorial Hospital, Albany, GA, USA

References

[1] Rodríguez-Morales AJ, Paniz-Mondolfi AE. Venezuela's failure in malaria control. Lancet 2014; 384(9944):663-664.

[2] Rodriguez-Morales AJ. Malaria: an eradicable threat? [Editorial]. J Infect Dev Ctries 2008 Feb; 2(1):1-2.

[3] Rodriguez-Morales AJ, Bolívar-Mejía A, Alarcón-Olave C, Calvo-Betancourt LS. Plasmodium vivax malaria in Latin America. In: C. Franco-Paredes, J.I. Santos-Preciado (eds.). Neglected Tropical Diseases – Latin America and the Caribbean, Neglected Tropical Diseases. Springer-Verlag Wien, 2015. doi: 10.1007/978-3-7091-1422-3_5. Pages 23. ISBN: 978-3-7091-1421-6. Pp: 89-111.

[4] World Health Organization. Severe malaria. Trop Med Int Health 2014; 19(Supp 1):S7-S131.

[5] World Health Organization. Severe falciparum malaria. Trans R Soc Trop Med Hyg 2000; 94(Supp 1):S1-S90.

[6] Gachot B, Ringwald P. Severe malaria. Rev Prat. 1998;48:273–8.

[7] Bartoloni A, Zammarchi L. Clinical aspects of uncomplicated and severe malaria. Mediterr J Hematol Infect Dis. 2012;4.

[8] Anstey NM, Douglas NM, Poespoprodjo JR, Price RN. *Plasmodium vivax*: Clinical Spectrum, Risk Factors and Pathogenesis [Internet]. Advances in Parasitology. Elsevier; 2012. Available from: http://dx.doi.org/10.1016/B978-0-12-397900-1.00003-7.

[9] Bassat Q, Alonso PL. Defying malaria: Fathoming severe Plasmodium vivax disease. Nat Med [Internet]. 2011;17(1):48–9. Available from: http://dx.doi.org/10.1038/nm0111-48.

[10] Bastidas AR, Quiroga LJ, Aponte JE, Aztorquiza MH, Perez CE. Multiorgan Failure caused by a splenic hematoma secondary to Plasmodium vivax infection. 2014;18(3): 116–9.

[11] Kevin BJ. Evidence and implications of mortality associated with acute Plasmodium vivax malaria. Clin Microbiol Rev. 2013;26(1):36–57.

[12] Kaushik JS, Gomber S, Dewan P. Clinical and epidemiological profiles of severe malaria in children from Delhi, India. J Heal Popul Nutr. 2012;30:113–6.

[13] Lança EFC, Magalhães BML, Vitor-Silva S, Siqueira AM, Benzecry SG, Alexandre MAA, et al. Risk factors and characterization of Plasmodium vivax-associated admissions to pediatric intensive care units in the Brazilian Amazon. PLoS One. 2012;7(4).

[14] Anstey NM, Russell B, Yeo TW, Price RN. The pathophysiology of vivax malaria. Trends Parasitol. 2009; 25(April):220–7.

[15] Anstey NM, Handojo T, Pain MCF, Kenangalem E, Price RN, Maguire GP. UKPMC Funders Group. Lung injury in vivax malaria: Pathophysiological evidence for pulmonary vascular sequestration and posttreatment alveolar-capillary inflammation. Baseline. 2008; 195 (May 2004):589–96.

[16] Karunaweera ND, Grau GE, Gamage P, Carter R, Mendis KN. Dynamics of fever and serum levels of tumor necrosis factor are closely associated during clinical paroxysms in Plasmodium vivax malaria. Proc Natl Acad Sci U S A. 1992; 89 (April): 3200–3.

[17] Raza A, Khan MS, Ghanchi NK, Raheem A, Beg M Tumour necrosis factor, interleukin-6 and interleukin-10 are possibly involved in Plasmodium vivax-associated thrombocytopaenia in southern Pakistani population. Malar J [Internet]. 2014;13:323. Available from: http://www.pubmedcentral.nih.gov/articlerender.fcgi?artid=4141950&tool=pmcentrez&rendertype=abstract.

[18] Rodriguez-Morales AJ, Benitez JA, Arria M. Malaria mortality in Venezuela: Focus on deaths due to Plasmodium vivax in children. J Trop Pediatr. 2008;54 (September 2005): 94–101.

[19] Douglas NM, Anstey NM, Buffet PA, Poespoprodjo JR, Yeo TW, White NJ, et al. The anaemia of Plasmodium vivax malaria. Malar J. 2012;11:1–14.

[20] Price RN, Douglas NM, Anstey NM. New developments in Plasmodium vivax malaria: severe disease and the rise of chloroquine resistance. Curr Opin Infect Dis [Internet]. 2009;22:430–5. Available from: http://www.ncbi.nlm.nih.gov/entrez/query.fcgi?cmd=Retrieve&db=PubMed&dopt=Citation&list_uids=19571748.

[21] O'Donnell A, Premawardhena A, Arambepola M, Samaranayake R, Allen SJ, Peto TEA, et al. Interaction of malaria with a common form of severe thalassemia in an Asian population. Proc Natl Acad Sci U S A [Internet]. 2009;106:18716–21. Available from: http://www.pnas.org/content/106/44/18716.full.

[22] Tan LK, Yacoub S, Scott S, Bhagani S, Jacobs M. Acute lung injury and other serious complications of Plasmodium vivax malaria. Lancet Infect Dis [Internet]. 2008;8:449–54. Available from: http://www.thelancet.com/journals/laninf/article/PIIS1473-3099(08)70153-1/fulltext\nhttp://www.ncbi.nlm.nih.gov/entrez/query.fcgi?cmd=Retrieve&db=PubMed&dopt=Citation&list_uids=18582837.

[23] Yadav D, Chandra J, Aneja S, Kumar V, Kumar P, Dutta AK. Changing profile of severe malaria in North Indian children. Indian J Pediatr. 2012;79 (April): 483–7.

[24] Taylor WRJ, Hanson J, Turner GDH, White NJ, Dondorp AM. Respiratory manifestations of Malaria. Chest. 2012; 142: 492–505.

[25] Kochar DK, Tanwar GS, Khatri PC, Kochar SK, Sengar GS, Gupta A, et al. Clinical features of children hospitalized with Malaria – A study from Bikaner, Northwest India. Am J Trop Med Hyg. 2010; 83(5):981–9.

[26] Andrade BBB, Reis-Filho A, Souza-Neto SMM, Clarêncio J, Camargo LMA, Barral A, et al. Severe *Plasmodium vivax* malaria exhibits marked inflammatory imbalance. Malar J. 2010; 9:13.

[27] Manning L, Laman M, Law I, Bona C, Aipit S, Teine D, et al. Features and prognosis of severe malaria caused by Plasmodium falciparum, Plasmodium vivax and mixed Plasmodium species in Papua New Guinean children. PLoS One. 2011; 6(12).

[28] Quispe AM, Pozo E, Guerrero E, Durand S, Baldeviano GC, Edgel KA., et al. Plasmodium vivax hospitalizations in a monoendemic malaria region: Severe vivax Malaria? Am J Trop Med Hyg. 2014; 91:11–7.

[29] Bhattacharya SK, Sur D, Dutta S, Kanungo S, Ochiai RL, Kim DR, et al. Vivax malaria and bacteraemia: a prospective study in Kolkata, India. Malar J [Internet]. Malaria J; 2013;12(1):176. Available from: http://www.pubmedcentral.nih.gov/articlerender.fcgi?artid=3691654&tool=pmcentrez&rendertype=abstract.

[30] Valecha N, Pinto RGW, Turner GDH, Kumar A, Rodrigues S, Dubhashi NG, et al. Case report: histopathology of fatal respiratory distress caused by Plasmodium vivax malaria. Am J Trop Med Hyg. 2009; 81(2):758–62.

[31] Imbert P, Rapp C, Buffet PA. Pathological rupture of the spleen in malaria: Analysis of 55 cases (1958–2008). Travel Med Infect Dis [Internet]. 2009; 7(3):147–59. Available from: http://dx.doi.org/10.1016/j.tmaid.2009.01.002.

[32] Ozsoy MF, Oncul O, Pekkafali Z, Pahsa A, Yenen OS. Splenic complications in malaria: Report of two cases from Turkey. J Med Microbiol. 2004; 53(May):1255–8.

[33] Nurleila S, Syafruddin D, Elyazar IRF, Baird E JK. Serious and fatal illness associated with falciparum and vivax malaria among patients admitted to hospital at West Sumba in Eastern Indonesia. Am J Trop Med Hyg. 2012; 87(69):41–9.

[34] Bassat Q. The use of artemether-lumefantrine for the treatment of uncomplicated Plasmodium vivax malaria. PLoS Negl Trop Dis. 2011; 5(12).

[35] McGready R, Boel M, Rijken MJ, Ashley EA, Cho T, Moo O, et al. Effect of early detection and treatment on malaria related maternal mortality on the north-western border of Thailand 1986–2010. PLoS One. 2012; 7(7).

[36] Tjitra E, Anstey NM, Sugiarto P, Warikar N, Kenangalem E, Karyana M, et al. Multidrug-resistant Plasmodium vivax associated with severe and fatal malaria: A prospective study in Papua, Indonesia. PLoS Med. 2008; 5(6):0890–9.

[37] Ministerio de la Protección Social de Colombia, Instituto Nacional de Salud, OPS. Guidelines for surveillance of malaria. 2011; 1–25.

[38] Rodríguez-Morales AJ, Sánchez E, Vargas M, Piccolo C, Colina R, Arria M, Franco-Paredes C. Is anemia in Plasmodium vivax malaria more frequent and severe than in Plasmodium falciparum? Am J Med 2006; 119(11):e9-e10.

[39] Rodríguez-Morales AJ, Giselle-Badillo A, Manrique-Castaño S, Yepes MC. Anemia and thrombocytopenia in Plasmodium vivax malaria is not unusual in patients from endemic and non-endemic settings. Travel Med Infect Dis 2014; 12(5):549-550.

2

Secondary Malaria Vectors of Sub-Saharan Africa: Threat to Malaria Elimination on the Continent?

Yaw Asare Afrane, Mariangela Bonizzoni and Guiyun Yan

Abstract

Secondary vectors of malaria include those anopheline species that are known to play minor part in malaria transmission. Primary vectors of malaria in Africa are *Anopheles gambiae* s.s, *Anopheles coluzzii, Anopheles arabiensis, Anopheles funestus, Anopheles moucheti* and *Anopheles nili*, while *Anopheles rivolorum, Anopheles pharoensis, Anopheles ziemanni*, among others are secondary vectors. They are recognized for their importance in malaria transmission, as they may help to augment or extend the malaria transmission period and potentially sustain malaria transmission after the main indoor resting and indoor biting vectors have been reduced by vector control measures such as indoor residual spraying or Long-lasting insecticidal nets (LLINs). Thus, the terminology "secondary" versus "primary" vector is fluid and forged by ecological conditions and malaria control strategies. Most secondary vectors are outdoor resting and outdoor biting are thus, not taken care of in the current control methods. High use of insecticides for vector control in Africa, climate change, unprecedented land use changes in Africa are some of the factors that could influence the conversion of secondary vectors to become main vectors in Africa. This chapter examines the role of secondary vectors in malaria transmission and the possibility of them becoming main vectors in future.

Keywords: secondary vectors, main vectors, exophilic, exophagic, malaria elimination, residual malaria transmission

1. Introduction

Malaria is still a major public health problem in sub-Saharan Africa despite the massive investment in intervention measures that have been rolled out within the last decade and have produced a decline of 37% of malaria cases [1]. Main interventions include the scaling up of vector control through long-lasting insecticidal nets (LLINs) and indoor residual spraying (IRS) [2], as well as the introduction of ACT and improved malaria diagnostic [1]. Malaria transmission dynamics within sub-Saharan African countries is highly variable. Transmission can occur throughout the year (in particular with areas that receive rainfall twice a year) or only during a few months in the year (in particular with areas that has only one transmission season) and even then heterogeneities in transmission are observed between years within the same area. Inoculation rates vary from 0 to over a 1000 infective bites per year. Some areas have sole vectors that are involved in transmission of parasites to the human population while others could have several vectors that will consist of main vectors and secondary vectors. Differences in ecological requirements, longevity and feeding behavior (e.g. anthropophily and endophily) account for the different roles played by main and secondary vectors in malaria transmission in Africa [3].

Secondary vectors of malaria include those anopheline species that are known to play or suspected of playing a minor part in malaria transmission. With over 140 species of anopheline species in sub-Saharan Africa, <20 of them are able to transmit malaria to humans [4]. There are some six species that are considered to be major malaria vectors that are responsible for 95% of the total malaria transmission on the continent [5]. These are *Anopheles gambiae* Giles, *Anopheles coluzzii* Coetzee & Wilkerson sp. n, *Anopheles arabiensis* Patton, *Anopheles funestus* Giles, *Anopheles moucheti* Evans and *Anopheles nili* Theobald [5, 6]. The remaining (5%) is transmitted by "secondary vectors" or "vectors that are normally of local importance" [5] that include *Anopheles rivolorum* Leeson [7], *Anopheles pharoensis* Theobald [8], *Anopheles coustani* Laveran [9], Anopheles *ziemanni* Grtünberg [10] *Anopheles squamosus* Theobald [11]. Secondary vectors have been recognized for their importance in malaria transmission, as they may help to augment or extend the malaria transmission period [12, 13]. Moreover, it is known that many of these secondary vectors are exophilic (outdoor resting) and exophagic (outdoor biting) and therefore has the potential to sustain transmission of malaria after the main vectors have been reduced by indoor control measures such as indoor residual spraying or insecticide-treated bednet (ITN) use [3, 8, 14].

The current malaria vector intervention tools are all indoor and insecticide based. This is because the main malaria vectors in Africa are majorly endophagic and endophilic. Secondary vectors that could be exophagic and exophilic or could bite earlier indoors before people sleep under their LLINs and those that move between being zoophilic (tendency to bite animals only) and anthropophilic (tendency to bite humans only) are left out of the current control methods. However, a few secondary vectors have been known historically to flourish and take over malaria transmission after the main vector(s) have been suppressed [7]. High use of insecticides for vector control in Africa, climate change, unprecedented land use and land cover changes that is ongoing in many parts of Africa are some of the factors that could influence the conversion of secondary vectors to become main vectors in sub-Saharan Africa.

Secondary vectors are species that frequently have relatively little contact with man and are perhaps less likely to be affected by house-spraying with residual insecticides and the use of insecticide impregnated bednets than are the primary vectors. This chapter emphasizes the importance of such secondary vectors. It examines the role of secondary vectors in malaria transmission and the possibility of them becoming main vectors in future, as many countries in sub-Saharan Africa drive towards the elimination of the disease. It highlights the overall malaria parasite transmission intensity by these secondary vectors in several sites across Africa. Historical evidence is presented in this chapter to underscore the possibility of secondary vectors becoming main vectors. For instance, *An. arabiensis* was considered a secondary vector of malaria some decades back but is now one of the most important vectors in Africa.

2. Contribution of secondary vectors to malaria transmission in different parts of sub-Saharan Africa

Secondary vectors just like the main vectors are distributed all over sub-Saharan Africa. From Senegal in the west of Africa through Cameroun to Ethiopia and down to Angola, each country has a few of them that could be either transmitting malaria or not and all of them contributes to 5% of malaria transmission on the continent. They are therefore of importance to the sustenance of malaria transmission. Some secondary vectors have historically been known to be transmitting sporozoites of malaria parasites, albeit, at a lower rate whilst some vectors have been known to bite man but have not been found carrying malaria parasites. For instance, the *An. coustani* have been reported to be carrying sporozoites of malaria parasites in Tanzania [8] and the Democratic Republic of Congo [10] in whilst *An. ziemanni* were found in Ethiopia and Cameroon in the 1950s to be infected with *Plasmodium* sporozoites [10]. *An. rivolorum* was also found in Kenya and Tanzania transmitting malaria in the late 1950s [7]. *An. pharoensis* was found with sporozoites in Tanzania [8] and Baukina Faso (formerly Upper Volta) [15]. *An. squamosus* sensu stricto Theobald was found with sporozoites in Muheza, Tanzania [11]. The following is an account of these secondary vectors and their contribution to malaria transmission according to the sub-regions of sub-Saharan Africa.

2.1. Western Africa

Around the Senegal River delta, *An. pharoensis* Theobald has been found to be the most prevalent man-biting anopheline mosquito. In one area, 5/912 of *An. pharoensis* examined were sporozoite positive [16], while in another area 3/396 were infected with *Plasmodium falciparum* sporozoites [17]. These were all living in sympatry with the main vector *An. gambiae* Giles sensu lato of which 98 were caught and none were positive for malaria sporozoites. Only 1/3076 of *An. funestus* was found to be with sporozoites. Other secondary vectors found there included, *An. coustani, Anopheles wellcomei* and *Anopheles rufipes*. These studies suggest that *An. pharoensis* has a bigger role to play in malaria transmission in this area of Senegal, than even the main malaria vectors.

In Gambia, presumed secondary vectors are *An. pharoensis, An. ziemanni, An. squamosus* and *An. rufipes,* which were caught in experimental huts. Their role in malaria transmission is still uncertain as Plasmodium infections were not checked [12, 13]. In Côte-d'Ivoire, *An. ziemanni* was the most abundant species (32.5% of the total vectors) caught as larvae in rice paddies in the western part of the country [14].

In Ghana, *An. pharoensis, An. coustani* and *An. rufipes* were the main secondary vectors that have been sampled. In the coastal savannah area of Kpone-on-Sea, *An. pharoensis* was sampled among other main malaria vectors using human landing catches (0.1 of 1233 vectors caught) [18]. *An. coustani* was also sampled (6/1642) in a nearby urban Accra also using human landing catches. In the forest-savannah transitional town of Kintampo, *An. rufipes* was sampled in night catches using CDC light traps and constituted 370/9391 of anophelines that were captured [19]. None of these vectors were tested by the authors for the presence of malaria sporozoites, and therefore, their contribution to malaria transmission in Ghana is not known; however, the fact that they were caught in human landing catches suggest their strong anthropophilic tendency.

In Baukina Faso, 3/3385 of *An. ziemanni* and *An. coustani* collected haboured sporozoites of malaria parasites [15]. In Benin, main secondary vectors were *An. pharoensis* and *An. coustani* in night catches in the northeastern Benin [20] whilst *An. ziemanni, An. pharoensis* and *An. coustani* have been sampled in southeastern Benin [21]. However, none were infected with Plasmodium parasites.

2.2. Central Africa

In irrigated rice fields in Goulmoun in south western Chad, four vectors were identified with a different human biting rate: *An. arabiensis* at 51 bites/human/night was the most efficient biting vector, followed by *An. pharoensis* (12.5), *An. funestus* (0.15 b/h/n) and *An. ziemanni* (1.3 b/h/n). The circumsporozoite protein rate was 1.4% for *An. arabiensis,* 1.4% for *An. funestus,* 0.8% for *An. pharoensis* and 0.5% for *An. ziemanni.* The overall annual EIR was estimated at 311 bites of infected anophelines/human/year, contributed mostly by *An. arabiensis* (84.5%) and *An. pharoensis* (12.2%) [22]. This study revealed the implication of *An. pharoensis* and to some extent *An. ziemanni* in malaria transmission in the area complementing the major role played by *An. arabiensis.*

Cameroun seems to be the country with most secondary vectors implicated in malaria transmission. In northwest of Cameroon, *An. ziemanni* was the main malaria vector. It was found in both outdoor and indoor catches with a range of 6.75–8.29 b/p/n and 0.063 infectious bites per person per night (ib/p/n) [23]. Studies have shown nine secondary vectors with history of carrying *Plasmodium sporozoites, namely*: An. *coustani* Laveran, *Anopheles ovengensis* Awono-Ambene et al., *Anopheles carnevalei* Brunhes et al., *Anopheles hancocki* Edwards, *Anopheles marshallii* (Theobald), *Anopheles paludis* Theobald, *An. pharoensis* Theobald, *An. wellcomei* Theobald and *An. ziemanni* Grtünberg [3, 12]. These constituted 11% of all anophelines sampled and with infection rate of 1.36% compared to 3.08% for the main vectors that live in sympatry with them. *An. pharoensis* and *An. ovengensis* were repeatedly found infected by *P. falciparum* and contributed substantially to the total malaria transmission intensity in some areas where they were abundant. Though these vectors showed strong exophilic and/or exophagic habits, they might elude vector control directed against endophilic and endophagic malaria vectors. In this same area, *An. pharoensis* has been reported since 1961 to be carrying Plasmodium infections [23, 24]. This shows that when conditions become favorable or when it becomes the most abundant vector in the area, it has the potential to assume the role of the main vector.

Anopheles coustani complex mosquitoes have been found harboring sporozoites in Katanga in the Democratic Republic of the Congo [10]. *An. paludis* Theobald, a member of the *An. coustani* group, has been reported as a vector in the Congo with sporozoite rates as high as 10% [25].

2.3. Eastern Africa

Anopheles pharoensis and *An. ziemanni* seems to be the most important secondary vectors in east Africa. In Ethiopia, *An. pharoensis* is the most prevalent secondary vector. It was the second most abundant malaria vector after *An. arabiensis* in irrigated rice paddies in central part of the country. *An. pharoensis* showed a slight preference for human blood (63.6%) over bovines (49.5%) and had 7.5 infective bites per person per year compared to 27.3 for *An. arabiensis. An. coustani* was also sampled in this study but none of them was infected with any Plasmodium parasites [26]. In an area close by in south-central Ethiopia, *An. pharoensis* was sampled with high human blood index (HBI) and carrying *Plasmodium vivax* [27]. *An. pharoensis* and *An. ziemanni* were also sampled in another study, most of which had taken human blood meals but none infected with Plasmodium parasites [28].

In Kenya, *An. pharoensis* was sampled from the Mwea irrigation scheme in Central Kenya, and it constituted 15.69% of the total anopheline catches, with *P. falciparum* sporozoite rates of 1.3% by ELISA and 0.68% by dissection, while those for *An. funestus* were 1.7% by ELISA and 1.25% by dissection [13]. In the same area, *Anopheles parensis* was the main member of the *An. funestus* species group found resting inside human dwellings in Mwea area of central Kenya. Even though none of them were positive for *P. falciparum* sporozoites, they had high human blood index (HBI) indicating that they have been biting humans indoors [29].

Anopheles ziemanni Grunberg was sampled resting inside several human dwellings in western Kenya. Although none of the *An. ziemanni* sampled were infected with *P. falciparum* sporozoites, the density of this species and their human blood index compared well with the other main vectors. This suggest that there is a possible role in malaria transmission [30]. Another study [31] also found *An. ziemanni* to have an HBI that was not significantly different from that of *An. arabiensis*, an important vector of malaria in Kenya and especially in rice irrigation schemes. Studies carried out in Ethiopia and Cameroon in the 1950s each found *An. ziemanni* mosquitoes to be infected with *Plasmodium* sporozoites [32], this suggests that this mosquito species is indeed susceptible to malaria parasites and can play a role in malaria transmission. Earlier studies in the same area also found proportions of *An. ziemanni* out of all mosquitoes collected that were higher than those of *An. gambiae s.l.* and *An. funestus* by factors of 2.6 and 43.7, respectively [33].

In Tanzania, *An. squamosus, An. coustani and An. ziemanni* have been historically implicated in malaria transmission [9].

2.4. Southern Africa

Anopheles coustani s.l. Laveran and *An. squamosus* Theobald have been reported in southern Zambia to demonstrate an unexpected high degree of anthropophilic tendencies, even though they have generally been of negligible importance to malaria transmission due to their overwhelmingly zoophilic behavior. They also have been found foraging during early evening and the majority of blood meals from these mosquito species were from human hosts. Although no *An. coustani s.l.* or *An. squamosus* were found to be positive for Plasmodium species, the demonstrated anthropophilic tendencies of these mosquitoes in southern Zambia suggest their potential as secondary vectors of malaria [34]. In eastern Zambia, Lobo et al. [9] also observed unexpected number of sporozoite positive mosquitoes in some secondary vectors, namely, *Anopheles rivulorum* (2/30), *Anopheles theileri* (2/14) and the *An. coustani* group (12/340). *An. coustani* was more anthropophilic than its siblings.

Similarly, studies from Mozambique displayed high anthropophilic behavior with early peaks in foraging activity with *An. coustani s.l.* There was a combination of outdoor and early evening foraging behavior for these species and this could increase their potential as secondary vectors in areas where indoor control measures such as indoor residual spraying or LLINs are employed [35].

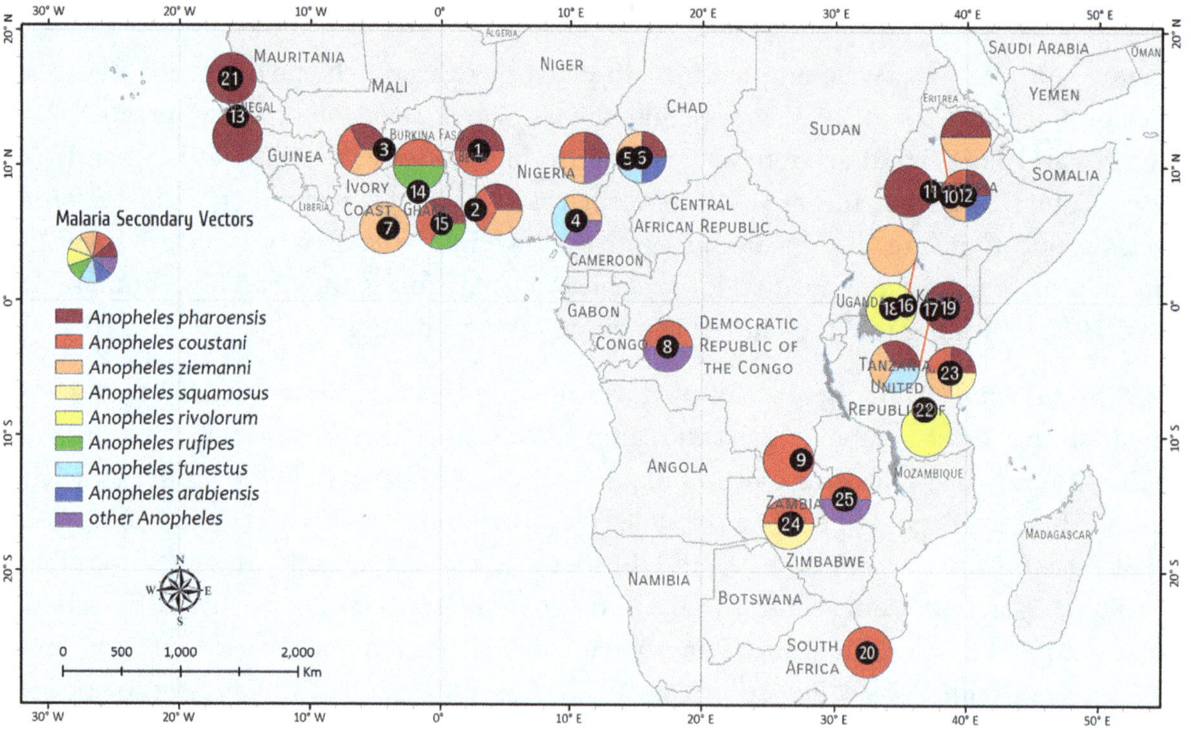

Figure 1. A map showing the distribution of the secondary vectors discussed from sub-Saharan Africa.

All these shows that these secondary vectors do assume anthropophilic behaviors, could get infected with plasmodium infection and could potentially become the main vector of malaria. **Figure 1** shows a map of the distribution of all the secondary vectors discussed here in this review from sub-Saharan Africa.

3. Impact of land use and land cover changes on mosquito species proliferation

Environmental change is driving the expansion of numerous vector species and the intensification of pathogen transmission in many places in the world [36] because vectors respond sharply to changes in the ecology of their breeding habitat. These ecological changes include land use and land cover changes [37–40] which can change the environment within which the vector prefers to breed or the microclimate of the area within which certain vectors would tolerate [40]. Malaria vectors could therefore invade a new area when the land use and land cover changes [41]. Land cover changes and human settlement subsequent to deforestation has prompted an increase in the human-biting rate of formerly zoophilic vectors in several parts of the tropics and the instigation of upsurges in malaria transmission and malaria epidemics [40, 42]. Human settlement can increase malaria transmission if there are malaria infected people in among the settlers. Mitigating against the impacts of environmental change on malaria transmission will be particularly difficult when public health goals conflict with economic development. Economic development in many places in Africa is associated with extension of agricultural practices such as rice and sugar cane that are associated with extensive water bodies that favor the establishment of breeding sites for malaria vectors. Economic development has also been associated with deforestation, where the forest is cut down for housing and agricultural purposes. For instance in Guiana, following the elimination of malaria in the Demerara River Estuary by DDT spraying, the human population grew rapidly and land use activities switched from livestock herding to more profitable rice farming. This caused the formerly zoophilic *Anopheles aquasalis* to switch from being zoophilic to an anthrophilic behavior. This change initiated the return of transmission into the area after 16 years of absence [43]. Again in Swaziland, resurgence of malaria cases after elimination in 1959 was due to agricultural developments during that time that involved irrigation projects for sugar cane cultivation, which created conditions conducive for malaria vectors to breed and flourish. Vector density increased, with subsequent increase in biting frequency, as no animals were around the area to serve as alternative hosts. The resurgence of malaria was also influenced by migrant workers who came to the area from disease-endemic areas of Mozambique, some of whom were parasite-carriers, in the 1960s and early 1970s [44].

In many areas of Africa, the type of land use activity and the ecological context created after deforestation, determines which species of mosquito are able to remain and adapt, which ones disappear, and which new species are able to invade the place, that find the new habitat congenial to their survival and proliferation [45]. Deforestation could enhance the vectorial capacity of malaria transmitting mosquitoes, and there was 29–106% increase in vectorial capacity for *An. gambiae* in deforested areas compared with forested areas in western Kenya [46]. In the same area, it was found that deforestation increases water temperature of larval habitat, hence increase larvae survival, population density and gametocytes development in adult mosquitoes [38, 46, 47]. In western Africa, deforestation and irrigation have been followed by an increase in *P. falciparum* malaria transmitted by *An. gambiae* in villages close to forest, *An. funestus* in the savannah, and *An. arabiensis* in urban and peri-urban areas [48]. In northern Cameroon, changes to the ecology of the area along the Bamendjim dam has resulted in high densities of *An. ziemanni*, a secondary vector that is now playing the role of a primary vector [49]. The changes to the ecological settings have enabled the proliferation of breeding sites contributing to its development.

Environmental pressures and climate change may bring about malaria vectors dynamism, which leads to some malaria vectors becoming more efficient in transmitting malaria [50]. Manga et al. [41], working in an area that has been deforested to build a new airport in Cameroon, observed that deforestation caused the introduction of *An. gambiae* into a habitat that was previously predominated by *An. moucheti*. Changes to the forest cover led to the subsequent replacement of the vectors in the area, which could worsen the malaria situation in the area.

Outside of the continent of Africa, Conn *et al.* [42] found in Amapa state, Brazil that *Anopheles marajoara,* has become the main malaria vector species in this area, when it previously was of minor importance. This species occurred in much greater abundance compared with the presumed vector *Anopheles darlingi*. Also, a significantly higher proportion of *An. marajoara* was infected with malaria parasites. This was attributed to increased alterations in land use, invasion of its primary breeding sites by human immigrants, and its anthropophilic behavior. This finding highlights a challenge in malaria control, that the targeting of specific vectors may be complicated by a changing mosaic of different locally important vectors and their interactions with human populations.

4. Proliferation of mosquito species to higher altitudes due to climate change and climate variability

The highlands of Africa, where malaria incidence is on the rise, represent an ecological zone of special concern [51]. The high rate of deforestation leads to rise in temperatures in highland areas [39, 52, 53]. Global climate warming could potentially make the high-altitude areas which used to be unsuitable for mosquito proliferation suitable for these mosquitoes to increase in density. Each vector has its own ecological niche requirement, and an important limiting factor for vector spatial distribution range is climate. A typical case in point, in the highlands of western Kenya, Zhou et al. [54] reported that the population of *An. arabiensis* rose from >1% in 2003 to 18.8% in 2009. Again, *An. arabiensis* have been absent in the highlands of central Kenya, however, studies by Chen et al. [55] reported the presence of *An. arabiensis* in these highlands which have elevation of 1720–1921 m above sea level for the first time. This suggests that the ecological conditions or local climate have become conducive to the proliferation of this vector species.

In the Amani hills of Tanzania, Matola et al. [56] reported that malaria vectors were scarce on the Amani hills until the late 1960s, and it was generally presumed that any cases of malaria transmission must have been contracted by people visiting surrounding lower altitudes where malaria is holoendemic. However, *An. funestus* and *An. gambiae* both became more abundant during the 1970s and 1980s with high sporozoite-positive specimens of both. Malaria asexual parasite rates increased dramatically in the early 1908s, with the percentage of children below 1 year who had parasitamia and whose parents reported not visiting lowland localities away from the Amani hills increased drastically, suggesting possible local malaria infection. The conclusion was that various factors including climatological changes, and increased deforestation for agricultural activities have contributed to this changed malaria endemicity and transmission.

Even though these vectors are main and not secondary vectors, the fact that the highlands became permissible to their proliferation leading to increases in malaria transmission suggest that this could happen with secondary vectors. Some of these secondary vectors already live in the highland areas [30, 57] and therefore when conditions such as land use changes, climate change and reduction in interspecific competition from main vectors as a result of elimination or reduction in their population could trigger their proliferation. Others could migrate into the highlands from surrounding lowland areas when conditions such as those already discussed become permissible to their survival. Malaria vectors and non-vectors could periodically extend their range beyond their normal area of distribution.

5. Impact of intensive use of insecticides for public health interventions

Insecticides are the primary weapon against malaria vectors in the current malaria intervention paradigm. However, their prolonged use have been associated with the development of resistance by malaria vectors. Their intensive application has evolutionary implications evident in the number, behavior and physiology of the vectors. For numeric responses to intensive insecticide use, mosquito populations typically decrease in density because their longevity is reduced very much [58, 59]. For instance, studies carried out in western Kenya showed that, *An. gambiae s.l.* and *An. funestus* population density declined markedly in treatment compared to control villages in a randomized trial of insecticide treated bed nets [60]. This effect persisted for 3 years after the trial ended [61]. For behavioral responses, females of some *Anopheline* vectors showed elevated activity due to excitation effects of the active ingredients in insecticide formulations of insecticide-treated bednets or indoor residual sprays, which resulted in their movement away from the insecticide source, irrespective of having obtained a human blood meal [62, 63]. Evolutionary responses typically involve changes in phenotypic sensitivity to the insecticides being used, when alleles associated with reduced target site sensitivity or enhanced metabolic detoxification increase in frequency [64].

The reduction in one target vector may trigger a cascade of ecological effects that could impede or enhance transmission by another. A notable examples include the apparent replacement of the highly anthropophilic and endophagic *An. funestus* by the less potent vectors *Anopheles rivolurum* Leeson and *An. parensis* in Kenya and Tanzania following house spraying campaigns in the 1950s [7]. *An. rivolurum* population rose up to about seven times its former density. During this period also, *An. gambiae s.s.* also declined markedly in their population. Quiet recently, there have also been reported increase in population size of *An. rivulorum* Leeson, in western Kenya lowland areas where there have been high coverage of LLIN distribution. This vector has shown early outdoor biting activity [65]. These changes could be attributed to a reduction in interspecific competition caused by the intervention that allowed these secondary vectors to move into the niche formerly occupied by *An. funestus*. In regions with sympatric vector species where insecticide-based vector control are used, malaria vectors that do not enter houses will have selective survival advantage over vectors that do enter houses, due to the latter's exposure to the insecticides used indoors. This will result in a selective decline in the density of house-entering endophagic vectors relative to more exophagic species. In such situations, exophagic vectors in the area which may be considered secondary in importance could maintain transmission [66].

Again, in Kenya, the inception of rigorous malaria control in the early part of the 2000s using LLINs saw dramatic changes of vector species. There has been a marked decline in the population of *An. gambiae s.s.* and an increase in the population of *An. arabiensis* as household ownership of bed nets rose over a 10-year period [54, 67]. Similarly, in Tanzania, there are shifts in species composition due to the use of ITNs, which resulted in a more dramatic drop in the density of highly anthropophagic and endophagic *An. gambiae s.s.* relative to the zoophagic and adaptable *An. Arabiensis* [68]. Most recently, there are reported new species that have emerged in western Kenya [69]. These species of mosquitoes did not match the morphologic descriptions of any of the more recently identified species. This demonstrates the presence of outdoor-active, early-biting potential malaria parasite vectors not previously described in Kenya. It has not yet been proven whether these vectors existed or are entirely new species. Their overall biology needs to be studied to understand their role in malaria transmission.

These scenarios demonstrate that secondary vectors have the potential to occupy the niche left by main vectors after the latter's elimination through intensive vector control in sub-Saharan Africa that relies solely on insecticides with the use of IRS and LLINs.

6. Commentary

Malaria transmission in Africa is a dynamic and complex system that is continuously changing. Despite the substantial amount of work done on malaria epidemiology and control in Africa, there remains gaps in our understanding of the ecology and biology of secondary vectors. Further knowledge is required to improve control of the disease especially as many countries embark on rigorous campaign to move from control to elimination phase of malaria transmission. Currently, much attention has been given to the main malaria vectors with the promotion of high LLIN use and IRS application which mainly tackle indoor transmitting vectors. However, a very big public health problem in recent years is residual malaria transmission. This has been reported to be increasing in many parts of sub-Saharan Africa [68, 70]. Most often studies on residual malaria transmission tend to focus on the main malaria vectors. However, the secondary vectors discussed here are mostly exophagic and exophilic and therefore would be more involved in residual transmission. The contribution of these secondary vectors should be seen much more in influencing residual malaria transmission. Moreso when there is currently no intervention in the vector control paradigm to take care of residual malaria transmitting vectors. Other measures such as larviciding or larval source reduction that could tackle secondary vectors and residual malaria transmission have not receive much attention. There is a great need to understand the bioecology of secondary vectors and their contribution to malaria epidemiology in order to program intervention for them.

From the above review, it was seen that *An. pharoensis, An. coustani* and *An. ziemanni* in particular are secondary vectors that are prevalent in almost every part of sub-Saharan Africa, right from Senegal in western Africa to Ethiopia in the east and down to Mozambique and Angola. They have shown in their ecology that, they could be anthropophilic since they were caught in human landing catches and also carried *P. falciparum* sporozoites as well as *P. vivax* in Ethiopia. Their exophilic behavior means they have the potential to increase residual malaria transmission wherever, they are found. The fact that in some instances they have been found in indoor collections [29, 49] shows that they could also become endophagic and endophilic and have the potential to occupy a new niche if the main vectors are eliminated or their population becomes suppressed. The ecology and population dynamics of these secondary vectors should be monitored as many countries in Africa move towards the elimination phase of malaria epidemiology.

Why the population densities of these secondary vectors have not been as much as the main vectors has received little attention in the research world. It could be that interspecific competition with the main vectors has not favored the secondary vectors. If this is true, then when main vectors are eliminated or their densities brought down by intervention, secondary vectors could assume the role of main vectors since there would not be any competition. However, Gillies [71] asserted that most secondary vectors do have a short lifespan with natural mortalities estimated to be around 50–60% per gonotrophic cycle. This could explain to an extent, why their population sizes have not been high in many places. However, it has been shown in several areas in sub-Saharan Africa that the rigorous LLIN distribution and IRS application for malaria control within the last decade has led to *An. arabiensis* becoming the main vector when the population of *An. gambiae s.s.* was suppressed by the high insecticide use for vector control. Also, in the late 1950s, *An. rivolorum* replaced *An. funestus* in east Africa after 18 months of indoor residual spraying with dieldrin [7]. Also in the late 1950s, *An. darlingi* which was the primary vector of malaria was eliminated from Venezuela, but malaria of low endemicity due to the secondary vectors *Anopheles albimanus* and *Anopheles nuneztovari* still persisted for many years in certain areas [66]. These show that it is possible for secondary vectors to become the main vectors as many countries in Africa move towards elimination of malaria through vector control.

Human behavior is identified to drive residual malaria transmission. In areas where it is warmer in some months of the year, some residents would want to sit outside of their house instead of being indoors for several hours of the night or sleep outside the whole night as happens in the north of Ghana [72]. In such areas, if the main vectors are eliminated, it is more likely that secondary vectors would replace them since blood meal will be available outdoors and possible pathogen transmission would be enhanced. It has also been suggested that since many secondary vectors are exophagic and exophilic, they could potentially sustain transmission of malaria after the main endophagic and endophilic vectors have been reduced by indoor control measures such as IRS and LLIN use [3, 8, 14].

However, it is worth noting that a possible reason why these vectors have not been able to actively transmit malaria might be that these secondary vectors may not be as refractory to the development of Plasmodium parasites as the main vectors are. If this is true, then no matter how abundant their population might be, they may not be able to assume the responsibility as main vectors and actively increase malaria transmission.

It is worth to note that the co-occurrence of primary and secondary vectors at the same sites may lead to an increased risk of malaria transmission. High infection rates in the secondary vectors could also arise as a result of high malaria transmission maintained by the primary vectors and increased density of humans who maybe carrying gametocytes [73].

The implementation of any successful vector-control measures requires knowledge of the biology of the anopheline species present in the area to be targeted. The scientific world needs to be concerned with the bionomics, morphology and genetics of these secondary vectors, to be ready when they also step up their game to become main vectors. In addition, malaria control measures needs to take into account secondary vectors most of whom are exophagic and exophilic.

Author details

Yaw Asare Afrane[1*], Mariangela Bonizzoni[2] and Guiyun Yan[3]

*Address all correspondence to: yaw_afrane@yahoo.com

1 Department of Medical Microbiology, College of Health Sciences, University of Ghana, Accra, Ghana

2 Department of Biology and Biotechnology, University of Pavia, Pavia, Italy

3 Program in Public Health, College of Health Sciences, University of California, Irvine, CA, USA

References

[1] WHO: World Malaria Report 2014. *WHO, Geneva* 2015.

[2] O'Meara WP, Bejon P, Mwangi TW, Okiro EA, Peshu N, Snow RW, Newton CR, Marsh K: Effect of a fall in malaria transmission on morbidity and mortality in Kilifi, Kenya. *Lancet* 2008, 372:1555–1562.

[3] Antonio-Nkondjio C, Kerah CH, Simard F, Awono-Ambene P, Chouaibou M, Tchuinkam T, Fontenille D: Complexity of the malaria vectorial system in Cameroon: contribution of secondary vectors to malaria transmission. *J Med Entomol* Nov; 2006, 43(6): 1215–1221.

[4] Hervy JF, Le Goff G, Geoffroy B, Hervé JP, Manga L, Brunhes J: Anopheles of the Afrotropical Region. *CD-ROM, ORSTOM editions*, 1998, Paris, France.

[5] Mouchet J, P. Carnevale, Coosemans M, Julvez J, Manguin S, Richard-Lenoble D, Sircoulon J: Biodiversity of malaria worldwide. *Editions John Libbey Eurotext, Montrouge, France* 2004.

[6] Coetzee M, Hunt RH, Wilkerson R, Della Torre A, Coulibaly MB, Besansky NJ: *Anopheles coluzzii* and *Anopheles amharicus*, new members of the *Anopheles gambiae* complex. *Zootaxa* 2013, 3619:246-274.

[7] Gillies MT, Smith A: Effect of a residual house spraying campaign on species balance in *Anopheles funestus* group: the replacement of *Anopheles funestus* Giles with *Anopheles rivulorum* Leeson. *Bull Entomol Res.* 1960, 51: 248-252.

[8] Gillies MT: The role of secondary vectors of malaria in North-East Tanganyika. *Trans R Soc Trop Med Hyg* 1964, 58:154–158.

[9] Lobo NF, Laurent BS, Sikaala CH, Hamainza B, Chanda J, Chinula D, Krishnankutty SM, Mueller JD, Deason NA, Hoang QT, et al: Unexpected diversity of *Anopheles* species in Eastern Zambia: implications for evaluating vector behavior and interventions using molecular tools. *Sci Rep* 2015, 5:17952. doi:10.1038/srep17952

[10] Vincke IH, Jadin JB. Contribution to the study of anophelism in altitude countries. *Ann Soc Belg Med Trop.* 1946;26:483–500.

[11] de Meillon B: The Anophelini of the Ethiopian geographical region. *Publ S Afr Inst Med Res* 1947, 10:1–272.

[12] Wanji S, Tanke T, Atanga SN, Ajonina C, Nicholas T, Fontenille D: *Anopheles* species of the mount Cameroon region: biting habits, feeding behaviour and entomological inoculation rates. *Trop Med Int Health* 2003, 8:643–649.

[13] Mukiama TK, Mwangi RW: Seasonal population changes and malaria transmission potential of *Anopheles pharoensis* and the minor anophelines in Mwea Irrigation Scheme, Kenya. *Acta Trop* May; 1989, 46(3):181–189.

[14] Wilkes TJ, Matola YG, Charlwood JD: *Anopheles rivulorum*, a vector of human malaria in Africa. *Med Vet Entomol* 1996, 10:108–110.

[15] Hamon J, Mouchet J: The secondary vectors of human malaria in Africa. In: Studies on malaria in Africa. *Médecine Tropicale*, 1961, 21:643–660.

[16] Carrara GC, Petrarca V, Niang M, Coluzzi M: *Anopheles pharoensis* and transmission of *Plasmodium falciparum* in the Senegal River delta, West Africa. *Med Vet Entomol* 1990, 4(4):421–424.

[17] Dia I, Konate L, Samb B, Sarr JB, Diop A, Rogerie F, Faye M, Riveau G, Remoue F, Diallo M, Fontenille D: Bionomics of malaria vectors and relationship with malaria transmission and epidemiology in three physiographic zones in the Senegal River Basin. *Acta Trop* 2008, 105(2):145–153. Epub 2007 Nov 4.

[18] Tchouassi DP, Quakyi IA, Addison EA, Bosompem KM, Wilson MD, Appawu MA, Brown CA, Boakye DA: Characterization of malaria transmission by vector populations for improved interventions during the dry season in the Kpone-on-Sea area of coastal Ghana. *Parasit Vectors* 2012, 5:212.

[19] Dery DB, Brown C, Asante KP, Adams M, Dosoo D, Amenga-Etego S, Wilson M, Chandramohan D, Greenwood B, Owusu-Agyei S: Patterns and seasonality of malaria transmission in the forest-savannah transitional zones of Ghana. *Malar J* 2010, 9:314. doi:10.1186/1475-2875-9-314

[20] Govoetchan R, Gnanguenon V, Azondékon R, Agossa RF, Sovi A, Oké-Agbo F, Ossè R, Akogbéto M: Evidence for perennial malaria in rural and urban areas under the Sudanian climate of Kandi, Northeastern Benin. *Parasit Vectors* 2014, 7:79. doi: 10.1186/1756-3305-7-79

[21] Sovi A, Govoétchan R, Tokponnon F, Hounkonnou H, Aïkpon R, Agossa F, Gnanguenon V, Salako AS, Agossou C, Ossè R, et al: Impact of land-use on malaria transmission in the Plateau region, southeastern Benin. Parasit Vectors 2013, 6:352. doi: 10.1186/1756-3305-6-352

[22] Kerah-Hinzoumbé C, Péka M, Antonio-Nkondjio C, Donan-Gouni I, Awono-Ambene P, Samè-Ekobo A, Simard F: Malaria vectors and transmission dynamics in Goulmoun, a rural city in south-western Chad. *BMC Infect Dis* 2009, 9:71. doi: 10.1186/1471-2334-9-71

[23] Robert V, Van den Broek A, Stevens P, Slootweg R, Petrarca V, Coluzzi M, Le Goff G, Di Deco MA, Carnevale P: Mosquitoes and malaria transmission in irrigated rice-Þelds in the Benoue valley of northern Cameroon. *Acta Tropica* 1992, 52:201–204.

[24] Cavalie P, Mouchet J: The malaria eradication campaign in the north of the republic of the Cameroon. *J Trop Med Hyg* 1961, 21:847–869.

[25] Lips M: Anopheles of Congo. 5. *A. brunnipes* Theobald 1910 and *A. paludis* Theobald, 1900, vector of human malaria. *Rivista di Parassitologia* 1961, 23:275–295.

[26] Kibret S, Wilson GG, Tekie H, Petros B: Increased malaria transmission around irrigation schemes in Ethiopia and the potential of canal water management for malaria vector control. *Malar J* 2014, 13:360.

[27] Animut A, Balkew M, Gebre-Michael T, Lindtjorn B: Blood meal sources and entomological inoculation rates of anophelines along a highland altitudinal transect in south-central Ethiopia. *Malar J* 2013, 12:76.

[28] Gari T, Kenea O, Loha E, Deressa W, Hailu A, Balkew M, Gebre-Michael T, Robberstad B, Overgaard HJ, Lindtjorn B: Malaria incidence and entomological findings in an area targeted for a cluster-randomized controlled trial to prevent malaria in Ethiopia: results from a pilot study. *Malar J* 2016, 15:145.

[29] Kamau L, Koekemoer LL, Hunt RH, Coetzee M: *Anopheles parensis*: the main member of the *Anopheles funfunestusestus* species group found resting inside human dwellings in Mwea area of central Kenya toward the end of the rainy season. *J Am Mosq Control Assoc* 2003, 19:130–133.

[30] Kamau L, Mulaya N, Vulule JM: Evaluation of potential role of *Anopheles ziemanni* in malaria transmission in western Kenya. *J Med Entomol* 2006, 43(4):774–776.

[31] Githeko AK, Service MW, Mbogo CM, Atieli FK: Resting behaviour, ecology and genetics of malaria vectors in large scale agricultural areas of western Kenya. *Parassitologia* 1990, 38:481–489.

[32] Gillies MT, De Meillon B, 1968. The Anophelinae of Africa South of the Sahara. Publication no. 54. Johannesburg, South Africa: South African Institute of Medical Research, 54; 1–343.

[33] Chandler JA, Highton RB, Hill MN: Mosquitoes of the Kano Plain, Kenya. I. Results of indoor collections in irrigated and nonirrigated areas using human bait and light traps. *J Med Entomol* 1975, 12(5):504–510.

[34] Fornadel CM, Norris LC, Franco V, Norris DE: Unexpected anthropophily in the potential secondary malaria vectors *Anopheles coustani s.l.* and *Anopheles squamosus* in Macha, Zambia. *Vector Borne Zoonotic Dis* 2011, 11(8):1173–1179.doi:10.1089/vbz.2010.0082 Epub 2010 Dec 13.

[35] Mendis C, Jacobsen JL, Gamage-Mendis A, Bule E, Dgedge M, Thompson R, Cuamba N, Barreto J, Begtrup K, Sinden RE, Hogh B: *Anopheles arabiensis* and *An. funestus* are equally important vectors of malaria in Matola coastal suburb of Maputo, southern Mozambique. *Med Vet Entomol* 2000, 14: 171–180.

[36] Patz JA, Olson SH, Uejio CK, Gibbs HK: Disease emergence from global climate and land use change. *Med Clin North Am* 2008, 92:1473–1491, xii.

[37] Afrane YA, Zhou G, Lawson BW, Githeko AK, Yan G: Life-table analysis of *Anopheles arabiensis* in western Kenya highlands: effects of land covers on larval and adult survivorship. *Am J Trop Med Hyg* 2007, 7:660–666.

[38] Munga S, Minakawa N, Zhou G, Mushinzimana E, Barrack OO, Githeko AK, Yan G: Association between land cover and habitat productivity of malaria vectors in western Kenyan highlands. *Am J Trop Med Hyg* 2006, 74:69–75.

[39] Afrane YA, Lawson BW, Githeko AK, and Yan G: Effects of microclimatic changes due to land use and land cover on the duration of gonotrophic cycles of *Anopheles gambiae* Giles (Diptera: Culicidae) in western Kenya Highlands. *J Med Entomol* 2005, 42:974–980.

[40] Lindblade KA, Walker ED, Onapa AW, Katungu J, and Wilson ML: Land use change alters malaria transmission parameters by modifying temperature in a highland area of Uganda. *Trop Med Int Health* 2000, 5:263–274.

[41] Manga L, Toto JC, Carnevale P: Malaria vectors and transmission in an area deforested for a new international airport in southern Cameroon. *Soc Bel Med Trop* 1995, 75:43–49.

[42] Conn JE, Wilkerson RC, Segura MN, de Souza RT, Schlichting CD, Wirtz RA, Povoa MM: Emergence of a new neotropical malaria vector facilitated by human migration and changes in land use. *Am J Trop Med Hyg* 2002, 66:18–22.

[43] Giglioli G: Ecological change as a factor in renewed malaria transmission in an eradicated area. *Bull World Health Organ* 1963, 29:131–145.

[44] Packard RM: Agricultural development, migrant labor and the resurgence of malaria in Swaziland. *Soc Sci Med* 1986, 22(8):861–867.

[45] Patz JA, Graczyk TK, Geller N, Vittor AY: Effects of environmental change on emerging parasitic diseases. *Int J Parasitol* 2000, 30:1395–1405.

[46] Afrane YA, Little TJ, Lawson BW, Githeko AK, Yan G: Deforestation increases the vectorial capacity of *Anopheles gamgambiaebiae* Giles to transmit malaria in the western Kenya Highlands. *Emerg Infect Dis* 2008, 10:1533–1538.

[47] Afrane YA, Zhou G, Lawson BW, Githeko AK, Yan G: Effects of microclimatic changes due to deforestation on the survivorship and reproductive fitness of *Anopheles gambiae* in western Kenya Highlands. *Am J Trop Med Hyg* 2006, 74:772–778.

[48] Patz JA, Lindsay SW: New challenges, new tools: the impact of climate change on infectious diseases. *Curr Opin Microbiol* 1999, 2:445–451.

[49] Tabue RN, Nem T, Atangana J, Bigoga JD, Patchoke S, Tchouine F, Fodjo BY, Leke RG, Fondjo E: *Anopheles ziemanni* a locally important malaria vector in Ndop health district, northwest region of Cameroon. *Parasit Vectors* 2014, 7:262. doi:10.1186/1756-3305-7-262

[50] Zhou G, Minakawa N, Githeko AK, Yan G: Association between climate variability and malaria epidemics in the East African highlands. *Proc Natl Acad Sci U S A* 2004, 101:2375–2380.

[51] Lindsay SW, Martens WJ: Malaria in the African highlands: past, present and future. *Bull World Health Organ* 1998, 76:33–45.

[52] Siraj AS, Santos-Vega M, Bouma MJ, Yadeta D, Ruiz Carrascal D, Pascual M: Altitudinal changes in malaria incidence in highlands of Ethiopia and Colombia. *Science* 2014, 343:1154–1158.

[53] Githeko AK, Ndegwa W: Predicting malaria epidemics in the Kenya highlands using climate data: a tool for decision makers. *Glob Chang Hum Health* 2001, 2:54–63.

[54] Zhou G, Afrane YA, Vardo-Zalik AM, Atieli H, Zhong D, Wamae P, Himeidan YE, Minakawa N, Githeko AK, Yan G: Changing patterns of malaria epidemiology between 2002 and 2010 in Western Kenya: the fall and rise of malaria. *PLoS One* 2011, 6(5):20318.

[55] Chen H, Githeko AK, Zhou G, Githure JI, Yan G: New records of *Anopheles arabiensis* breeding on the Mount Kenya highlands indicate indigenous malaria transmission. *Malar J* 2006, 7:17.

[56] Matola YG, White GB, Magayuka SA: The changed pattern of malaria endemicity and transmission at Amani in the eastern Usambara mountains, north-eastern Tanzania. *J Trop Med Hyg* 1987, 90:127–134.

[57] Mulambalah C, Ngeiywa MM, Siamba DN, Vulule JM: Diversity of *anopheles* species and prevalence of malaria in a highland area of western Kenya. *J Parasitol Vector Biol* 2011, 3:33–39.

[58] MacDonald G: The epidemiology and control of malaria. *Oxford University Press, Oxford* 1957.

[59] Gratz NR: The future of vector biology and control in the World Health Organization. *J Am Mosq Control Assoc* 1985, 1:273–278.

[60] Gimnig JE, Vulule JM, Lo TQ, Kamau L, Kolczak MS, Phillips-Howard PA, Mathenge EM, ter Kuile FO, Nahlen BL, Hightower AW, Hawley WA: Impact of permethrin-treated bed nets on entomologic indices in an area of intense year-round malaria transmission. *Am J Trop Med Hyg* 2003, 68:16–22.

[61] Lindblade KA, Gimnig JE, Kamau L, Hawley WA, Odhiambo F, Olang G, ter Kuile Fo, Vulule JM, Slutsker L: Impact of sustained use of insecticide-treated bednets on malaria vector species distribution and culicine mosquitoes. *J Med Entomol* 2006, 43:428–432.

[62] Taylor RN, Hill MD, Stewart DC, Slatter R, Gichanga M: A field evaluation of permethrin (OMS-1821) and Nrdc 161 (OMS-1998) for residual control of mosquitoes. *Mosq News* 1981, 41:423–433.

[63] Miller JR, Siegert P, Amimo F, Walker E: Designation of chemicals in terms of the locomotor responses they elicit from insects: an update of Dethier et al. (1960). *J Econ Entomol* 2009, 102:2056–2060.

[64] Hemingway J, Ranson H: Insecticide resistance in insect vectors of human disease. *Ann Rev Entomol* 2000, 45:371–391.

[65] Kawada H, Dida GO, Ohashi K, Sonye G, Njenga SM, Mwandawiro C, Minakawa N, Takagi M: Preliminary evaluation of insecticide-impregnated ceiling nets with coarse mesh size as a barrier against the invasion of malaria vectors. *Jpn J Infect Dis* 2012, 65(3): 243–246.

[66] Reid JA: Secondary vectors, an obstacle to malaria eradication. *Med J Malaya* 1960, 14:228–231.

[67] Bayoh MN, Mathias DK, Odiere MR, Mutuku FM, Kamau L, Gimnig JE, Vulule JM, Hawley WA, Hamel MJ, Walker ED: *Anopheles gambiae*: historical population decline associated with regional distribution of insecticide-treated bed nets in western Nyanza Province, Kenya. *Malar J* 2010, 9:62.

[68] Russell TL, Govella NJ, Azizi S, Drakeley CJ, Kachur SP, Killeen GF: Increased proportions of outdoor feeding among residual malaria vector populations following increased use of insecticide-treated nets in rural Tanzania. *Malar J* 2011, 10:80.

[69] Stevenson J, St Laurent B, Lobo NF, Cooke MK, Kahindi SC, Oriango RM, Harbach RE, Cox J, Drakeley C. Novel vectors of malaria parasites in the western highlands of Kenya. Emerg Infect Dis. 2012 Sep;18(9):1547–9. doi: 10.3201/eid1809.120283.

[70] Durnez L, Coosemans M. Residual transmission of malaria: an old issue for new approaches. In Anopheles mosquitoes – New insights into malaria vectors. Edited by Manguin S., ISBN 978-953-51-1188-7-S.I., Intech; 2013: 671–704. Available at: http://www.intechopen.com/books/anopheles-mosquitoes-new-insights-into-malaria-vectors

[71] Gillies MT. Observations on nulliparous and parous rates in some common East African mosquitoes. *Ann Trop Med Parasitol.* 1963 Dec;57:435–442.

[72] Monroe A, Asamoah O, Lam Y, Koenker H, Psychas P, Lynch M, Ricotta E, Hornston S, Berman A, Harvey SA: Outdoor-sleeping and other night-time activities in northern Ghana: implications for residual transmission and malaria prevention. *Malar J* 2015, 14:35.

[73] Quakyi IA, Leke RG, Befidi-Mengue R, Tsafack M, Bomba-Nkolo D, Manga L, Tchinda V, Njeungue E, Kouontchou S, Fogako J, et al: The epidemiology of *Plasmodium falciparum* malaria in two Cameroonian villages: Simbok and Etoa. *Am J Trop Med Hyg* 2000, 63:222–230.

3

Challenges of Managing Childhood Malaria in a Developing Country: The Case of Nigeria

Tagbo Oguonu and Benedict O. Edelu

Abstract

Malaria still remains one of the highest childhood killer diseases, especially in the developing countries of Africa, Southeast Asia, and Eastern Mediterranean regions. With an estimated 100 million cases and 300,000 deaths from malaria annually, Nigeria has one of the highest burdens of malaria in the world, with children mostly affected. It accounts for 60% of outpatient visits, 30% hospitalization among children under 5 years of age. Great efforts and huge funding have been committed globally towards the fight for malaria, but malaria continues to be a major challenge in these developing countries, especially countries in Sub-Saharan Africa. The World Health Organisation adopted a cost-effective intervention strategy, which comprises a three-pronged approach: vector control, chemoprophylaxis, and case management. Case management involves early diagnosis and treatment. This chapter looks at the challenges militating against the achievement of this important aspect of malaria control in children as well as efforts that have been made or not made to overcome these challenges using Nigeria as a case study.

Keywords: malaria, childhood, challenges, managing, Nigeria

1. Introduction

Malaria still remains one of the highest childhood killer diseases, especially in the developing countries of Africa, Southeast Asia, and Eastern Mediterranean regions. In Africa, it is estimated that malaria kills one child every 2 minutes [1]. According to the latest estimates from the World Health Organisation (WHO), there were 214 million new cases of malaria worldwide in 2015 with an estimated 438 000 malaria deaths [1]. Most of these cases (88%) and deaths (90%) were recorded in the African region [1]. Nigeria and the Democratic Republic of Congo, both in African region, accounted for about 40% of the total estimated malaria deaths worldwide. The Southeast Asia and the Eastern Mediterranean regions account for the few remaining cases in that order. The denominator in all these regions, apart from the favourable weather conditions for the breeding of malaria parasite-carrying mosquitoes, is the widespread poverty and systemic inadequacies: lack of political will and poor health systems in many of the countries that make up the regions. In parts of the world where malaria is endemic, severe malaria is mainly a disease of children under the age of 5 years due to the acquisition of specific immunity against plasmodium; the malaria-causing parasite as the child gets older, providing some protection (though incomplete) against malaria [2]. Malaria is endemic in most countries of Sub-Saharan Africa with the children and pregnant women population being the most vulnerable to the disease. Of the estimated 438,000 malaria deaths worldwide, children under the age of 5 years constitute 306,000 (70%) [1].

Despite these seemingly very high figures, there has been marked decline in the mortality from malaria. The global cases of malaria declined by 18% from an estimated 262 million in the year 2000 to 214 million in 2015. The death rate decreased by 48% from a global estimate of 839,000 in year 2000 to 438,000 in 2015. In children under the age of 5 years, the number of malaria deaths fell from an estimated 723,000 in year2000 to 306,000 in 2015, a decrease of about 58% (**Table 1**). This has come through the combined efforts of the World Health Organisation, its Rollback Malaria Partners and the various governments in the different countries afflicted by the malaria scourge.

WHO region	**Estimated malaria deaths by year**				**Percentage reduction**
	2000	**2005**	**2010**	**2015**	**2000–2015**
Africa	694,000	5910,000	410,000	292,000	–58%
Americas	400	300	300	100	–66%
Eastern Mediterranean	5300	5200	2000	2200	–58%
European	0	0	0	0	0
Southeast Asia	19,000	16,000	14,000	10,000	–49%
Western Pacific	4,700	2,000	1,600	1,500	–68%
World	723,000	614,000	428,000	306,000	–58%

Source: World Malaria Report 2015.

Table 1. Estimated number of malaria deaths in children under the age of 5 years from year 2000 to 2015 by the WHO region.

To achieve this, the WHO adopted a cost-effective intervention strategy, which comprises a three-pronged approach: vector control, chemoprophylaxis, and case management. The vector control involves the prevention of mosquitoes from acquiring or transmitting infection through the use of long lasting insecticidal nets (LLIN) and indoor residual spray (IRS). Chemoprophylaxis involves the use of antimalarial drugs to suppress and prevent the establishment of infection in the human, whereas case management involves the prompt diagnosis and treatment of malaria.

Although these strategies are said to be cost effective, the achievements recorded in the fight against malaria has not come at a cheap price. The global cost of fighting malaria increased from the sum of US$ 960 million in year 2000 to a whopping US$ 2.5 billion in 2014 [1]. The majority of these funds were contributed by international partners (donor agencies). In spite of these global efforts and huge funding for malaria control, malaria continues to be a major challenge in these developing countries, especially countries in Sub-Saharan Africa. These challenges in the fight against malaria, with particular attention to case management, are discussed below using Nigeria as a case study.

2. Nigeria and malaria burden

As the most populous country in Africa, Nigeria contributes the majority of the Africa malaria burden. The country has an estimated total population of approximately 172 million (2014 estimate) with an annual growth rate of about 2.7% and a GDP per capita of US$1091.64 (2014) and inflation rate of 9.0% (2015) [3]. The public health sector in Nigeria is run by the three tiers of government: federal, state, and local governments. The federal government co-ordinates the affairs of the tertiary health facilities and provides overall policy and technical support to the health sector. The state government co-ordinates those of the secondary centres and some state-owned tertiary centres and also lend support to the primary health sector. The local government takes care of the primary health centres, which have gone moribund in many parts of the country. The annual health budget is usually well below 10% of the total budget. For instance; in 2015, it was 6.3%, whereas in 2016, it dropped to about 3.7%. In general, the country's health system may be described as weak due to inadequate funding and supervision.

Nigeria, being a tropical country, has one of the best combinations of adequate rainfall, temperature, and humidity, allowing for the breeding and survival of the female anopheline mosquitoes, the malaria vector. Most (97%) of the malaria in Nigeria are mainly due to *Plasmodium falciparum*, with *Plasmodium ovale* and *Plasmodium malariae* affecting only a few persons. Although, severe malaria is mostly caused by *P. falciparum*, *Plasmodium vivax*,and *Plasmodium knowlesi* have also been indicated in causing severe disease [2]. However, *P. vivax* does not occur in indigenous Nigerians [4], and there is no documentation of *P. knowlesi* in any Nigeria.

Malaria remains a major public health problem in Nigeria. It accounts for more cases and deaths than in any other country in the world. There are an estimated 100 million malaria cases with over 300,000 deaths per year in Nigeria [5]. Malaria accounts for 60% of outpatient visits and 30% of hospitalizations among children under 5 years of age in Nigeria [5]. This implies a huge loss in terms of financial resources and man hours and in the case of the school age child, loss of school hours [6–8].

In line with the World Health Organization recommendation, the country has adopted the Test, Treat, and Track (3T) strategy with all suspected cases of malaria properly diagnosed using Rapid Diagnostic Tests or microscopy, treated promptly with recommended artemisinin-based combination therapy (ACT) if the result is positive and documented [4].

3. Malaria diagnosis

3.1. Clinical diagnosis

WHO has identified early diagnosis as the first step in the treatment of malaria. This is necessary to prevent progression of the disease to severe forms. Malaria does not have any specific symptoms and signs and as such may mimic several tropical childhood illnesses [9]. These include bacterial sepsis, enteric fever, pneumonia, meningitis, urinary tract infection, otitis media, and pharyngitis. This makes the specificity of clinical diagnosis of malaria very poor and thus gives room for indiscriminate use of antimalarials especially in endemic areas. In some cases, malaria may co-exist with any of these other conditions [10–13], necessitating more competent health personnel in the management. Studies [14–16] have shown that treatment based on clinical information alone leads to over diagnosis and over treatment of malaria. In addition, there may be increased morbidity and possible death from the neglected disease causing the child's symptoms.

Even with the unreliability and consequences of reliance on clinical information alone for malaria diagnosis, a large proportion of healthcare providers in Nigeria still treat malaria presumptively [14, 17, 18]. The 2013 Nigeria Demographic and Health Survey indicated that the average rate of antigen or parasite detection in children before treatment was 11.1% [19]. Reasons adduced for the presumptive diagnosis by the healthcare providers included delay in getting a blood microscopy from hospital laboratories, unavailability of malaria rapid diagnostic test (mRDT), reliance on blood tests create an impression of incompetence of the health personnel, as well as malaria being the first suspect in any child with fever since malaria is endemic in Nigeria [17]. According to WHO, less than half of the suspected malaria cases in most malaria endemic regions are truly infected with malaria parasite, hence their insistence on laboratory confirmation before treatment [1].

3.2. Parasite detection

In line with the WHO policy, the national malaria guideline of Nigeria recommends the confirmation of all suspected cases of malaria by parasitological testing either with microscopy or by the use of mRDT. This is particularly important as accurate diagnosis before treatment will enhance a more targeted therapy, reduce the duration of illness, and may even prevent death from treatment of another disease as malaria. It will help prevent drug resistance and also enhance the diagnosis and case management of other diseases that may mimic malaria in children since the exclusion of malaria will mean a search for the cause of illness. Apart from saving lives, both money and man hours are saved.

The challenge with this confirmation test is mainly that of availability and willingness to go for test before treatment. Microscopy, which still remains the gold standard, is fast disappearing from many health facilities. The reasons range from inability to acquire new or replace old and damaged microscopes to absence of a qualified microscopist. In addition, ready availability of reagents and slides for use with the microscopes, where available may be a problem. There is also the need for quality assurance, which is virtually non-existence in most health facilities in the country. Another important consideration is the need for electrical power, which is a big issue in the country. The alternative is the mRDT, which is an antigen detection test. Three antigens: *Plasmodium falciparum* histidine-rich protein 2 (*Pf*HRP2), plasmodial aldolase, and plasmodial lactate dehydrogenase (pLDH) are currently used for mRDTs. The *pf*HRP2 mRDTs are the most commonly available types in Nigeria and seem most suited for the country as up to 97% of the malaria cases are due to *P. falciparum*. The test is easier to conduct and requires neither power supply nor any expertise. It is usually available as a pre-packed ready-to-use kit with a single container of buffer solution in every box of kits. Since the adoption of the mRDT by the WHO, the number of the products has continued to increase rapidly with over 200 different products available in the market worldwide [20]. This rapid proliferation of brands also lead to increase in the number of substandard products, which easily find their way into developing countries like Nigeria with less stringent quality control. Reviews and studies show that the commercially available MRDTs show wide variability in diagnostic sensitivity and specificity [21–25]. To stem this "influx," WHO has continued to conduct testing of the products and issuing guidelines to assist countries adopt the mRDT for use [20].

Since the introduction of RDT kits, there has been increased knowledge of mRDT by healthcare givers and increasing availability at health facilities, but its regular utilization to confirm suspected cases of malaria by these health workers prior to treatment is not encouraging [17, 26]. Another major concern is the fact that a good number of these mRDTs have high false negative results at lower antigen titre (200–500 parasites/ml) [20, 23]. For the detection of *P. falciparum* in all transmission settings, WHO recommended the panel detection score against *P. falciparum* samples should be at least 75% at 200 parasites/μL [27]. The Nigerian malaria treatment guideline recommends the use of an alternate diagnostic test where continued suspicion exists after a negative test [4]. Some authors have recommended the combined use of two methods to confirm the diagnosis of malaria [22]. This invariably adds to the cost of treatment as well as time spent at the health facility, which many healthcare givers and patients will evade. Also, quality and performance check of the mRDTs is partly absent or non-existent in malaria-endemic countries, including Nigeria [20]. The quality of the mRDT may be affected the very high temperatures (above 40°C) such as can be found in some parts of the country. It is important to note that although mRDT may constitute an extra cost to the case management of malaria, it is no doubt a cost-effective innovation, even more cost effective than microscopy [28]. Despite these challenges with the use of mRDT and microscopy, they are still very useful components of malaria case management.

4. Malaria treatment

In consonance with the WHO recommendation on the treatment of malaria, the Nigerian government adopted the use of artemether-lumefantrine (AL) for the treatment of uncomplicated malaria and artesunate-amodiaquine (AA) as alternative [4]. For severe falciparum malaria treatment, the drug of choice is intravenous artesunate with parenteral artemether or quinine as alternatives where intravenous artesunate is not available. For settings where a complete treatment of severe malaria is not feasible, a pre-referral treatment with intramuscular or rectal artesunate or intramuscular quinine in this order of preference is recommended.

Although the Nigerian government had adopted AL and AA as the first and second line respectively, several brands of other ACTs are widely available and used in the country. These include artesunate-mefloquine, dihydroartemisinin-piperaquine, artemisinin-piperaquine, and artesunate-sulfadoxine pyrimethamine. Regardless of the constellation of ACT antimalarial drugs available, many children still receive monotherapy notably chloroquine and sulfadoxine-pyrimethamine especially among the lower socioeconomic class and those with uneducated or under educated parents [17, 29]. Other commonly used antimalarial monotherapy in children include oral artesunate, amodiaquine, halofantrine, and oral quinine and paludrine [29, 30]. The drawback in this practice is the progression to severe malaria with its consequences, which include prolonged hospitalization, increased cost of treatment, avoidable blood transfusions, and even death. The frequent prescription of concomitant medications in the form of different antipyretics, sometimes multiple, haematinics, multivitamin preparations, and antibiotics, which are mostly inappropriate also add to the cost of treatment and burden of medications for the child [29]. In Sub-Saharan Africa, the proportion of children aged under 5 years, who received an ACT, is estimated to have increased from less than 1% in 2005 to 16% in 2014, but still falls substantially short of the target of universal access for malaria case management [1]. One important reason for this poor situation is that a greater proportion of children with fever are treated outside the health sector.

In Nigeria, only about 35% of children receive treatment at government health facilities [19]. The rest are treated by the patent medicine vendors (PMV), pharmacy shops, private health facilities, or by traditional medicine practitioners. In the light of this, the government of Nigeria with the assistance of Roll back Malaria partners and donor agencies tried to scale up the treatment of malaria through the engagement of the private sectors, especially the PMVs whom they have trained in some states of the federation and the provision of pre-packaged, age-specific antimalarials for easier dosing [19]. A study by Berendes et al. [31] in the northern part of Nigeria showed that patent medicine vendors are not reliable in the treatment of malaria because most PMVs were ignorant of and lacked training about new treatment guidelines that had endorsed ACTs as first-line treatment for uncomplicated malaria. They stocked and dispensed monotherapy to patients with suspected malaria. However, another study [32] in the southern part of the country showed an improved knowledge of ACT by PMVs, but yet other non-recommended antimalarial drugs such as chloroquine were still sold to customers without prescription. Another worrisome trend is the prevalent use of various forms of herbal medications in the treatment of malaria even in urban areas [7, 33, 34]. Some of these herbal preparations, which mostly do not have standard dosage, have the potential to cause liver or kidney damage [35].

The cost of malaria treatment is also a contributing factor to the non-use of ACT because this remains high for the average Nigerian. In 2009, the cost of treating a child was about US$6.58, which was mostly on out of pocket expenses [8]. Although a national health insurance scheme is available, only a very small percentage of the population, mainly federal civil servants and staff of big companies, have access to it.

Another major challenge with the treatment of malaria in Nigerian children is the high rate of fake and substandard antimalarial drugs [36, 37]. This brought about a lot of confusion to the healthcare provider regarding the possibility of co-morbidities when the child failed to respond to the proper treatment. This may lead to the administration of unwarranted antibiotics while the child deteriorates from untreated malaria. However, the situation has improved significantly in recent times [36]. The rate of fake and substandard drugs in the country improved from about 41% in 2002 to about 10% in 2010 [36]. The fight is still ongoing by the country's National Agency for Food and Drug Administration and Control (NAFDAC) to eradicate fake drugs from the country.

5. Other challenges

5.1. Co-morbidity with chronic diseases

Nigeria being a developing country has its fair share of children with chronic diseases, such as malnutrition, HIV/AIDS, and sickle cell anaemia. These children equally suffer from malaria, which is usually more severe than in the normal child [38–40]. Managing such children could pose a great challenge. Apart from the complications such as severe anaemia, which are more prevalent in these children [38–40], concurrent management of the underlying disease in the face of challenging finances often result in difficult decisions.

5.2. Blood transfusion

Children with severe malaria anaemia suffer greatly due to the difficulty in obtaining safe blood for transfusion. The primary health facilities and many private facilities do not have logistics to store blood. Patients requiring blood transfusions in these facilities are either referred to tertiary centres or made to purchase blood from private blood banks at very exorbitant prizes, some of which the safety are not guaranteed. In some cases, the child may be unable to make it alive to the referred centre. Those who do often face many logistic challenges ranging from cost of processing to provision of donor to replace the transfused blood.

5.3. Delayed presentation

Late presentation usually results in delay in initiation of the right and adequate treatment. No doubt this contributes significantly to the malaria mortality in children. Factors responsible may include poverty, inadequate home treatment, and lack of access to standard treatment centres. Certain traditional beliefs such as association of fever with teething and growth may also delay presentation. Likewise, the increasing belief in unorthodox treatment such as herbal medications and faith-based healing may also lead to delays in presentation.

5.4. Geographic inequality of health facilities and personnel

Although majority of Nigerians reside in the rural areas, only a small proportion of health facilities are located there and these are mainly primary and secondary care facilities. Likewise, fewer personnel are available in these rural communities. As a result, most patients with severe forms of malaria will need to travel some distance with all the attendant challenges such as bad roads.

6. Conclusion

Despite all these numerous challenges plaguing the management of malaria in Nigerian children, there have been significant gains in the fight against malaria as evidenced by the improved indices. Thanks to all the Rollback Malaria partners operating in the country. However, a lot of commitment and willingness to translate what is on paper to action is still expected from the Nigerian government.

First is to strengthen the health systems at all levels from primary to tertiary in order to restore the hopes of the numerous Nigerians who die because they cannot afford standard private health facility treatments. This should include the recruitment and adequate training and retraining of healthcare personnel in all the primary and secondary care centres to be able to make proper diagnosis and treat malaria cases. Also, adequate equipping of all the government health facilities with diagnostic facilities and eradication of the "out of stock syndrome" for antimalarial drugs.

There should be strengthening of the already on-going awareness creation through the media to sensitize the public on the need to seek care early and at government approved health facilities.

There should be continuous appraisal of the antimalarial drugs and mRDTs in the country with a view of identifying and expunging the substandard and fake ones. The large number of different brands of ACTs and in the country need to be pruned down to just a few quality and trusted brands.

Author details

Tagbo Oguonu* and Benedict O. Edelu

*Address all correspondence to: tagbo.oguonu@unn.edu.ng

Department of Paediatrics, College of Medicine, University of Nigeria, Enugu Campus, Enugu State, Nigeria

References

[1] WHO Global Malaria Programme. World Malaria Report 2015. Geneva: World Health Organization, 2015.

[2] World Health Organisation. Severe malaria. Tropical Medicine &International Health 2014;19 (suppl):7. doi:10.1111/tmi.12313.

[3] World Bank. Data on Nigeria 2015. Available from: http://www.worldbank.org/en/country/nigeria

[4] Federal Ministry of Health National Malaria and Vector Control Division. National Guidelines for Diagnosis and Treatment of Malaria. Third ed. Federal Ministry of Health, Abuja Nigeria 2015.

[5] United States Embassy in Nigeria. Nigeria Malaria Facts Sheet. 2011. Available from: http://www.nmcp.gov.ng/Downloads

[6] Uguru NP, Onwujekwe OE, Uzochukwu BS, Igiliegbe GC Eze SB. Inequities in incidence, morbidity and expenditures on prevention and treatment of malaria in Southeast Nigeria. BMC International Health and Human Rights 2009;9: 21. doi: 10.1186/1472-698X-9-21.

[7] Salihu OM, Sanni NA. Malaria burden and the effectiveness of malaria control measures in Nigeria: A case study of Asa Local Government Area of Kwara State. Journal of Sustainable Development 2013;4:295-308

[8] Onwujekwe O, Hanson K, Uzochukwu B, Ichoku H, Ike E, Onwughalu B. Are malaria treatment expenditures catastrophic to different socio-economic and geographic groups and how do they cope with payment? A study in southeast Nigeria. Tropical Medicine &International Health 2010;15 (1):18-25.

[9] D'Acremont V, Kilowoko M, Kyungu E, Philipina S, Sangu W, Kahama-Maro J, et al. Beyond malaria—causes of fever in outpatient Tanzanian children. The New England Journal of Medicine 2014;370:809-817

[10] Okunola PO, Ibadin MO, Ofovwe GE, Ukoh G. Co-existence of urinary tract infection and malaria among children under five years old: A report from Benin City, Nigeria. Saudi Journal of Kidney Diseases and Transplantation 2012;23(3):629-634

[11] Ukwaja KN, Aina OB, Talabi AA. Clinical overlap between malaria and pneumonia: Can malaria rapid diagnostic test play a role? The Journal of Infection in Developing Countries 2011;5(3):199-203.

[12] Uneke CJ. Concurrent malaria and typhoid fever in the tropics: The diagnostic challenges and public health implications. Journal of Vector Borne Diseases 2008;45:133–142.

[13] Berkley JA, Maitland K, Mwangi I, Ngetsa C, Mwarumba S, Lowe BS. Use of clinical syndromes to target antibiotic prescribing in seriously ill children in malaria endemic

area: Observational study. British Medical Journal 2009. doi:10.1136/bmj. 38408.471991.8F.

[14] Oladosu OO, Oyibo WA. Overdiagnosis and overtreatment of malaria in children that presented with fever in Lagos, Nigeria. ISRN Infectious Diseases. 2012 Jul 19;2013.

[15] Reyburn H, Mbatia R, Drakeley C, et al. Overdiagnosis of malaria in patients with severe febrile illness in Tanzania: A prospective study. British Medical Journal 2004;329:1212–1217.

[16] D'Acremont V, Kahama-Maro J, Swai N, Mtasiwa D, Genton B, Lengele C. Reduction of anti-malarial consumption after rapid diagnostic tests implementation in Dar es Salaam: A before-after and cluster randomized controlled study. Malaria Journal 2011;10:107.

[17] Ughasoro MD, Okoli CC, Uzochukwu BSC. Qualitative study of presumptive treatment of childhood malaria in third tier tertiary hospitals in southeast Nigeria: A focus group and in-depth study. Malaria Journal 2013;12:436.

[18] Mangham LJ, Cundill B, Ezeoke O, Nwala E, Uzochukwu BSC, Wiseman V, et al. Treatment of uncomplicated malaria at public health facilities and medicine retailers in south-eastern Nigeria. Malaria Journal 2011;10:155.

[19] National Population Commission Nigeria, ICF International. Nigeria Demographic and Health Survey 2013. Abuja, Nigeria, and Rockville, Maryland, USA: NPC and ICF International. 2014; p. 217.

[20] WHO. Malaria Rapid Diagnostic Test Performance Results of WHO Product Testing of Malaria RDTs: Round 6 (2014-2015). Geneva: World Health Organization, 2011.

[21] Wilson ML. Malaria rapid diagnostic tests. Medical Microbiology 2012;54:1637-1641.

[22] Oguonu T, Okafor HU. Comparison of clinical, microscopic and rapid diagnostic test methods in the diagnosis of *Plasmodium falciparum* malaria in Enugu, Nigeria. The Nigerian Postgraduate Medical Journal 2007;14(4):285-289.

[23] Jeremiah ZA, Uko EK, Buseri FI, Jeremiah TA. Field evaluation of SD Bioline rapid diagnostic test among asymptomatic malaria infected children in Port Harcourt, Nigeria. Research Journal of Parasitology 2007;2:37-44.

[24] Mouatcho JC, Dean Goldring JP. Malaria rapid diagnostic tests: Challenges and prospects. Journal of Medical Microbiology 2013;62:1491–1505.

[25] Ezeudu CE, Ebenebe JC, Ugochukwu EF, Chukwuka JO, Amilo GI, Okorie OI. The performance of an histidine rich protein-2 rapid diagnostic test (RDT) against the standard microscopy in the diagnosis of malaria parasitaemia among febrile under-five children at Nnewi. Nigerian Journal of Paediatrics 2015;42(1):59-63.

[26] Uzochukwu BSC, Chiegboka LO, Enwereuzo C, Nwosu U, Okorafor D, Onwujekwe OE, et al. Examining appropriate diagnosis and treatment of malaria: Availability

and use of rapid diagnostic tests and artemisinin-based combination therapy in public and private health facilities in southeast Nigeria. BMC Public Health 2010;10:486.

[27] Global Malaria Programme. Recommended Selection Criteria for Procurement of4 Malaria Rapid Diagnostic Tests. World Health Organization Geneva, Switzerland. 2016. Available from:5 www.who.int/malaria/publications/atoz/rdt_selection_criteria/en6

[28] Batwala V, Magnussen P, Hansen KS, Nuwaha F. Cost-effectiveness of malaria microscopy and rapid diagnostic tests versus presumptive diagnosis: Implications for malaria control in Uganda. Malaria Journal 2011;10:372.

[29] Ezenduka CC, Ogbonna BO, Ekwunife OI, Okonta MJ, Esimone CO. Drugs use pattern for uncomplicated malaria in medicine retail outlets in Enugu urban, southeast Nigeria: Implications for malaria treatment policy. Malaria Journal. 2014;13(1):1.

[30] Edelu BO. Home treatment of presumed malaria in children attending outpatient clinic at the University of Nigeria Teaching Hospital, Enugu, Nigeria. Nigerian Medical Journal. 2011;52 (2):99–103.

[31] Berendes S, Adeyemi O, Oladele EA, Oresanya OB, Okoh F, Valadez JJ. Are patent medicine vendors effective agents in malaria control? Using lot quality assurance sampling to assess quality of practice in Jigawa, Nigeria. PLoS One 2012; 7(9): e44775. doi:10.1371/journal.pone.0044775.

[32] Chukwuocha UM, Nwakwuo GC, Mmerole I. Artemisinin- based combination therapy: Knowledge and perceptions of patent medicine dealers in Owerri metropolis, Imo State, Nigeria and implications for compliance with the current malaria treatment protocol. The Journal of Community Health 2013;38:759-765.

[33] Oreagba IA, Oshikoya KA, Amachree M. Herbal medicine use among urban residents in Lagos, Nigeria. BMC Complementary and Alternative Medicine. 2011;11(1):117.

[34] Ene AC, Atawodi SE, Ameh DA, Kwanashie HO, Agomo PU. Locally used plants for malaria therapy amongst the Hausa, Yoruba and Ibo Communities in Maiduguri, North-Eastern Nigeria. Indian Journal of Traditional Knowledge. 2010;9(3):486-490.

[35] Posadzki P, Watson LK, Ernst E. Adverse effects of herbal medicines: an overview of systematic reviews. Clinical Medicine. 2013;13(1):7-12.

[36] Bate R, Hess K. Anti-malarial drug quality in Lagos and Accra—a comparison of various quality assessments. Malaria Journal 2010;9:157.

[37] Newton PN, Green MD, Mildenhall DC, Plançon A, Nettey H, Nyadong L, et al. Poor quality vital anti-malarials in Africa—an urgent neglected public health priority. Malaria Journal. 2011;10(1):1.

[38] Sanyaolu AO, Fagbenro-Beyioku AF, Oyibo WA, Badaru OS, Onyeabor OS, Nnaemeka CI. Malaria and HIV co-infection and their effect on haemoglobin levels from three

healthcare institutions in Lagos, southwest Nigeria. African Health Sciences. 2013;13(2): 295-300.

[39] Makani J, Komba AN, Cox SE, Oruo J, Mwamtemi K, Kitundu J, Magesa P, Rwezaula S, Meda E, Mgaya J, Pallangyo K. Malaria in patients with sickle cell anemia: Burden, risk factors, and outcome at the outpatient clinic and during hospitalization. Blood. 2010;115(2):215-220.

[40] Osazuwa F, Ayo OM. Contribution of malnutrition and malaria to anemia in children in rural communities of Edo State, Nigeria. North American Journal of Medical Sciences. 2010;2(11):532.

4

Exploiting the Potential of Integrated Vector Management for Combating Malaria in Africa

Emmanuel Chanda

Abstract

Integrated Vector Management (IVM) is advocated by the World Health Organization (WHO) as the pivotal platform for vector control. The threat for malaria and emerging and re-emerging vector borne diseases is increasing. However, adoption and deployment of the IVM strategy has been minimal. Though malaria endemic countries are embracing and consolidating the IVM approach, real time entomological data on transmission risk and targeting the right vector with the appropriate intervention is lacking. IVM could be harnessed for circumventing operational constraints for vector control. Herein IVM for combating malaria and other insect-borne diseases is reviewed and ways to maximize its potential and benefits are proposed. IVM promotes operational research for evidence-based, cost-effective and optimally sustainable vector control with judicious integration of available options, improves management of insecticides, and effective mitigation of potential negative health and environmental impacts. IVM enhances institutional arrangements including accountability, collaboration and coordination of stakeholders. IVM will require policies and frameworks to maximize intervention impact; and infrastructure and human resources capacity, community involvement and information sharing, strengthened regulation for registration and quality assurance, procurement, financial management and supply chain management for commodities. However, national health system-based response among stakeholders and political commitment is needed for optimal IVM implementation.

Keywords: integrated vector management, malaria transmitting mosquitoes, insect-borne diseases, strategic planning, operational frameworks, evidence-informed decisions, intersectoral collaboration, capacity building

1. Introduction

Malaria remains the biggest health threat among vector-borne diseases (VBDs) with approximately 214 million annual cases and a related 438,000 deaths occurring worldwide in 2015, particularly in sub-Saharan Africa [1, 2]. Though vector control is a proven approach for controlling and eliminating disease, its continued efficacy is likely to be compromised by a multiplicity of constraints [3]. To mitigate the problem, endemic countries in collaboration with the World Health Organization (WHO) have implemented various vector control tools over the years. The quest by WHO for rational evidence-based vector control approaches can be traced through several conceptual stages as: integrated vector control strategy, 'utilization of all appropriate, safe and compatible means of control to bring about an effective degree of vector suppression in a cost-effective manner' [4]; selective vector control, 'application of targeted, site specific and cost-effective activities to reduce disease morbidity and mortality' [5]; and comprehensive vector control, 'control of the vectors of two or more co-prevalent diseases through a unified managerial structure using similar or different vector control methods' [6]. Until recently, management of some vector control programmes have mostly been vertical in disposition. To maintain the effectiveness of vector control, the integrated vector management (IVM) strategy was established and advocated by the WHO as a pivotal and recommended platform for combating VBDs [7]. As such, vector control programmes in endemic countries are encouraged to adopt, establish and implement national policies for the approach. By definition IVM is 'a rational decision-making process for optimal use of resources for vector control' [8]. The IVM strategy is based on the premise that effective control is not the sole preserve of the health sector but of various public and private agencies, including communities. It uses sound principles of management and allows full consideration of the determinants of disease transmission and control [8].

Effective IVM policies incorporate available health resources and infrastructure, uses methods based on knowledge of factors influencing local vector biology; disease transmission and morbidity, deploys a multi-disease approach, integrates recommended environmental, biological or chemical interventions, often in combination and synergistically, includes inter-sectoral collaboration within the health sector and with other public and private sectors that impact on vectors; engagement of local communities and other stakeholders; and a public health regulatory and legislative framework , and reinforces vector control management systems [7]. To circumvent vector control-related constraints in the face of dwindling public-sector human and financial resources, the WHO provides technical assistance [8] and documents, guidance on policy-making [9], structure for training [10], handbook for IVM [11] and monitoring and evaluation [12] to facilitate implementation processes. Unfortunately, only a limited number of countries have harnessed IVM to operationalize efficacious VBD control. The IVM approach has five key strategic elements: advocacy, social mobilization and legislation; collaboration within the health sector and with other sectors; integrated approach; evidence-based decision-making; and capacity building [7]. Notably, an IVM-based process should be underpinned by operational research and monitoring and evaluation of impact on vectors and disease transmission, cost-effective, encompassing requisite infrastructure, financial resources and adequate human resources to manage and implement vector control [13]. Nevertheless, substantial challenges for implementation exist at national and local levels and operational experience for the strategy is still limited to relatively few countries.

While vector control has potential to control and eliminate VBDs [2], it has been invariably compromised by: the emergency of insecticide resistance in disease vectors coupled with the lack of sustainable financial resources to sustain control programmes [7], scarcity of personnel with requisite skills and minimal or lack of collaboration between health and other relevant sectors (e.g. infrastructure development, agriculture, environment and educational sectors) to effectively monitor and manage it [5]. Other constraints include residual and outdoor malaria transmission, nominal real-time entomological and epidemiological information to understand transmission risk and to target the right vector with the right control method at the right time; environmental, socio-cultural, socio-economic, technical and programmatic setbacks; weak health systems; limited access to health services; lack of pesticide and resistance management plans; weak planning and coordination amongst disease control programmes. Equally, population increase, returnees, internally displaced and nomadic behaviour of people preclude effective deployment of interventions, particularly in emergencies. The situation is further aggravated by the absence of guidance on IVM in humanitarian emergencies and exclusion of emergency situations in the WHO Handbook for IVM [11].

The need for strengthened human and infrastructural resources to improve vector control has been a topical issue deliberated upon at various forums [14]. Accordingly, appeals and proposals to address inherent challenges have invariably been made to bilateral and multilateral organizations, funding and implementing partners [15]. Nevertheless, limitations that are operationally crucial and with potential to compromise effective programming locally still remain minimally addressed. Though highly divergent at country levels, in the face of shrinking resources, the need to adequately circumvent these pertinent shortcomings is obvious and inevitable. Well-implemented IVM provides a potential platform that could be exploited for enhanced entomological monitoring and surveillance, strategic insecticide resistance management (IRM) planning and rational VBD control and elimination of transmission [16]. In this chapter, an attempt is made to critically review and appraise information on malaria vectors and other insect-borne diseases that could potentially be controlled in tandem, using available tools and management strategies for their control and bringing to the fore some of the pertinent challenges experienced in operational settings. A framework of policies and strategies to facilitate the implementation of the IVM approach is presented and will accentuate coordinated responses amongst stakeholders and political commitment for effective policy execution within the context of national health systems.

2. Methods and literature search strategy

The need to streamline vector control efforts for mosquito-borne diseases, particularly malaria is the case for this review describing a 'literature overview' about implementation of IVM for combating diseases. Information sources for this review included all available data and accessible archived documentary records on malaria vector control. Structured literature searches of published, peer-reviewed sources using online scientific bibliographic databases were utilized to gather pertinent data from endemic countries. This was conducted via systematic literature search of Library catalogues and online electronic databases, particularly PubMed [17], WHO Library Database [18], Google Scholar [19], African Journals Online [20], Armed Forces Pest Management Board [21], and research for life database HINARI [22] were used to search for the relevant literature. All digital electronic database searches for peer-reviewed, published work used a combination of key search terms: (1) complex of *Anopheles* malaria vectors and one of the following terms; (1) 'IRS' and IVM; (2) ITNs/LLINs and IVM; (3) LSM and 'vector control' and 'prevention' and 'surveillance'; (4) malaria epidemiology; (1) and (4); (2) and (4); and (3) and (4); vector control, epidemiology, malaria, house improvement, *Bacillus thuringiensis* var. *israelensis* and *Bacillus sphaericus*, biological control for malaria control and innovative malaria vector control tools, dengue fever, chikungunya, yellow fever, lymphatic filariasis, Western equine encephalomyelitis, St. Louis encephalitis virus (SLE), human African trypanosomiasis, South American trypanosomiasis (Chagas disease), leishmaniasis, onchocerciasis, Zika and trachoma. Literature was also reviewed from settings with similar framework strengthening approaches. Reference sections of all relevant articles were also reviewed to identify more literature. Additional non-peer reviewed literature including strategic and implementation plans and annual reports were examined for information related to the subject. The inclusion criteria considered all manuscripts and publications in English language that report on malaria vector control and IVM. The literature was reviewed and applicable research findings and key concepts from other countries in different regions were considered for inclusion and translation into this framework.

3. Important insect-borne diseases and responsible vectors

The threat of malaria [14] and emerging and re-emerging VBDs such as dengue fever [23], chikungunya [24], yellow fever [25] and lymphatic filariasis [26], most of which are mosquito-borne, is increasing. Vector control need assessments for IVM conducted in several countries indicate the presence of multiple VBDs with divergent endemicities and spatial distribution. Globally, there are many important vectors of malaria parasites such as *Anopheles gambiae* s.s., *Anopheles arabiensis* and *Anopheles funestus* in Africa; *Anopheles stephensi* and *Anopheles culicifacies* in Asia; *Anopheles albimanus* and *Anopheles darlingi* in the New World tropics; and *A. labranciae* and *Anopheles sacharovi* in Europe. Detailed descriptions of the updated global distribution of malaria vectors are provided elsewhere [27, 28]. Many species of *Aedes* and *Culex* are vectors of arboviruses that infect various vertebrates, including humans. *Aedes aegypti* is a principal urban vector of the yellow fever virus and is the primary vector of the dengue viruses. *Aedes albopictus* is a primary vector of forest yellow fever and a secondary vector for dengue fever in most regions. Chikungunya vectored by *Ae. albopictus* and *Ae. aegypti* has increasingly been reported [24]. *Culex quinquefasciatus* is a vector of the nematode worms causing lymphatic filariasis (LF) and of several arboviruses. LF is also transmitted by *An. gambiae, An. arabiensis* and *An. funestus* mosquitoes in several countries. *Culex pipiens* is the vector of Tahyna virus in Europe, St. Louis encephalitis virus (SLE) in North America, and West Nile virus in several continents. *Culex tritaeniorhynchus* is the primary vector of Japanese encephalitis virus in Asia, and *Culex tarsalis* is the primary vector of Western equine encephalomyelitis and SLE in western North America. *Aedes* (*Neomalaniconion*) *mcintoshi* and related species are important enzootic transmitters of Rift Valley fever virus in Africa [29]. Human African trypanosomiasis is vectored by *Glossina fuscipes, Glossina tachinoides, Glossina palpalis, Glossina pallidipes* and *Glossina morsitans* species of tsetse flies. South American trypanosomiasis (Chagas disease) vectored by *Triatoma infestans, Panstrongylus megistus, Rhodnius prolixus, Triatoma brasiliensis* and *Triatoma dimidiata*. Leishmaniasis (kala-azar) is transmitted by *Phlebotomus orientalis, P. argentipes, P. papatasi, P. longipes, P. sergenti, P. martini* and *P. celiae* species of sand flies. Onchocerciasis (River Blindness) is vectored by *Simulium damnosum* complex and *Simulium neavei* group black flies in Africa, and *Simulium ochraceum, Simulium metallicum* and *Simulium exiguum* complexes in Central and South America. Other commonly endemic diseases include trachoma vectored by *Musca sorbens* bazaar flies [30]. Recently, outbreaks of yellow fever were reported in Ethiopia, South Sudan [31], Zambia [25], DRC and Angola [32]. Notably, the global scale of insect-borne diseases is enormous despite most of them having World Health Assembly resolutions passed on combating them [32, 33].

4. Epidemiological context of malaria

The global burden of malaria remains threateningly high, especially in Sub-Saharan Africa where the disease is endemic in most areas and the region is responsible for about 90% of all malaria deaths globally [2]. The majority of people reside in areas with relatively stable malaria transmission with few inhabiting areas supporting seasonal and less predictable transmission, because of either altitude or rainfall patterns. In areas of stable malaria transmission, the disease burden is highest amongst very young children and pregnant women within the population. An estimated one million people in Africa die from malaria each year and most of these are children under 5-year old [34, 35]. The consensus view of empirical studies, reviews and well informed expert opinion is that malaria causes at least 20% of all deaths in children under 5 years of age in Africa [36]. In most areas, malaria transmission is high, defined as greater than one case per 1000 residents and perennial with substantial seasonal variation in intensity [37]. *An. gambiae* s.s., *An. funestus* and *An. arabiensis* are the main vectors with marked temporal and spatial distribution variation at certain times of the year [38]. Vectorial capacity is high due to abundant rainfall (>2000 mm/annum), elevated year-round temperatures and high humidity [39]. Approximately 98% of malaria cases are due to *Plasmodium falciparum* and is responsible for all severe forms of the disease and deaths [2].

In 1998, the Roll Back Malaria (RBM) partnership revived global malaria control efforts [34]. By 2007, these efforts were invigorated following a call for global malaria eradication [35, 40]. While substantial global progress has been made with 34 countries advancing towards elimination, 64 countries remain in the control phase, mainly in Africa where malaria remains endemic [2]. Examples of countries that successfully eliminated malaria include: Australia in 1960, Taiwan in 1965, Mauritius in 1998, Morocco in 2002 and the United Arab Emirates in 2007

[41]. Between 2000 and 2010, malaria mortality rates fell by 26% globally and by 33% in the World Health Organization (WHO) African Region with approximately 1.1 million malaria deaths averted [2]. Pivotal to these gains, principally in Africa, has been the expansive scale-up of insecticide-based interventions against malaria vectors [42]. From 2008 to 2012, USD 5.83 billion was spent for malaria control in Africa by international donors, and endemic countries scaled up WHO proven interventions including vector control [2]. Generally, attempts to control the anopheline vectors have been limited and intermittent and have had little apparent impact on the huge overall malaria burden [43]. However, the epidemiological trend of malaria disease in the WHO African region has changed significantly over the past years, particularly, due to improved vector control using indoor residual spraying (IRS), long-lasting insecticidal nets (LLINs) and larval source management (LSM), in addition to effective treatment with *artemether-lumefantrine* [43]. There has been a sustained impact on malaria disease burden, evidenced through the reduction in the morbidity and mortality in Namibia, Swaziland, Botswana and Eritrea thus paving the way for them to potentially achieve elimination [44]. However, progresses made in the last 50 years in restricting the geographical areas affected by malaria are being eroded recently, due to changes in land use, global climate changes, armed conflicts/movement of refugees, international travel and emergency of insecticide-resistant vectors.

Vector control is the only available intervention able to reduce transmission at the inception stages of malaria elimination and plays a pivotal role during the attack phase [41]. Vector control remains vital in knocking out the remaining foci of transmission during the later stages of elimination; post-elimination, its role is reducing outbreak risk and as a defence against reinvasion [41, 45]. However, transmission-reducing interventions must be cognizant of behavioural and bionomic attributes of the local vector species including the geography and epidemiology of the malaria foci to be attacked. Therefore, the formulation of plans of action for vector control activities within the malaria elimination strategy should take this information into consideration [45, 46]. The attack phase will aim at maximum intensity and complete coverage throughout to interrupt transmission entirely using selective IRS and universal coverage with LLINs for utmost impact [41, 47]. Nevertheless, there is need to guard against potential challenges such as technical and operational obstacles, procurement, forest malaria, human resource, sustainability, limited data on vector bionomics, insecticide resistance in malaria vectors and gradual declines in both the technical quality of spraying operations and acceptance by target communities. In this regard, capacity building will be critical for successful delivery and effectiveness of the vector control programme [41, 47]. Currently, the global technical strategy for malaria is prioritizing vector control and surveillance. New strategies for vector control are emphasizing IVM [48].

As countries pursue malaria elimination, with strong indications that many, will achieve their goal, IVM approaches will be critical. In countries with well- established IVM, intensive health promotional campaigns and provision of necessary materials have resulted in active participation of communities in vector control activities [44, 49]. To best achieve set goals, an integrated approach in controlling the diseases is recommended wherever feasible given the endemicity overlaps and transmission similarities of some VBDs. This requires adherence to all the five key strategic elements of the approach. Recognizing that the IVM approach has been adopted and implemented as the main platform for vector control that include deployment of IRS and LLINs supplemented by LSM [49, 50], there is need for countries to set out to update, revise and widen the scope of their IVM strategies, because of increasing malaria transmission and challenges in vector control. However, the most useful and feasible options for IVM to be applied to the IVM frameworks are: capacity building, integration across diseases, different sectors and communities, evidence-based approach, and collaboration within the health sector and other sectors [42]. This is critical and on effective and efficient deployment of existing and new vector control interventions, to generate and share evidence on integration of all vector control tools and to work with all RBM partners to build entomology and vector control capacity in endemic countries.

5. Rational for integrated vector management

More than half of the world's population is at risk of VBDs, and over one billion people are infected and more than one million die from these diseases annually [1, 2]. In tropical and subtropical regions, climate is most favourable to major VBDs. High diversity of vector-species complexes has the potential to redistribute themselves to new climate or intervention-driven habitats leading to new disease patterns [3]. Up to now, effective reduction of VBDs burden has primarily been ascribed to well-planned and implemented vector control [48], nevertheless, its full potential benefits have not been exhaustively exploited due to limited capacity to manage and deploy vector control; nominal collaboration between infrastructure development and the health sectors; and the detrimental effects of insecticide resistance in disease vectors [51]. To this effect, a Global Strategic Framework setting out the principles and approaches to IVM was developed by WHO [7, 48]. Though IVM forms the cornerstone of contemporary efforts for the prevention and control of VBDs, the approach has only been operationally harnessed in settings with relatively well-established health systems [44, 49]. Only 62% of 113 endemic countries globally and 53% of countries in Africa have national IVM policies and implemented the strategy [52]. IVM has been prompted in part by limited knowledge about deployment in post-conflict settings, where delivery structures are lacking or less developed; very little efforts towards integrating control of multiple VBDs and use of various tools with vector control targeting a single disease and are not fully integrated into health systems, thus compromising their sustainability.

Despite developing multiple global strategies to combat VBDs with renewed emphasis on vector control, high rates of morbidity and mortality are still ascribed to malaria [2, 7]. Vector control need assessments have demonstrated a variety of key factors that undermine the effectiveness of vector control, including: sub-optimal choice or improper timing of interventions and subsequent waste of valuable resources resulting from inadequate capacity for evidence-based decision-making to guide vector control strategies at national, regional, district and community levels; the effect of climate change, environmental degradation and urbanization on malaria and other VBDs, necessitating an adaptive management approach to vector control underpinned by local evidence; lack of collaboration and coordination with other pertinent sectors such as agriculture, industrial works and construction including communities, culminating in limited awareness of the consequences of their actions on the incidence of VBDs; the development of resistance that could potentially undermine effectiveness of insecticide-based vector control efforts [53]. The Stockholm Convention on Persistent Organic Pollutants (POPs) [54] and World Health Assembly resolution WHA50.13 [55] call on countries to design sustainable strategies for vector control. These opportunities, coupled with the presence of arboviral diseases also transmitted by mosquitoes, substantiate the need for an IVM approach to vector control and the development of guidelines that apply, in principle, to all VBDs but focus mainly on malaria control. The IVM strategic plans would require regular adaptation to changes in local eco-epidemiological or socio-economic conditions. IVM provides a unique opportunity to develop cross-disease control programmes, thus facilitating generation and establishment of entomological and epidemiological baseline data for future tracking of performance of interventions. The IVM also plays a pivotal role in mitigating the impact of resistance on vector control interventions as part of resistance management approaches and their inherent effect on control tools [53].

6. Malaria vector control interventions

The arsenal for insecticide-based contemporary malaria vector control is unnervingly limited to a small number of insecticide classes. Furthermore, extensive exposure of malaria vectors to insecticides eventually selects for resistance to them. This necessitates thorough appreciation of available chemical classes, their mode of action, and resistance mechanisms to facilitate utilization of chemical control either in isolation or as part of an IVM approach [56]. Insecticides are classified into four main classes according to their chemical structure. These include chlorinated hydrocarbons (organochlorines) that act by inhibiting the normal functioning of the nervous system. Examples encompass DDT and its analogues that act on the sodium channels of the nerve membrane, benzene hexachloride (BHC) and cyclodienes such as dieldrin acting on the GABA receptors. These insecticides are cheap and easy to manufacture, but their persistence in the environment, wildlife and humans has reduced their use drastically [56]. The second class comprises phosphorothioate insecticides (organophosphates) that include fenitrothion, malathion, pirimiphos methyl and temephos. These insecticides act by binding the enzyme acetylcholinesterase at the nerve junction, and thus commonly called cholinesterase inhibitors. Once bound, this enzyme can no longer remove acetylcholine from the nerve-membrane junction, and the nerve continues to fire in an uncontrolled manner, eventually leading to paralysis and death of the insect. The third class consists of carbamates that have a similar mode of action to that of phosphorothioate insecticides, but they are used in their insecticidally active form as opposed to organophosphates that are invariably administered as the insecticidally inactive phosphorothioate. Examples of carbamates used in vector control are bendiocarb and to a limited extent propoxur. The fourth class is referred to as pyrethroid insecticides. Examples of pyrethroids are deltamethrin, lambda-cyhalothrin and permethrin. Pyrethroids were developed from insecticidally active components of pyrethrum flowers (pyrethrins). These insecticides act in exactly the same way as DDT and its analogues.

Their lack of persistence makes them good, safe 'knock-down' agents, and they are often still used in aerosols, frequently with the Monooxygenase synergist piperonyl butoxide, which increases their insecticidal activity and reduces their cost. Other insecticides include: insect growth regulators (IGRs) which are compounds that act on the highly species-specific insect hormonal systems (juvenile hormone) that control moulting and metamorphosis. Examples of IGRs are pyriproxyfen and buprofezin; and chitin synthesis inhibitors (benzoylphenylureas) that interfere with the formation of chitin, a major constituent of the exoskeleton of insects. An example of this chemical group is diflubenzuron. The other group involves bio-rationals (bacteria pathogens) that produce toxins capable of disrupting the midgut lining of mosquito and blackfly larvae. The toxins produced by bacteria such as *Bacillus thuringiensis* var. *israelensis* and *B. sphaericus* can be considered as insecticides although they are usually regarded as biological control agents. Detailed descriptions of contemporary and innovative malaria vector control approaches are elaborated elsewhere [57, 58]. A summary is presented below:

6.1. Chemical control

The control of arthropod-borne diseases is anchored by vector control, personal protection and community participation as key WHO strategies. In this regard, vector control aims to reduce and/or interrupt transmission of malaria by preventing human contact with malaria-bearing mosquitoes, reducing the longevity of adult mosquitoes, eliminating breeding sites or killing the mosquito larvae [59]. Contemporary interventions for malaria vector control and elimination encompasses: effective indoor residual spraying; community-wide coverage and use of LLINs; LSM interventions where applicable; and window screens, protective clothing, repellents, etc. The use of IRS and LLINs remains the mainstream malaria vector control tools [60, 61]. Their efficacy has been evaluated widely in different epidemiological settings [62] at community-wide levels [63, 64] and experimental field trials [65, 66]. In reducing abundance and infectivity of malaria vectors, IRS and LLINs reduce overall transmission and confer community-wide protection to all individuals [65], albeit with variation in responsiveness amongst vector populations. Evidence is mounting that combining IRS and insecticide-treated nets (ITNs) affords enhanced protection to exposed populations compared to using one method alone [67]. As such, their deployment together in high malaria risk areas has been advocated [65, 68, 69]. However, the optimal policy for the co-implementation of the two interventions still remains to be determined. Moreover, the development of insecticide resistance in malaria vectors remains a major cause for concern and an increasing threat to these efficacious interventions [70]. Given the inherent diversity in the responsiveness of malaria vectors to control, the core interventions can be supplemented in specific locations by LSM strategies, e.g. larviciding with temephos, biological control and environmental management (EM) in the context of IVM [71].

6.2. Environmental management

The environment plays a particularly important role in determining the distribution of VBDs. Factors that are critical to the survival of different species of disease-carrying vectors include water and temperature, other factors such as humidity, vegetation density, patterns of crop cultivation and housing. In this regard, managing the environment of the vectors that transmit diseases can be harnessed for controlling VBDs. Environmental management (EM) methods that are particularly applicable to malaria may include destruction of breeding sites by drainage, filling, impounding, or channelling streams and rivers into canals or by altering the vegetation and shade characteristics of the sites favoured by the vectors. However, it should be noted that different species of mosquitoes have distinct larval and pupal water quality requirements. The basic definition of EM for vector control is 'the planning, organization, carrying out, and monitoring of activities for the modification and/or manipulation of environmental factors or their interaction with humans with a view to preventing or minimizing vector propagation and reducing human-vector-pathogen contact' [72–75]. Owing to extreme lack of resources and dependency of vector control programmes on insecticide based interventions, EM has not been widely adopted in Africa, where it could potentially have the greatest impact on vector-borne diseases. However, EM should be part of integrated control programmes devoid of net economic drain on individuals of the community. Notably EM practices have potential to adversely affect the flora and fauna of an area [76], necessitating consideration of environmental impact assessments during the planning stage. Several important species of *Anopheles* that serve as vectors of malaria are able to breed in paddy fields. An environmental control method employed successfully in several countries to control mosquitoes breeding in paddy fields is intermittent irrigation. Intermittent irrigation successfully controlled the malaria vector *Anopheles labranchiae* in rice growing regions of Portugal, the malaria vector *Anopheles sinensis*, and some members of the *An. culicifacies* complex in India [77]. A number of important mosquito species breed in the brackish water of coastal marshes. These include: *Anopheles melas* and *Anopheles merus* in Africa; *An. sacharovi* around the Mediterranean; and *An. albimanus*, *Anopheles aquasalis* and *Anopheles grabhamii* in the Americas [78]. One approach to controlling mosquitoes breeding in salt marshes is to drain the marsh and remove the breeding sites [79]. This method, particularly marsh alteration by ditching, is now largely abandoned for more environmentally friendly methods of control. The other successful approach was exclusion of salt water, which prevented marshes from becoming brackish. Though not universally applicable, this method was effective in controlling *Anopheles sundaicus* in Malaya and *An. sacharovi* in Italy [80]. Some mosquito species, such as *An. albimanus*, can breed in fresh water as well as in brackish water, and the existence of fresh water in marshes may provide the water quality required by local fresh water-breeding vectors. All future salt marsh mosquito control programmes based on EM will, therefore, have to be aware not only of the effect that mosquitoes have on people living in and around the salt marsh but also of the impact that any proposed measures will have on salt marsh ecosystems. Environmental methods for vector control in water impoundments, such as the damming of rivers and streams, and the construction of irrigation systems, can dramatically alter the environment both in and around them. In particular, they can provide or enlarge the environment suitable for the breeding of major invertebrate disease vectors. This is exemplified by the Tennessee Valley Authority project that resulted in an outbreak of malaria caused by the vector, *Anopheles quadrimaculatus*, breeding in them [81]. It should be noted that the environmental methods to prevent malaria may also include elimination of breeding sites by drainage or by applying locally grown plants [78].

6.3. Biological control

Biological control involves the reduction of a target vector population by a predator, pathogen, parasite, competitor or toxin produced by a microorganism. Biological control usually has the advantage, over conventional broad-spectrum insecticides, of target host specificity with corresponding little disruption of non-target organisms in the environment. It is also capable of providing long-term control after a single introduction. The fundamental principles of biological control encompass two aspects: population ecology and mosquito ecology. In population ecology, most populations do not fluctuate around their carrying capacity that the environment can support due to the presence of other mortality factors. Mortality factors are mostly classified as density dependent (DD) or density independent (DI). With DD factors, mortality increases as the population becomes denser and decreases as the population becomes less dense. Density-dependent mortality factors tend to regulate a population around an average size and to resist change to that average size, and are characterized by mortality that is not proportionate to the population density. Therefore, with both DD and DI mortality, biological control will be successful only if the vectorial capacity of the adult vector population declines to an acceptable level [82].

As regards mosquitoes, ecology differs considerably by species, although some generalizations can be made. Mosquito populations are often characterized by rapid increases and precipitous declines. The females are highly fecund, and most species have short generation times under tropical conditions. Thus, most populations can quickly increase when the breeding season begins or rapidly rebound after a catastrophic event. Furthermore, the adults of many species disperse well and the females quickly re-colonize habitats. Larval habitats are diverse, ranging from ephemeral to permanent, from artificial to completely natural, from hoof prints to rice fields, although most species occupy only a well-defined subset of these breeding sites. Different mortality factors predominate in different habitats. DD factors in mosquito populations include predators in permanent ponds of rice fields, overcrowding and competition and, more rarely from predators or pathogens in small-containers, such as tree holes. DI mortality factors such as flooding, temperature extremes and desiccation can be important in any of these habitats. However, the ideal mosquito biological control agent probably does not exist, as it should respond to any vector population increase by rapidly colonizing its habitat and quickly producing numerous progeny. It should be able to efficiently find all vectors, survive periods of mosquito absence, and function well in any habitat. Mosquito natural enemies usually affect the larval stages. The diversity of larval habitats, feeding behaviour and physiology probably provides an insurmountable challenge to the development of a single control agent for all mosquito species [82, 83].

Biological control can be broadly categorized into two divisions: natural biological control which is vector reduction caused by naturally occurring biotic agents, and applied biological control which refers to planned human intervention to deliberately add natural enemies to a habitat to reduce vector population (augmentation) or to protect the agents already present (conservation) by manipulating the environment to optimize natural biological control through minimizing detrimental effects on natural enemies or by enhancing their efficacy. Biological control agents are more likely to cause significant mortality in permanent habitats than in ephemeral habitats. However, natural biological control alone does not usually reduce vector populations sufficiently to interrupt disease transmission. Two major types of augmentation are inoculation and inundation. With *inoculative* releases, small numbers of natural enemies are introduced that are expected to reproduce in the environment and provide long-term vector suppression over successive generations. For inundative releases, overwhelming numbers of organisms are released to produce an immediate decline in a vector population. Invertebrate pathogens include viruses, bacteria (*Bacillus thuringiensis israelensis* and *B. sphaericus*), protists (*Nosema algerae, Vavraia* spp. and *Amblyospora connecticus*), fungi (*Lagenidium giganteum, Coelomomyces* spp., and *Culicinomyces clavisporus*) and nematodes (*Romanomermis culicivorax*). Also, invertebrate predators (*Toxorhynchites* spp. and the copepod *Mesocyclops aspericornis*) and to a lesser extent vertebrates such as larvivorous fish (*Gambusia affinis, Poecilia reticulata* and *Aphyocypris chinensis*) have been experimented upon and/or utilized for biological vector control [84]. However, both abiotic (temperature, pH, salinity, organic matter, oxygen levels, toxic agents, habitat type and size and water depth) and biotic (ecology, target species, host specificity and adaptation, dispersal and host-finding abilities, infectivity or capture ability, persistence mechanisms, generation time and population age structure) factors can affect the efficacy and sustainability of biological control, and the suitability of a habitat must be verified at each new location. Biological control has many perceived advantages. It is relatively natural and host specific, it can be self-perpetuating, and it does not adversely affect beneficial invertebrates. As attractive as biological control is in principal, in practice this technique has had limited success in malaria vector control [82, 83].

7. Innovative tools for malaria vector control

Vector suppression plays a pivotal role in the control of mosquito-borne infectious agents. In light of contemporary control constraints, novel approaches are required to achieve effective protection against malaria vectors. Several innovative genetic approaches are being applied to microbial organisms to extend their usefulness as vector control agents. Implementation of IVM requires combinations of control measures that are critical in providing optimal control with minimal detrimental environmental outcomes. With the selection of resistance, new insecticides and novel approaches to vector control are being developed [85]. Innovative approaches invariably being harnessed for contemporary vector control include Durable wall linings, attractive toxic sugar baits, long-lasting topical repellents, spatial repellents, entomopathogenic bacteria traps, fungus-impregnated targets, eave tubes and new molecules for IRS, i.e. chlorfenapyr, including improved housing [42, 86–88].

7.1. Genetic control

Reviews of potential genetic control approaches have invariably included discussion of their operational feasibility against vectors of disease, progress made in population suppression of an increasing number of vectors and population replacement of disease vectors with harmless forms of the same species. Population replacement involves modification of the genetic structure of a disease vector in a way that favours human benefit. The desired modification ('useful gene') would be one that prevents disease transmission, either by altering vector behaviour or by producing some physiological change in parasite-vector interaction. The species specificity and non-polluting properties of genetic methods, in contrast to insecticides make the approach attractive. The choice of genetic method for a given species depends on the control strategy to be adopted, whether focal, i.e. adjusted to local needs, or in an area wide rolling programme [89]. The sterile-insect technique (SIT) or sterile-insect release method (SIRM) is the only genetic approach to control that has succeeded on an extensive practical scale with operational effectiveness. SIT is based on the release into the natural habitat of large numbers of the target vector, sterilized in a breeding factory. The released insects carry dominant lethal mutations in their reproductive cells, due to treatment with ionizing radiation or chemical mutagens. All wild female mating with such a male lays sterile eggs. The success of SIT depends on the sterile male's capacity to locate, attract and mate with wild females, in direct competition with wild males. Field trials of SIT against mosquitoes have been conducted on *Culex pipiens quinquefasciatus* in Florida, USA, *An. albimanus* in El Salvador, *An. stephensi* in southern India and *An. arabiensis* in Sudan [89]. The feasibility of integrating sterile-insect technique (SIT), for population reduction of *Ae. albopictus* to prevent and control of chikungunya and dengue, has been considered in the context of IVM in Mauritius [90]. The major technical aspects of mass rearing to be evaluated and improved in mosquitoes are: (1) automated mass rearing, (2) genetic sexing, (3) rapid sterilization, (4) quality control, (5) transportation and release and (6) trapping to evaluate progress [91]. The infection of mosquitoes with *Wolbachia* spp. has been considered to carry a gene for vector competence but would depend on (1) introducing such an 'incompetence' gene into *Wolbachia*, (2) associating *Wolbachia* with *Anopheles* and (3) ensuring that the 'incompetence' gene product, expressed in *Wolbachia*, reaches the gut or salivary glands, which are sites occupied by the malarial parasites [92]. Among all potential methods of genetic control of vectors of disease, SIT has the greatest potential of being effective and economically viable. SIT is at its most effective in combination with other control measures, and it probably extends the effective life of insecticides by slowing down the evolution of resistance [93]. Population replacement remains a distant dream, although research on it provides a rich source of new information on vector physiology and genomics [94, 95].

7.2. Immunological control

Immunological approaches have also been harnessed for the control of malaria vectors. Development of anti-mosquito vaccines reduces blood-feeding and/or pathogen transmission. Their advantages include specificity, safety and cost, ease of administration, long-term protection and absence of residues in the environment. The practicality of vector-blocking vaccines has been given a significant boost by studies that provide protection against pathogen transmission. Advances in immunobiology, genomics, proteomics, DNA immunization and other vaccine-related technologies provide a foundation for new ways to control vectors mosquitoes and malaria [96]. Anti-mosquito vaccines could be designed to disrupt blood feeding, impair reproduction and block development and transmission of mosquito-borne infectious agents. Important resources for anti-mosquito vaccines have been generated from mosquito expressed sequence tags and genome sequencing projects. Attempts have been made to vaccinate against malaria parasites transmitting mosquitoes such as *An. quadrimaculatus* [97], *An. stephensi* [98–100], *Anopheles tessellates* [100, 101], *Anopheles farauti* [102] and multiple *Anopheles* spp. [103, 104].

Most of these contemporary vector control methods have shown to be successful only in small scale- and, more rarely, in large-scale- and country wide programmes. The IVM strategy provides a platform for integrating these into vector control programmes across the malaria-endemic countries in the tropics. However, clear commitment from national authorities including long-term support from funding partners will be required for effective and sustained malaria vector control [105]. Prompted by fragmentary empirical evidence to inform policy formulation for rational vector control, malaria control programmes are encouraged to adopt the WHO-led IVM strategy [49] underpinned by evidence-based decision-making process and a coherent monitoring and evaluation component [13]. The approach should incorporate routine insecticide resistance surveillance and inherent resistance mechanisms to inform decisions and policy changes on insecticide resistance management operations [106].

8. Status of IVM implementation for combating malaria

Integrated vector management has been harnessed for the control of malaria vectors in various endemic countries according to the five key elements of the strategy. In response to the call by the WHO for member states to implement IVM, most VBD-endemic countries have adopted IVM as a pivotal approach to vector control and developed relevant policy documents particularly for malaria vector control. In Mauritius, IVM is one of the three principal components of preventing reintroduction of malaria. The strategy focuses on bi-weekly routine island-wide larviciding with temephos based on entomological surveillance, and indoor and outdoor residual spraying at and around the port and airport with DDT or lambda-cyhalothrin every six months [90]. IVM targets former malaria foci and high-risk areas around migrant workers' residences [107]. Tanzania has been implementing IVM with ITNs, IRS and LSM including environmental management and larviciding using Bti [108, 109]. Notably, IVM has mostly been harnessed for malaria vector control with minimal utilization as an overarching strategy for VBDs. This is exemplified by Kenya [110], Malawi [15], Mozambique [111], Namibia [44], Tanzania [108], Zambia [49], Zimbabwe [112], most of which were pioneers in implementing the approach. The utilization of IVM for multiple VBD control has been compromised by a lack of requisite resources and the inherent cross-sectoral collaboration. It is noteworthy that in some countries such as Swaziland, Botswana, Lesotho, Namibia, Seychelles, Madagascar and South Africa, the presence of VBDs is almost negligible.

With the increasing emergence (dengue, Zika) and re-emergence (chikungunya, yellow fever) of VBDs, countries have embarked on consolidating their IVM policy and strategic documents. In the Comoros, further to the low levels of insecticide resistance observed in the main mosquito vectors of the island (*Cx. p. quinquefasciatus, An. gambiae, Ae. aegypti and Ae. albopictus*), the optimism is high to implement IVM as a more realistic and feasible approach for the control of malaria, bancroftian filariasis, dengue, chikungunya and rift valley fever [113]. Rwanda has developed a comprehensive IVM strategic plan to improve the ecological soundness, cost-effectiveness and sustainability of vector control interventions. The strategy incorporates interventions with clear implementation and collaborative arrangements, strengthened entomological monitoring and surveillance including resistance management [114]. To improve control of VBDs, Uganda has successfully consolidated strategic planning and operational frameworks for VBD disease control and established an evidence-based IVM approach. The country envisions improved VBD control by operationalizing implementation arrangements as outlined in the IVM strategic guidelines [115, 116]. Equally, South Sudan has developed a draft strategic plan for control of VBDs [117] and has embarked on strengthening frameworks for implementation [51]. Eritrea has updated, revised and widened the scope of its IVM strategy due to increasing malaria transmission and challenges in vector control [118]. Ethiopia has developed an IVM strategy and plan of action to include dengue fever and other VBDs; and establishing a coordination mechanism with relevant sectors, including a multi-sectoral task force for capacity building in IVM and surveillance; and to actively engage in advocacy, communication and social mobilization.

IVM strategies have been implemented in Mosquito Control Programmes (MCPs), which aim to reduce the cost and optimize protection of the populations against VBDs in the Americas, and research has been conducted to evaluate MCPs strategies to improve vector control activities [119]. Reviews and case studies have been conducted to discuss and analyse the major strategies currently employed in an effort to minimize the burden of VBDs, and the major progress and achievements resulting from international as well as local efforts [120]. Studies considering how one or more interventions can impact multiple VBDs have been conducted to guide the development of an IVM programme to assist the elimination of malaria and lymphatic filariasis [121]. The contribution of vector management methods has also been critically reviewed to prevent and control outbreaks of West Nile virus infection and to present the challenges for Europe [122]. Expansion of IVM to promote healthy environments has been proposed to control pests, improve cleanliness of communities, increase structural soundness and decrease health disparities that arise from external hazards [123].

9. Challenges and opportunities for establishing viable IVM strategies

While the expectation to reduce the burden of VBDs in endemic countries is high, the operational challenges to effective vector control are enormous. Integrated management of malaria vectors still remains an underdeveloped component of malaria control policies in most programmes. This could in part be attributed to the shortage of health workers in general, but other key contributors are technical, operational, political and social economic in nature. Major challenges to malaria control include very high malaria transmission intensity, low coverage of proven malaria control interventions, inadequate health care resources, a weak health system, inadequate understanding of malaria epidemiology, the impact of control interventions and insecticide resistance development in mosquito vectors. The key challenges are categorized and elaborated further as outlined below:

Limited ability to fully utilize the available tools: In most programmes, vector control is managed by naïve, low calibre and mediocre level public health workers devoid of field experience or is hijacked by clinicians, who are mostly less competent in entomology and vector control. Such programme managers are not receptive to well-informed expert technical advice and are naïve to fully participate in the discourse on vector control and are not open to innovative ideas. The competent public health entomologist and vector control specialists are by and large left frustrated. While surveillance monitoring and evaluation, and operational research are key components of malaria control strategies, activities in the area of vector control are always less prioritized as clinically inclined managers tend to have a predilection for drug efficacy studies. The lack of skills and knowledge has resulted in apathy and unreceptiveness towards scientific results generated by field teams, poor utilization of available tools, low up take of available innovative vectors control tools, vector surveillance, and resistance monitoring and management guidance. While non-governmental organizations (NGOs) play a key role in complementing public sector endeavours in health service delivery, in post-conflict environments, most NGOs have engaged vector control people with minimal or no field experience to effectively transfer competences to the local cadre. Consequently, the IVM strategy has not been fully harnessed for strengthening vector control. However, this trend should be guarded against if meaningful gains are to be attained from contemporary vector control efforts.

Lack or minimal inter-sectoral collaboration amongst stakeholders: Across-sector collaboration amongst stakeholders-public and private sectors—including community empowerment, involvement and participation—and integration amongst VBDs remains an obvert constraint to effective vector control. Even in situations where various partners exist and are working on VBDs control, coordination remains negligible. The situation is aggravated in emergency situations, particularly by the notable absence of entomologists at central level to adequately coordinate entomological resources. There are nominal levels of utilization of available guidance from the WHO and other collaborating stakeholders, as well as limited sharing of experiences by programmes. In recent years, cross-border collaboration and inter-sectoral collaboration on VBDs have been inefficient relative to collaboration on other diseases such as polio elimination [124].

Minimal or absent operational research competences: Efforts to revamp insectaria and entomology laboratories have been embarked upon by various funding organizations. However, entomological infrastructures in most countries are either lying in a state of dilapidation or operating at sub-optimal scale to be useful in any way. They lack requisite equipment and commodities, including a minimal number of dedicated personnel. In certain cases, central laboratories do exist with adequate numbers of staff but lack field laboratory at regional or local levels, making data collection inefficient and thus eroding the potential of existing entomological competencies. There is minimal evidence-based decision-making to provide technical guidance to policy makers and programme managers. Limited operational research and country-wide spatio-temporal mapping of VBDs are also amongst the major challenges. The situation is aggravated by inadequate in-country information systems, lack of geo-coding of relevant attributes and centralized data bases for easy information retrieval as and when it is required.

Emergency situations, environmental and climate changes: In conflict and post-conflict environments, security is the major impediment to successful vector control. There is lack of technical and physical infrastructure and personnel are mostly of mediocre caliber. The situation is compounded by high personnel turn over and a lack of touch with the latest information. While these settings experience human resource crises and competent skills are scarce, flexible people who are not possessive about 'the way things are done around here' are needed. Most vector control issues are left in the hands of non-professionals who tend not to be open to constructive criticism. Appropriate requisite regulatory and legislative framework for public health is also non-existent. Equally, the changing climate and land use patterns are having a toll on the efficacy of the once effective vector control interventions. This necessitates innovation and implementation of local situation amenable interventions.

Community sensitization, mobilization and information sharing: There is inadequate and inconsistent social mobilization and community sensitization and insufficient participation and ownership resulting in low compliance with existing interventions. Mass media and interpersonal communication channels have been used to disseminate advocacy, behavioural change and information and education communications to enhance community participation. Unfortunately, such communications never run consistently annually due to limited resources for requisite activities and are hampered by issues of socio-economic and political factors, cultural aspects and alleged abuse of vector control interventions. There is minimal innovative ways to engage the communities in vector control activities including entomological surveillance and resistance monitoring, including information on country and multi-country level experiences with IVM and IRM. Documentation and sharing of lessons learnt from the field will be essential and will to some extent offset the dependency on the overstretched international technical assistance. However, this requires availability of local competences for documenting the experiences.

Funding and operational constraints: Vector control is mostly donor driven, but the funding is often restricted and with prescribed activities. This tends to have detrimental effects on the ambitious and innovative programme officers who may want to adapt the interventions to the local situation. Most development partners have neglected health system strengthening. Therefore, collaborative approaches and strong political commitment and consistent financial support are required to scale up cost-effective interventions for vector control, including focused research and inter-country cooperation and exchange to share best practices. Effective deployment of vector control interventions including entomological monitoring is hinged on efficient operational logistics including transport systems. Programmes in most settings do not have transport dedicated to entomology and vector control but do have pool vehicles, which in most cases are not easy to access as transport officers often lack an understanding of vector control.

10. Recommendations for moving forward

Notably, tackling contemporary vector control challenges will require strategic efforts beyond those aimed at addressing the human resources crisis. Opportunities for strengthening vector control exist and could be harnessed for effective VBD control. Looking forward; the following are proposed priority actions for advancing IVM implementation within the context of its five key strategic elements and the inherent effective monitoring and evaluation in line with the WHO recommendations:

Development of IVM policy frameworks: To improve national vector-borne disease control programmes, countries should develop national IVM policy and national policy on pesticide management. Development of relevant strategic documents and improving the uptake and use of policy documents produced by the WHO will be critical to achieving this end [8]. Particularly in emergency situations that should include the provision of guidance on IVM in humanitarian emergencies.

Institutional arrangements and Inter-sectoral collaboration: Successful inter-country and inter-sectoral collaborations and vector control initiatives are needed to achieve effective control. However, this will require establishing national steering committees on IVM and national coordinating units on vector control, together with developing and field testing approaches for engaging community organizations in an effective partnership with the operational and regulatory personnel of health and local government departments to improve implementation. Although engagement of sectors other than health is important for vector control, the success of inter-sectoral collaboration will be determined by the extent to which other sectors impact vector proliferation [124].

Vector surveillance and insecticide resistance monitoring: Effective IVM strategies need improved entomological surveillance, risk assessment, preparedness and response; including plans for IRM. Therefore, planning and implementation will require the epidemiological surveillance system on vector-borne diseases, and setting up sentinel sites for vector surveillance and insecticide resistance monitoring. In this regard, countries should (1) develop, evaluate, and promote the effective use of vector control methods, in the context of IVM; (2) support improvements in surveillance, including the collection and use of case reports, environmental and demographic data, and other information to better understand disease distribution patterns and strengthen disease control programmes [125].

Operational research agenda on vector-borne disease control: Planning and implementation will require operational research priorities and expected outcomes on vector control to be used in deployment of programmes. In areas prone to malaria epidemics, understanding the local distribution of the disease and its relation to environmental and demographic factors will help public health officials improve the prevention and control activities they direct. The role of operational research and the interactions between research institutions, vector control programmes, civil society organizations, and of financial and technical partners to address challenges and to accelerate translation of research into policies and programmes should be considered [14]. Therefore, strengthening the capacity of vector control programmes to conduct operational research, publish its findings and improving linkages between them and research institutes may aid progress towards effective control [126].

Standard operating procedures or protocols need to be developed for entomology teams to collect specimens and map their locations, including insecticide susceptibility status. For the purposes of mapping the presence or absence of a vector, a much more targeted and streamlined sampling strategy with optimal collection methods, e.g. animal-baited traps, light traps, should be determined. Programmes need to plan operational, or implementation research activities for increasing effectiveness of current vector control tools and to better engage specific groups such as the military, mobile and migrant workers and marginalized populations to improve access and appropriated interventions.

Community sensitization, mobilization and information sharing: Advocacy communication and social mobilization would be important in putting national strategic and implementation plans on IVM in place. There should be consistent community sensitization via mass media and interpersonal communication channels to disseminate advocacy, behavioural change and information and education communications and address issues of socio-economic-political factors, cultural aspects, urbanization or climate and abuse of vector control tools and enhance community participation. The key messages, based on scientific evidence and information available and disseminated without delay, are crucial for an effective and urgent response [14]. Campaigns on behavioural change and community mobilization on vector control should be conducted. Lessons learned from programmes will provide the requisite platform for accelerated implementation of IVM.

Capacity building: Developing greater capacity in vector control programmes for collecting, managing and analysing malaria case reports and environmental data is useful for planning control operations. Professional training and experience in entomology and vector control are critical for running an IVM programme that makes appropriate use of all available control methods. Certified training courses on IVM and judicious use of pesticides should be in place at national or regional level. Organization and management of IVM requires standards for professions and careers in vector control and public health entomology to be established [127]. Organizing and implementing regional training programmes, professional associations and technical assistance networks that can operate over the long term to build and sustain the human resource capacity needed for effective vector control programmes. Making headways would require enhancing national vector control capacities in terms of human and infrastructural resources to enable efficient monitoring and management of malaria vectors [128]. Governments in malaria-endemic countries should mobilize enough local resources to supplement the limited and restricted donor funding. As efforts are made towards addressing inherent limitations, seeking rare and often overstretched external technical assistance by control programmes will be critical. This will necessitate institution of local training programmes.

11. Discussion

Most malaria-endemic countries have adopted and implemented the IVM strategy. Although the approach has primarily been harnessed for malaria control, countries are presently consolidating their strategic plans and operational frameworks to incorporate other VBDs in the IVM approach. Efforts are being expended towards establishing requisite infrastructure and human resources for vector control. However, control programmes are still faced with several limitations. Successful IVM would require circumventing contemporary challenges to ensure universal access to interventions.

Effective vector control demands for diligent entomological capacity and necessitate adequate requisite financial and human resources and pertinent physical infrastructural strengthening at national and local levels [7]. The major limitations for capacity-building for IVM are lack of essential physical infrastructure (insectaries, laboratories and equipment), financial resources and technical resources (qualified vector control human resources-medical entomologists and vector control specialists) to support entomological monitoring and evaluation of vector control interventions and to manage and implement IVM. The technical assistance provided by the very few resources that exist is extremely strained. Addressing deficiencies in all these areas of public health capacity would be necessary for the successful implementation of IVM. This would need strengthened collaboration with stake holders including local and international academic and scientific institutions and line ministries such as environment and agriculture.

An IVM-based process should be cost-effective, guided by operational research and subject to routine monitoring and evaluation of impact on vector populations and disease transmission [13]. Evidence-based vector control requires regular collection of comprehensive entomological data from spatially segregated geo-locations to adequately inform decision-making on effective targeting, deployment and monitoring of interventions. Monitoring by countries should incorporate key elements of entomological surveillance, including determining species composition, establishing vector distribution and seasonality, collecting vector behaviour data, conducting insecticide susceptibility testing and establishing underlying mechanisms of resistance. Mosquito vectors have developed insecticide resistance to all four classes of public health insecticides, which are spreading with great potential to compromise vector control efforts [70]. Research on innovative vector control tools should be enhanced to provide adequate convincing evidence that can compel and foster donor flexibility. This will be critical in light of selection of insecticide resistance and outdoor/residual transmission. Otherwise vector control will remain dependent on the archaic tool box full of ineffective interventions. Countries should improve global insecticide resistance tracking and get support for developing management plans and the development of an online interactive platform for mapping level resistance [129].

The WHO recommends IVM as a pivotal platform for combating vector-borne diseases. To this effect, several policy and strategic documents as well as training materials have been developed, including a Global Strategic Framework that sets out the principles and approaches to IVM. For effective vector control, endemic countries need to develop three key documents: (1)

an IVM-based vector control strategy; (2) a resistance monitoring and management plan; and (3) vector surveillance guidelines, according to WHO recommendations. There is significant opportunity to integrate vector control for VBDs because in many areas either the same vectors transmit more than one disease, or the local vectors share common ecology. Therefore, IVM should focus on redesigning programmes in the context of vector surveillance, insecticide resistance response, environmental and climate change, cross-border initiatives and IVM in emergency situations [129]. The WHO Emergency Response Framework also stresses the need of sufficient risk reduction and preparedness capacities in member states; and institutional readiness of WHO in ensuring that adapted disease surveillance, early warning and response systems are in place. Risk assessments for yellow fever, chikungunya, dengue and Zika should be prioritized in all settings with the presence of *Aedes* spp. mosquitoes.

Successful implementation of IVM requires adequate financial, human and technical resources, a robust entomological monitoring and resistance surveillance and management system, and demands for meticulous operational considerations and preparedness: strengthened operational research to generate data for decision-making and evaluation of new vector control tools; establishing pertinent physical infrastructure-sentinel sites and laboratory and insectary facilities; adherence to WHOPES specifications and WHO recommendations for procurement; institutionalize data repositories and capacity to implement the interventions. Countries should develop strategic and operational frameworks and maximize impact of current tools. This necessitates adequate planning including detailed situation analyses to obtain relevant local data and implementation frameworks (adherence to pertinent regulatory obligations for registration of insecticides, developing overall multi-year budgets for operations). It will need strengthened collaborations with all stakeholders with vested interest in vector control and insecticide resistance including the funders.

12. Conclusion

Despite the slow pace, malaria-endemic counties are embracing and consolidating the IVM approach. The development and implementation of IVM with strict adherence to the five key elements of the approach are crucial for effective operational malaria vector control. Regular need assessments for vector control human and infrastructural resources and technical support to facilitate capacity building in entomological surveillance and monitoring for evidence-based decision-making in vector control are critical for successful IVM, including guiding development of IVM strategic plans, country IRM plans and vector surveillance plans, advocacy for the global plan for IRM (GPIRM), guidance on IVM in humanitarian emergencies, and supporting entomological surveillance, risk assessment, preparedness and response. Effective IVM necessitates strengthening of research, studies of the efficacy and cost-effectiveness of IVM, knowledge, attitude and practice, community participation, and development and harmonization of BCC/IEC messages and effective delivery of materials. Insecticide resistance requires an emergence approach and IVM in humanitarian emergencies need appropriate guidance. The IVM approach can be harnessed as a platform for strategic planning and deployment of vector surveillance, resistance monitoring and management. Thus, rational

IVM strategies should be a pivotal platform for malaria vector control in endemic countries, particularly in conflict and post-conflict or emergency situations. Countries should develop policies, standard operational procedures, country specific guidelines; strengthen human resource capacity, inter-sectoral collaborations, advocacy, legislation and regulation, including community sensitization and engagement. However, significant coordinated response amongst stakeholders and political commitment is needed for timely and effective policy implementation within the context of a national health system. This will require a realization that IVM will yield a positive return for investment in terms of reduced disease burden and the resulting social and economic gains.

Acknowledgements

The author is grateful to the anonymous reviewers for the constructive comments on the manuscript. EC conceptualized this manuscript, formulated the ideas, collected and analysed the data and wrote the manuscript.

Author details

Emmanuel Chanda

Address all correspondence to: emmanuel_chanda@yahoo.co.uk

Department of Biomedical Sciences, School of Medicine, University of Zambia, Lusaka, Zambia

References

[1] Townson H, Nathan MB, Zaim M, Guillet P, Manga L, Bos R, Kindhauser M. Exploiting the potential of vector control for disease prevention. Bull World Health Organ. 2005; 83: 942–947.

[2] WHO. World Malaria Report. Geneva: World Health Organization; 2015. Available from: http://apps.who.int>iris>9789241565158_eng.pdf [cited 2016 Apr 11].

[3] Eisen L, Coleman M, Lozano-Fuentes S, McEachen N, Orlans M, Coleman M. Multi-disease data management system platform for vector-borne diseases. PLoS Negl Trop Dis. 2011; 5:e1016.

[4] WHO. Integrated vector control. Report of the WHO Expert Committee on Vector Biology and Control. WHO Technical Report Series, No. 688. Geneva: World Health Organization; 1983.

[5] WHO. Vector control for malaria and other mosquito-borne diseases. Report of a WHO Study Group. WHO Technical Report Series, No. 857. Geneva: World Health Organization; 1995.

[6] WHO. Second Regional Training Course on Comprehensive Vector Control. Regional Office for South East Asia, World Health Organization; 2001.

[7] WHO. Global Strategic Framework for Integrated Vector Management. WHO/CDS/CPE/PVC/2004.10. Geneva: World Health Organization; 2004. http://whqlibdoc.who.int/hq/2004/WHO_CDS_CPE_PVC_2004_10.pdf

[8] WHO. Position statement on integrated vector management. Geneva: World Health Organization; 2008. http://whqlibdoc.who.int/hq/2008/WHO_HTM_NTD_VEM_2008.2_eng.pdf

[9] WHO. Guidance on policy-making for Integrated Vector Management. Geneva: World Health Organization; 2012.

[10] WHO. Core Structure for training curricula on Integrated Vector Management. Geneva: World Health Organization; 2012. http://whqlibdoc.who.int/publications/2012/9789241502788_eng.pdf.

[11] WHO. Handbook for Integrated Vector Management WHO/HTM/NTD/VEM/2012.3. Geneva: World Health Organization; *2012.* http://whqlibdoc.who.int/publications/2012/9789241502801_eng.pdf.

[12] WHO. Monitoring and Evaluation indicators for Integrated Vector Management. Geneva: World Health Organization; 2012. http://www.who.int/iris/bitstream/10665/76504/1/9789241504027_eng.pdf.

[13] Beier JC, Keating J, Githure JI, Macdonald MB, Impoinvil DE, Novak LR: Integrated vector management for malaria control. Malar J. 2008; 7(Suppl 1):S4.

[14] Guyant P, Corbel V, Guérin PJ, Lautissier A, Nosten F, Boyer S, Coosemans M, Dondorp AM, Sinou V, Yeung S, White N. Past and new challenges for malaria control and elimination: the role of operational research for innovation in designing interventions. Malar J. 2015; 14:279.

[15] Chanda E, Mzilahowa T, Chipwanya J, Mulenga C, Ali D, Troell P, Dodoli W, Govere JM, Gimini J. Preventing malaria transmission by indoor residual spraying in Malawi: grappling with the challenge of uncertain sustainability. Malar J. 2015; 14:254.

[16] Chanda E, Ameneshewa B, Mihreteab S, Berhane A, Zehaie A, Ghebrat Y and Usman A. Consolidating strategic planning and operational frameworks for integrated vector management in Eritrea. Malar J. 2015; 14:488

[17] PubMed Central. www.ncbi.nlm.nih.gov/pubmed.

[18] World Health Organization Website. http://www.who.int/.

[19] Google Scholar. http://www.google.com.

[20] African Journals Online (AJOL). http://www.ajol.info

[21] Armed Forces Pest Management Board http://www.afpmb.org/publications.htm

[22] HINARI http://www.who.int/hinari

[23] MOH. Dengue fever out-breaks in Eritrea, 2005–2015: a case for strengthening control, surveillance and reporting. Asmara, Eritrea: Ministry of Health, 2016.

[24] Sundarama SG, Vijayalakshmia M, Chaaitanyab IK, Nagarajanb M, Sunandhajeevab-harathi G. Research on reemerging of chikungunya - virus disease. J. Chem Pharm Res. 2010; 2:766–773.

[25] Babaniyi OA, Mwaba P, Mulenga D, Monze M, Songolo P, Mazaba-Liwewe ML, Mweene-Ndumba I, Masaninga F, Chizema E, Eshetu-Shibeshi M, Malama C, Rudat-sikira E, Siziya S. Risk assessment for yellow fever in western and North-Western provinces of Zambia. J Global Infect Dis. 2015; 7:11–17.

[26] Simonsen PE, Makelela MN, Michael E, Mackenzie CD (Editors). Lymphatic filariasis: research and control in East and Southern Africa. Denmark: DBL-Centre for Health Research and Development. 2008.

[27] Harbach RE. The Phylogeny and Classification of Anopheles. In Anopheles mosquitoes – New insights into malaria vectors (Sylvie Manguin, ed.). InTech. 2013. pp.3–55. Janeza Trdine 9, 51000 Rijeka, Croatia.

[28] Harbach RE. Mosquito Taxonomic Inventory. http://mosquito-taxonomic-inventory.in-fo/ (accessed on 30 April 2016).

[29] Elbridge BF. Mosquitoes, the Culicidae. In Biology of Disease vectors (William C. Marquardt, ed.). Amsterdam: Elsevier Academic Press, 2005, pp.95–111.

[30] Service MW. Medical Entomology for Students. 5th edition. Cambridge University Press, New York, New York, USA; 2012 ISBN: 978-1107668188 Pages: 317.

[31] OCHA. UN Office for the Coordination of Humanitarian Affairs (OCHA), 2013.

[32] WHO. Sustaining the drive to overcome the global impact of neglected tropical diseases. Second WHO Report on Neglected Tropical Diseases. Geneva, Switzerland: World Health Organization, 2013.

[33] WHO. Working to overcome the global impact of neglected tropical diseases. First WHO Report on Neglected Tropical Diseases. Geneva, Switzerland: World Health Organization; 2012.

[34] WHO. Promise for Progress. Geneva: World Health Organization. Document WHO/CDS/RBM/2000.17; 2000.

[35] Gates B. Malaria forum keynote address. Oct 17, 2007. http://www.gatesfoundation.org/media-center/speeches/2007/10/melinda-frenchgatesmalariaforum (accessed on April 30, 2016).

[36] WHO. Mental health: new understanding, new hope. The World Health Report 2001. Geneva: World Health Organization; 2001.

[37] Mathanga DP, Walker ED, Wilson ML, Ali D, Taylor TE, Laufer MK. Malaria control in Malawi: current status and directions for the future. Acta Trop. 2012; 121: 212–217.

[38] Sinka ME, Bangs MJ, Manguin S, Rubio-Palis Y, Chareonviriyaphap T, Coetzee M et al. A global map of dominant malaria vectors. Parasit Vectors. 2012; 5:69.

[39] Hay SI, Smith DL, Snow RW. Measuring malaria endemicity from intense to interrupted transmission. Lancet Infect Dis. 2008; 8(6): 369–378.

[40] Roll Back Malaria Partnership. Global malaria action plan (2008) http://www.rbm.who.int/gmap/ (accessed on July 27, 2013).

[41] Enayati AA, Lines J, Maharaj R, Hemingway J. Suppressing the vector. In Shrinking the Malaria Map a Prospectus on Malaria Elimination (RGM Feachem, AA Phillips, GA Targett, eds.), San Francisco: Global Health Group. 2009, pp.140–154.

[42] Thomas MB, Godfray HCJ, Read AF, van den Berg H, Tabashnik BE, et al. Lessons from agriculture for the Sustainable Management of Malaria Vectors. PLoS Med. 2012; 9(7): e1001262.

[43] Korenromp EL, Hosseini M, Newman RD, Cibulskis RE. Progress towards malaria control targets in relation to national malaria programme funding. Malar J. 2013; 12:18.

[44] Chanda E, Ameneshewa B, Angula HA, Uusiku P, Iitula I, Trune D, et al. Strengthening tactical planning and operational frameworks for vector control: the roadmap for malaria elimination in Namibia. Malar J. 2015; 14:302.

[45] WHO. Global Malaria Control and Elimination. Report of the Technical Review. Geneva, Switzerland: World Health Organization; 2008.

[46] WHO. Malaria elimination: a field manual for low and moderate endemic countries. Geneva, Switzerland: World Health Organization; 2007.

[47] WHO. Disease surveillance for malaria elimination: an operational manual. Geneva, Switzerland: World Health Organization; 2012.

[48] WHO. Position statement on integrated vector management. Geneva: World Health Organization; 2008. http://whqlibdoc.who.int/hq/2008/WHO_HTM_NTD_VEM_2008.2_eng.pdf.

[49] Chanda E, Masaninga, F, Coleman, M, Sikaala, C, Katebe, C, MacDonald, M, Baboo KS, Govere J, Manga L. Integrated vector management: the Zambian experience. Malar. J. 2008; 7: 164.

[50] Mnzava AP, Michael B. Macdonald, Tessa B. Knox, Emmanuel A. Temu, Clive J. Shiff. Malaria vector control at crossroads: public health entomology and the drive to elimination. Trans R Soc Trop Med Hyg. 2014; 108(9):550–554.

[51] Chanda E, Govere JM, Macdonald MB, Lako RL, Haque U, Baba SP, et al. Integrated vector management: a critical strategy for combating vector-borne diseases in South Sudan. Mal J. 2013; 12:369.

[52] RBM. Roll Back Malaria Vector Control Working Group (VCWG) 10th Annual Meeting, 28th–30th January 2015. Geneva, Switzerland.

[53] Okia M, Okui P, Lugemwa M, Govere JM, Katamba V, Rwakimari JB, Mpeka B, Chanda E. Consolidating tactical planning and implementation frameworks for integrated vector management in Uganda. Malar J. 2015; 15:214

[54] The Stockholm Convention on Persistent Organic Pollutants, May 2001.

[55] WHOPES. Decision-making for the judicious use of insecticides. WHO/CDS/WHOPES/2004.9a. Geneva, Switzerland: World Health Organization; 2004. http://whqlibdoc.who.int/hq/2004/WHO_CDS_WHOPES_2004.9a.pdf

[56] Hemmingway J, Ranson H. Chemical control of vectors and mechanisms of resistance. In Biology of Disease Vectors (William C. Marquardt, ed.). Amsterdam: Elsevier Academic Press. 2005. pp.627–647.

[57] Marquardt WC. Biology of Disease Vectors. Amsterdam: Elsevier Academic Press, 2nd edition, 2005.

[58] Berker N. et al. Mosquitoes and their Control. Heidelberg, Dordrecht, London, New York: Springer. 2nd edition, 2010.

[59] van den Berg H. Global status of DDT and its alternatives for use in vector control to prevent disease. Environ Health Perspect. 2009; 117: 1656–1663.

[60] Pluess B, Tanser FC, Lengeler C, Sharp BL. Indoor residual spraying for preventing malaria. Cochrane. Database Syst Rev. 2010; 4: CD006657.

[61] Lindsay SW, Snow RW, Broomfield GL, Janneh MS, Wirtz RA, Greenwood BM. Impact of permethrin-treated bednets on malaria transmission by the Anopheles gambiae complex in the Gambia. Med Vet Entomol. 1989; 3(3): 263–271.

[62] Lengeler C, Sharp B. Indoor residual spraying and insecticide-treated nets, In Reducing Malaria's Burden: Evidence of Effectiveness for Decision Makers. Global Health Council Technical Report. December 2003, pp.17–24.

[63] Lines J, Lengeler C, Cham K, de Savigny D, Chimumbwa J, Langi P, Carroll D, Mills A, Hanson K, Webster J, Lynch M, Addington W, Hill J, Rowland M, Worrall E, MacDonald M, Kilian A. Scaling-up and sustaining insecticide-treated net coverage. Lancet Infect Dis. 2003; 3(8): 465–466.

[64] Curtis CF, Mnzava AE. Comparison of house spraying and insecticide-treated nets for malaria control. Bull World Health Organ. 2000; 78(12): 1389–1400.

[65] Lengeler C. Insecticide-treated bed nets and curtains for preventing malaria. Cochrane. Database Syst Rev. 2004; (2): CD000363.

[66] Mabaso ML, Sharp B, Lengeler C. Historical review of malarial control in southern African with emphasis on the use of indoor residual house-spraying. Trop Med Int Health. 2004; 9(8): 846–856.

[67] Kleinschmidt I, Schwabe C, Shiva M, Segura JL, Sima V, Mabunda SJ, Coleman M. Combining indoor residual spraying and insecticide-treated net interventions. Am J Trop Med Hyg. 2009; 81(3): 519–524.

[68] Kleinschmidt I, Sharp B, Benavente LE, Schwabe C, Torrez M, Kuklinski J, Morris N, Raman J, Carter J. Reduction in infection with *Plasmodium falciparum* one year after the introduction of malaria control interventions on Bioko Island, Equatorial Guinea. Am J Trop Med Hyg. 2006; 74(6): 972–978.

[69] Protopopoff N, Van BW, Marcotty T, Van HM, Maes P, Baza D, D'Alessandro U, Coosemans M. Spatial targeted vector control is able to reduce malaria prevalence in the highlands of Burundi. Am J Trop Med Hyg. 2008; 79(1): 12–18.

[70] N'guessan R, Corbel V, Akogbeto M, Rowland M. Reduced efficacy of insecticide-treated nets and indoor residual spraying for malaria control in pyrethroid resistance area, Benin Emerg Infect Dis. 2007; 13: 199–206.

[71] Keiser J, Singer BH, Utzinger J. Reducing the burden of malaria in different eco-epidemiological settings with environmental management: a systematic review. Lancet Infect. Dis. 2005; 5(11): 695–708.

[72] World Health Organization. Environmental Management for Vector Control. WHO Technical Report Series, No. 649. Geneva. Switzerland: World Health Organization; 1980.

[73] Ault, S.K. Environmental management: a re-emerging vector control strategy. Am J Trop Med Hyg. 1995; 50: 35–49.

[74] Cutis, C.F. et al. Insect proofing of sanitation systems. In: Appropriate Technology in Vector Control (C.F. Cutis ed.). Boca Raton, FL: CRC Press. 1990, pp.173–186.

[75] Mather, TH, That, TT. Environmental Management for Vector Control in Rice Fields. Rome: Food and Agriculture Organization of the United Nations; 1984.

[76] Provost, MW. Environmental hazards in the control of disease vectors. Environ Entomol. 1972; 1:333–339.

[77] Rajagopalan, P.K. et al. Environmental and Water Management in mosquito control. In Appropriate Technology in Vector Control (C.F. Cutis ed.). Boca Raton, FL: CRC Press. 1990, pp.121-138

[78] Small GJ. Environmental management for vector control. In Biology of Disease vectors (William C. Marquardt, ed.). Amsterdam: Elsevier Academic Press, 2005, pp.639–647.

[79] Reimold, RJ. Mangals and salt marshes of eastern United States. In Wet Coastal Ecosystems. Ecosystems of the World: Vol. 1 (V.J. Chapman, ed). Amsterdam: Elsevier Scientific. 1977, pp.157–166.

[80] Mitchell CJ. Environmental management for vector control. In Biology of Disease vectors (Barry J Betty, and William C. Marquardt, eds.). Niwot: University Press of Colarado. 1996, pp.492–501.

[81] U.S. Public Health Services and Tennessee Valley Authority. Malaria Control on Impounded Water. Washington, DC: Government Printing Office; 1947.

[82] Hemmingway, J. Biological control of mosquitoes. In Biology of Disease Vectors (William C. Marquardt, ed.). Amsterdam: Elsevier Academic Press. 2005. pp. 649–660.

[83] Service, MW. Some ecological considerations basic to bio-control of culicidae and other medically important insects. In Integrated Control of Vectors, Vol. 1. (M. Laird, and J. W. Miles, eds.). London: Academic Press. 1985, pp.9–30.

[84] Walker K, Lynch M. Contributions of Anopheles larval control to malaria suppression in tropical Africa: review of achievements and potential. Med Vet Entomol. 2007; 21(1): 2–21.

[85] Higgs, S. Special methods as applied to vectors of disease agents. In Biology of Disease Vectors (William C. Marquardt, ed.). Amsterdam: Elsevier Academic Press. 2005, pp. 684–692.

[86] Oxborough RM, N'Guessan R, Jones R, Kitau J, Ngufor C, et al. The activity of the pyrrole insecticide chlorfenapyr in mosquito bioassay: towards a more rational testing and screening of non-neurotoxic insecticides for malaria vector control. Malar J. 2015; 14: 124.

[87] Tusting LS, Ippolito MM, Willey BA, Kleinschmidt I, Dorsey G, et al. The evidence for improving housing to reduce malaria: a systematic review and meta-analysis. Malar J. 2015; 14: 209.

[88] Nnankya M, Matthews G. Malaria control, Better Health, Better Future. Out looks Pest Manage. 2015; 26: 1–2.

[89] Wood RJ. Genetic control of vectors. In Biology of Disease Vectors (William C. Marquardt, ed.). Amsterdam: Elsevier Academic Press. 2005, pp.661–669.

[90] Lyaloo DP, Elahee KB, Bheecarry A, Lees RS. Guidelines to site selection for population surveillance and mosquito control trials: a case study from Mauritius. Acta Tropica 132S. 2014; S140–S149.

[91] Townson H. SIT for African malaria vectors: epilogue. Malar J. 2009; 8(Suppl 2):S10.

[92] Curtis CF, Sinkins SP. *Wolbachia* as a possible means of driving genes into populations. Parasitology. 1998; 116: 371–374.

[93] Curtis CF, Townson, H. Malaria: existing methods of vector control and molecular entomology. Br Med Bull. 1998; 54:311–325.

[94] Seawright JA, Keiser PE, Dame DA, Lofgren, CS. Genetic method for preferential elimination of females of *Anopheles albimanus*. Science. 1978; 300: 1303–1304.

[95] Thomas DD, Donnelly CA, Wood RJ, Alphey LS. Insect population control using a dominant, repressed lethal genetic system. Science. 2000; 287: 2474–2476.

[96] Wikel SK, Alarcon-Chaidez F, Muller-Doblies U. Immunological control of vectors. In Biology of Disease Vectors (William C. Marquardt, ed.). Amsterdam: Elsevier Academic Press. 2005, pp.671–682.

[97] Dubin IN, Reese JD, Seamans LA. Attempt to produce protection against mosquitoes by active immunization. J Immunol. 1948; 58: 293–297.

[98] Alger NE, Cabrera, EJ. An increase in death rate of *Anopheles stephensi* fed on rabbits immunized with mosquito antigen. J Econ Entomol. 1972; 65: 165–168.

[99] Almeida, AP, Billingsley, PF. Induced immunity against the mosquito *Anopheles stephensi* Liston (Diptera: Culicidae): effect on mosquito survival and fecundity. Int I Parasitol. 1998; 28: 1721–1731.

[100] Lal AA, Schriefer ME, Sacci JB, Goldman IF, Louis-Wileman V, Collins WE, Azad, AF. Inhibition of malaria parasite development in mosquitoes by antimosquito midgut antibodies. Infect Immun. 1994; 62: 316–318.

[101] Ramasamy MS, Raschid L, Srikrishnaraj KA, Ramasamy R. Antimidgut antibodies inhibit peritrophic membrane formation in the posterior midgut of *Anopheles tessellates* (Diptera: Culicidae). J Med Entomol. 1996; 33: 162–164.

[102] Srikrishnaraj KA, Ramasamy R, Ramasamy MS. Antibodies to *Anopheles* midgut reduces vector competence for *Plasmodium vivax* malaria. Med Vet Entomol.1995; 9: 353–357.

[103] Ramasamy MS, Ramasamy R. Effect of antimosquito antibodies on the infectivity of the rodent malaria parasite *Plasmodium berghei* to *Anopheles farauti*. Med Vet Entomol. 1990; 4: 161–166.

[104] Lal AA, Patterson PS, Sacci JB, Vaughan JA, Paul C, Collins WE, Wirtz RA, Azad, AF. Antimosquito midgut antibodies block development of *Plasmodium falciparum* and *Plasmodium vivax* in multiple species of *Anopheles* mosquitoes and reduce vector fecundity and survivorship. Proc Natl Acad Sci U.S.A. 2001; 98: 5228–5233.

[105] Komatsu R, Korenromp EL, Low-Beer D, Watt C, Dye C, Steketee RW, Nahlen BL, Lyerla R, Garcia-Calleja JM, Cutler J, Schwartlander B. Lives saved by global fund-supported HIV/AIDS, tuberculosis and malaria programs: estimation approach and results between 2003 and end-2007. BMC Infect Dis. 2010; 10: 109.

[106] Coleman M, Hemingway J. Insecticide resistance monitoring and evaluation in disease transmitting mosquitoes. J Pestic Sci. 2007; 32: 69–76

[107] Tatarsky A, Aboobakar S, Cohen JM, Gopee N, Bheecarry A, et al. Preventing the reintroduction of malaria in Mauritius: a programmatic and financial assessment. PLoS One. 2011; 6(9): e23832.

[108] Geissbühler, Y. Ecology and Epidemiology of Integrated Malaria Vector Management in Dar es Salaam, Tanzania. Doctoral Thesis, University of Basel; 2008.

[109] Mboera LEG, Mazigo HD, Rumisha SF, Kramer RA. Towards malaria elimination and its implication for vector control, disease management and livelihoods in Tanzania. MWJ. 2013, 4:19.

[110] Mutero CM, Mbogo C, Mwangangi J, Imbahale S, Kibe L, Orindi B, Girma M, Njui A, Lwande W, Affognon H, Gichuki C, Mukabana WR. An assessment of participatory integrated vector management for malaria control in Kenya. Environ Health Perspect. 2015; 123:1145–1151

[111] Abilio AP, Kleinschmidt I, Rehman AM, Cuamba N, Ramdeen V, et al. The emergence of insecticide resistance in central Mozambique and potential threat to the successful indoor residual spraying malaria control programme. Malar J. 2011; 10: 110. doi: 10.1186/1475-2875-10-110.

[112] MOH. National malaria control programme strategy. 2008–2013. Harare, Zimbabwe: Ministry of Health and Child Welfare, 2007.

[113] Pocquet N, Darriet F, Zumbo B, Milesi P, Thiria J, Bernard V, Toty C, Labbé P, Chandre F. Insecticide resistance in disease vectors from Mayotte: an opportunity for integrated vector management. Parasites Vectors. 2014; 7:299.

[114] Ministry of Health. National Strategic Plan on Integrated Vector Management (IVM) (2012–2017). Kigali: Republic of Rwanda; 2012.

[115] Mutero CM, Schlodder D, Kabatereine N, Kramer R. Integrated vector management for malaria control in Uganda: knowledge, perceptions and policy development. Malar J. 2012; 11:21.

[116] MoH. Integrated Vector Management Strategic Guidelines for Uganda. Ministry of Health; 2014.

[117] GoSS. Integrated Vector Management Strategic Plan for Southern Sudan 2007–2012. Juba: Government of Southern Sudan: Ministry of Health; 2006.

[118] MoH. Malaria and other vector-borne diseases control strategy 2015-2019 in Eritrea. The State of Eritrea: The National Malaria Control Program; 2014.

[119] Naranjo DP, Qualls WA, Jurado H, Perez JC, Xue RD, Gomez E, Beier JC. Vector control programs in Saint Johns County, Florida and Guayas, Ecuador: successes and barriers to integrated vector management. BMC Public Health. 2014; 14:674.

[120] Zofou D, Nyasa RB, Nsagha DS, Ntie-Kang F, Meriki HD, Assob JCN, Kuete V. Control of malaria and other vector-borne protozoan diseases in the tropics: enduring challenges despite considerable progress and achievements. Infect Dis Poverty 2014, 3:1.

[121] Stone CM, Lindsay SW, Chitnis N. How effective is integrated vector management against malaria and lymphatic filariasis where the diseases are transmitted by the same vector? PLoS Negl Trop Dis. 2014; 8(12): e3393.

[122] Bellini R, Zeller H, Bortel WV. A review of the vector management methods to prevent and control outbreaks of West Nile virus infection and the challenge for Europe. Parasites Vectors 2014, 7:323.

[123] Lizzi KM, Qualls WA, Brown SC, Beier JC. Expanding integrated vector management to promote healthy environments. Trends Parasitol. 2014;30(8): 394–400.

[124] The malERA Consultative Group on Health Systems and Operational Research. A research agenda for malaria eradication: health systems and operational research. PLoS Med. 2011; 8(1): e1000397.

[125] Environmental Health Project. Improving Vector Control and Surveillance for Malaria and Other Vector-Borne Diseases. Environmental Health Project. 2005. www.ehproject.org

[126] Zhou S, Rietveld AEC, Velarde-Rodriguez M, Ramsay AR, Zhang S, Zhou X, Cibulskis RE. Operational research on malaria control and elimination: a review of projects published between 2008 and 2013. Malar J. 2014; 13:473.

[127] WHO. Monitoring and Evaluation indicators for Integrated Vector Management. Geneva: World Health Organization; 2012. http://www.who.int/iris/bitstream/10665/76504/1/9789241504027_eng.pdf

[128] Mnzava AP, Knox TB, Temu EA, Trett A, Fornadel C, Hemingway J, Renshaw M. Implementation of the global plan for insecticide resistance management in malaria vectors: progress, challenges and the way forward. Malar J. 2015; 14:173.

[129] Roll Back Malaria Vector Control Working Group 10th Annual and Work Stream Meetings, 28th-30th January 2015. (http://www.rollbackmalaria.org/files/files/working-groups/VCWG/VCWG-10%20Meeting%20Report%20final.pdf).

5

Declining Transmission of Malaria in India: Accelerating Towards Elimination

Sunil Dhiman, Vijay Veer and Vas Dev

Abstract

India is ecologically vast and has close to a billion-population living at risk of malaria. Given the evidence-based present-day intervention tools and large-scale implementation, India has recorded declining trends in disease transmission from 2 million cases in 2001 to close to a million cases in 2017 and embarked upon malaria elimination in keeping with the Global Technical Strategy by 2030. India is malaria endemic, but transmission intensities varied across its landscape with just few States of the east, central and northeast contributing bulk (80%) of total positive cases. *Plasmodium falciparum* and *P. vivax* are the predominant infections of which there has been steady increase in proportions of the former for constituting >60% of total cases what was 50:50 in 2001, a phenomenon attributed to emerging drug resistance. With the rolling out of the available intervention tools, malaria elimination is foreseeable yet there are multiple challenges which must be addressed to overcome the constraints. We strongly advocate continued disease surveillance and monitoring, universal coverage and intensification of core-interventions for prevention and treatment prioritizing high-risk States, strengthening cross-border collaborations for information sharing and coordinated activities, and above all sustained allocation of resources, creating the enabling environment to end malaria transmission.

Keywords: malaria elimination, epidemiology, *Plasmodium falciparum*, drug-resistance, mosquito vectors, insecticide resistance, Southeast Asia

1. Introduction

The advent of new intervention tools including Noble prize-winning discovery of Artemisinin by Tu Youyou for treatment of malaria combined with large-scale implementation of insecticide-treated netting materials for vector containment has once again renewed the optimism of malaria elimination globally. Malaria map is shrinking with more than 35 countries certified to be malaria free, and another 21 countries that are likely to reach zero indigenous transmission (categorized as E-2020) are set to be declared malaria free by 2020 [1, 2]. Many more countries are moving forward from control to elimination. The Global Technical Strategy for Malaria 2016–2030 envisages: (i) to reduce global malaria mortality rates and case incidence by at least 90% compared to 2015 levels, (ii) to make at least 35 countries malaria free that reported cases in 2015 and (iii) preventing re-establishment in countries with no indigenous transmission [3]. Among member countries of the Southeast Asia Region of WHO (SEAR), Maldives and Sri Lanka have already been certified malaria free in 2015 and 2016, respectively, and Bhutan is targeting elimination in the foreseeable future. In the past decade, India has registered drastic decrease in cases and have formulated National Framework for Malaria Elimination (2016–2030) in close alignment with the Global Technical Strategy for Malaria, Roll Back Malaria Action (RBM), Investment to defeat Malaria (AIM) and the Asia Pacific Leaders Malaria Alliance (APLMA) for shared experiences and coordinated action to eliminate malaria (zero indigenous cases) throughout the country by 2030 [4]. The said task is set to be accomplished in phased manner with the following objectives: (i) eliminate malaria in all 26 low-to-moderate transmission States/Union Territories (UTs) by 2022, (ii) reduce the case incidence to <1 per 1000 population by 2024 in all States/UTs, (iii) interrupt indigenous transmission throughout the country by 2027 and (iv) prevent re-establishment of local transmission and maintain malaria-free status by 2030 and beyond.

India is historically endemic for both *Plasmodium vivax* and *P. falciparum* malaria and has history of successes and resurgences [5, 6]. Malaria was on the verge of elimination post-independence in 1960s with 0.1 million cases and no death, yet it reared its ugly head again in 1970s with record number of six million cases and many deaths attributed to technical and operational constraints. Transmission is largely seasonal corresponding to rainy season with record of focal disease outbreaks characterized by high rise in cases and attributable deaths. In 2017, India reported 0.84 million cases, the highest disease burden in SEAR member countries of WHO [4, 7]. Almost all Indian States and UTs are reporting cases, which can be broadly stratified into three different categories based on Annual Parasite Incidence (API) per 1000 population, that is, Category—I (total of 15 States/UTs including districts with API < 1) that are targeted for elimination phase, Category—II (total of 11 States/UTs with API < 1 with one or more districts reporting > 1 API) marked for pre-elimination phase and Category—III (total of 10 States/UTs with > 1 API) targeted for intensified control operations. With the rolling out of the present day evidence-based intervention tools, disease transmission is on the steady decline presenting window of opportunity to accelerate toward universal coverage for malaria prevention and treatment. India is a huge country (population 1.3 billion) with majority populous (80%) living at risk of malaria. The task is enormous and daunting. Given the political commitment and National Framework developed by the National Vector Borne Disease Control Programme (NVBDCP) of Government of India, malaria elimination is foreseeable, yet there are multiple challenges which must be addressed to overcome the constraints. In this chapter, we attempt to enumerate some of these issues helping strengthen healthcare services in combating malaria menace enabling elimination by due date.

2. Malaria transmission in India: current distribution and parasite formula

Malaria transmission is heterogenous across Indian landscape for its diverse ecology and multiplicity of disease vectors [8]. Malaria is a serious public health concern and almost all 36 States/UTs are consistently contributing cases, but transmission intensities varied ranging from low-to-moderate (**Table 1**). Among these, north-eastern, eastern and central Indian States consistently contributed 80% of the total disease burden having concentration of cases (API > 10) associated with large forest cover, ethnic tribes, poverty and high rainfall (**Figure 1**). These included States of Odisha (formerly Orissa) and Jharkhand (eastern India), Chhattisgarh and Madhya Pradesh (central India) and Meghalaya and Tripura (northeast India), which together contributed >65% of *P. falciparum* cases. Approximately a billion population of India resides in malaria endemic areas, however, 80% of malaria cases are reported by just 20% of the population living in the forest-fringe, tribal and foothills hard-to-reach areas of the country little aware of disease prevention and access to treatment [9]. These areas are prone to periodic disease outbreaks resulting in flare up of cases and attributable mortality accounting for inter-annual variation in reported morbidity. From the epidemiological data for the past 17 years (2001–2017), disease transmission trends are observed to be declining from two million cases in 2001 to close to a million cases in 2017 (**Figure 2**). However, consequent to the introduction of artemisinin-based combination therapy (ACT) beginning 2010 coupled with insecticide-treated netting materials (ITNs); there has been drastic decrease in cases and deaths. *P. falciparum* and *P. vivax* are the predominant infections of which there has been steady increase in proportions of the former parasite species presently constituting >60% of total cases what was 50:50 in 2001. Every single death was attributed to *P. falciparum*, majority of which were contributed by high-risk States of north-eastern, eastern and central India (**Figure 3**). The distribution of *P. malariae* is patchy, recorded in indigenous tribes of eastern, north-eastern and central India [10–12], but transmission of *P. ovale* except for few sporadic reports could not be clearly ascertained [13–15]. There exists no record of *P. knowlesi* malaria in India making inroads in other Southeast Asian countries [16].

The reported cases and deaths; however, are far from acccurate for disease surveillance that can be best described as fragmented and there is no system in place to capture data from private and public sectors alike, least the asymptomatic cases [17]; WHO estimates are much higher to the tune of >10 million cases and deaths manifold [1]. Nevertheless, the presented data showed disease transmisison trends in relation to existing interventions, and monitoring and evaluation in practice.

No	State/Union Territories	2014			2015			2016			2017		
		Total malaria cases	*Plasmodium falciparum* cases	Deaths	Total malaria cases	*Plasmodium falciparum* cases	Deaths	Total malaria cases	*Plasmodium falciparum* cases	Deaths	Total malaria cases	*Plasmodium falciparum* cases	Deaths
1	Andhra Pradesh	21,077	15,511	0	25,042	18,709	0	23,613	17,443	0	16,913	11,944	0
2	Arunachal Pradesh	6082	2338	9	5088	1714	7	3144	911	2	1538	487	0
3	Assam	14,540	11,210	11	15,557	11,675	4	7826	5686	6	5473	4131	0
4	Bihar	2043	699	0	4006	1286	1	5205	895	0	3175	356	2
5	Chhattisgarh	128,993	108,874	53	144,886	123,839	21	148,220	121,503	61	141,310	115,153	0
6	Goa	824	42	0	651	75	1	742	130	0	653	75	2
7	Gujarat	41,608	6253	16	41,566	7232	7	44,783	6298	6	37,801	3502	2
8	Haryana	4485	45	1	9308	726	3	7866	552	0	6887	904	0
9	Himachal Pradesh	102	1	0	60	1	0	121	19	0	95	9	0
10	Jammu & Kashmir	291	21	0	216	8	0	242	11	0	226	0	0
11	Jharkhand	103,735	46,448	8	104,800	54,993	6	141,414	83,232	15	92,770	42,047	1
12	Karnataka	14,794	1329	2	12,445	1598	0	11,078	1746	0	6529	1118	0
13	Kerala	1751	305	6	1549	400	4	1547	419	2	1194	317	2
14	Madhya Pradesh	96,879	41,638	26	100,597	39,125	24	69,106	22,304	3	46,176	15,554	3
15	Maharashtra	53,385	25,770	68	56,603	31,139	59	23,983	7815	26	18,133	5929	19
16	Manipur	145	72	0	216	119	0	122	58	0	80	22	0
17	Meghalaya	39,168	37,149	73	48,603	43,828	79	35,147	31,867	45	16,433	14,974	11
18	Mizoram	23,145	21,083	31	28,593	24,602	21	7583	5907	9	5710	4978	0

No	State/Union Territories	2014			2015			2016			2017		
		Total malaria cases	*Plasmodium falciparum* cases	Deaths	Total malaria cases	*Plasmodium falciparum* cases	Deaths	Total malaria cases	*Plasmodium falciparum* cases	Deaths	Total malaria cases	*Plasmodium falciparum* cases	Deaths
19	Nagaland	1936	647	2	1527	532	3	828	316	0	394	188	1
20	Orissa	395,035	342,280	89	436,850	369,533	80	449,697	389,332	77	352,140	297,554	25
21	Punjab	1036	14	0	596	13	0	693	8	0	808	12	0
22	Rajasthan	15,118	603	4	11,796	662	3	12,741	1031	5	6837	377	0
23	Sikkim	35	18	0	27	11	0	15	5	0	12	3	0
24	Tamil Nadu	8729	339	0	5587	355	0	4341	242	0	5449	197	0
25	Telangana	5189	4602	0	10,951	10,206	4	3512	2617	1	2688	2170	0
26	Tripura	51,240	49,653	96	32,525	30,074	21	10,546	9545	14	7040	6572	6
27	Uttarakhand	1171	89	0	1466	73	0	961	47	0	532	14	0
28	Uttar Pradesh	41,612	326	0	42,767	371	0	39,238	158	0	32,345	159	0
29	West Bengal	26,484	4981	66	24,208	5775	34	35,236	5928	59	30,008	4632	29
30	A.N. Islands	557	109	0	409	77	0	485	140	0	404	67	0
31	Chandigarh	114	0	0	152	1	1	157	0	0	114	1	0
32	D & N Haveli	669	90	1	418	46	0	375	30	0	297	16	0
33	Daman & Diu	56	4	0	84	18	0	48	7	0	37	4	0
34	Delhi	98	0	0	54	0	0	31	0	0	577	2	0
35	Lakshadweep	0	0	0	4	0	0	2	0	0	1	0	0
36	Puducherry	79	3	0	54	5	1	76	11	0	59	13	0
All India total		1,102,205	722,546	562	1,169,261	778,821	384	1,090,724	716,213	331	840,838	533,481	103

[*]*Source*: Ref. [7].

Table 1. Malaria-attributable morbidity and mortality in different States and Union Territories (UTs) of India during 2014–2017[*].

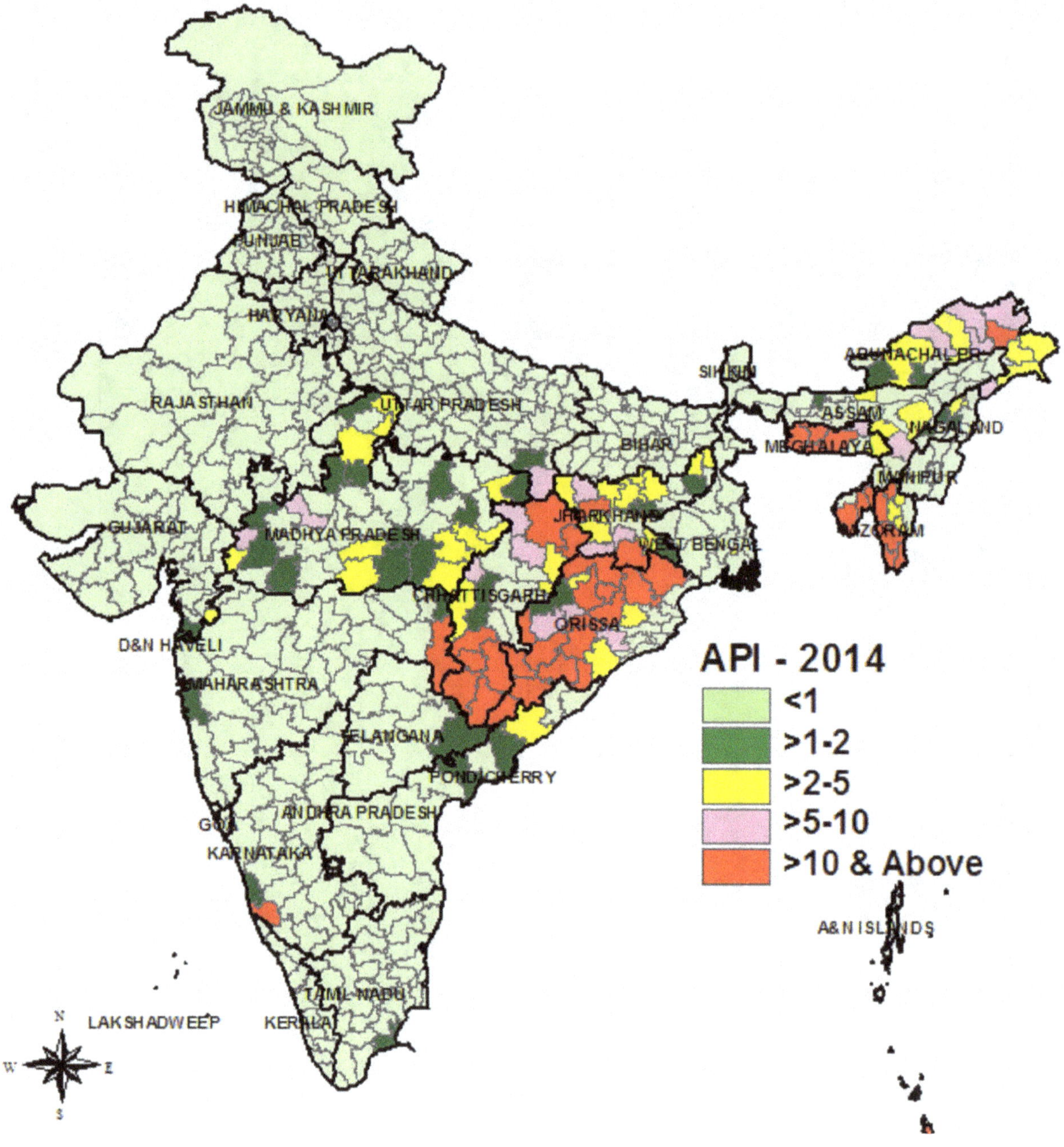

Figure 1. Malaria stratification by Annual Parasite Incidence (API) in Indian States for data based on 2014. API 10 corresponds to 10 confirmed cases per 1000 population. *Source*: Ref. [4].

3. Multiple disease vectors and insecticide resistance

India holds the distinction in malaria epidemiological research for Noble prize-winning discovery that malaria is transmitted by mosquitoes by Sir Ronald Ross on the day of August 20, 1897, and for monumental work on faunistic surveys dating back to 1930s [18]. Of the 58 anopheline species recorded in India [19], six major vector taxa are implicated in malaria transmission, including *Anopheles culicifacies s.l., An. fluviatilis s.l., An. minimus s.l., An. dirus s.l., An. sundaicus s.l.* and *An. stephensi* [20]. All of these, except *An. stephensi*, are species complexes among which members

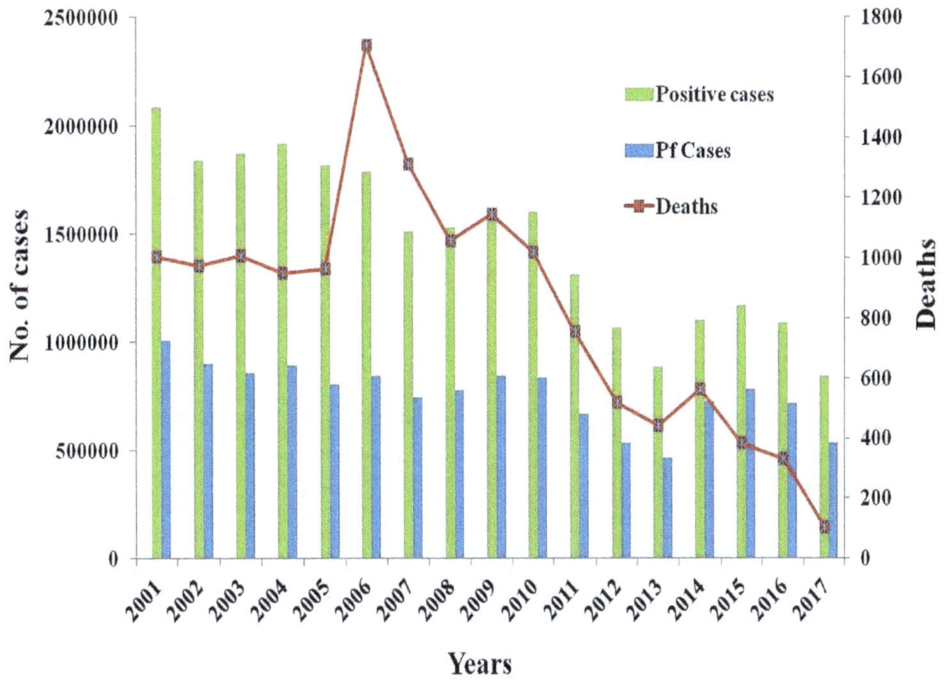

Figure 2. Malaria-attributable morbidity and mortality in India during 2001–2017. Malaria positive cases denote confirmed diagnosis by presence of malarial parasite in finger-prick blood-smears; Pf cases denote positivity for *Plasmodium falciparum;* death cases are attributed to confirmed falciparum malarial infection. *Source*: Ref. [7].

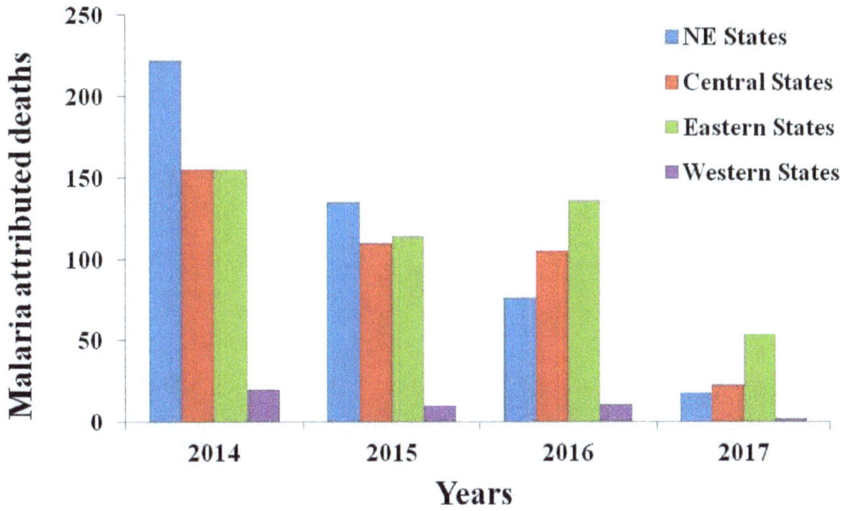

Figure 3. Distribution of malaria-attributed deaths in different geoepidemiological regions of India for data based on 2014–2017. NE refers to group of seven sister States of northeast India including Arunachal Pradesh, Assam, Meghalaya, Manipur, Mizoram, Nagaland and Tripura; Central States include Madhya Pradesh and Chhattisgarh; Eastern States include Bihar, Jharkhand, Odisha (formerly Orissa) and West Bengal; Western States include Maharashtra, Goa, Gujarat and Rajasthan. In the remaining Indian States and Union Territories, death cases were few and far (not shown). *Source*: Ref. [7].

were repeatedly incriminated as vectors evidenced by detection of live sporozoites in salivary glands across range of their distribution [21, 22]. With added tools of molecular taxonomy; however, there have been significant advances in understanding sibling-species composition of these taxa [23–25], distribution and their bionomics helping target species-specific control interventions in place and time (**Table 2**). Among these, *An. culicifacies* is the most widespread and extensively

Anopheles species/ taxa	Sibling species prevalent in India (total identified)	Diagnostic cytotaxonomic/ molecular tools	Breeding habitats	Feeding behavior (peak biting activity)	Resting habitats	Sporozoite infectivity (%)	Insecticide susceptibility status	Distribution range
An. culicifacies s.l.	A,B,C,D and E (5)	Fixed paracentric inversions, PCR based sequencing of 28S-D3 domain; ITS2-PCR-RFLP; rDNA ITS2	Rain water collections, riverine pools, rice fields, seepage water, streams, borrow pits, irrigation channels	Predominantly zoophilic except 'E' (A and B: 22:00–23:00; C and D: 18:00–21:00; no data for E)	Human-dwellings indoors and cattle sheds	Incriminated (0.3–20)	Resistant to DDT, malathion and pyrethroids	Throughout rural India
An. fluviatilis s.l.	S, T, U and Form 'V' (4)	Fixed paracentric inversions; PCR based sequencing of rDNA ITS2; 28S rDNA-D3	Seepage water foothill streams, irrigation channels, river ecology, shallow wells	Sibling species 'S'—highly anthropophilic (20:00–24:00); 'T'—zoophilic	S—human dwellings indoors; T—cattle sheds	Incriminated	Highly susceptible to all residual insecticides	Throughout India except north-eastern States
An. minimus s.l.	*An. minimus s.s.* (3)	rDNA ITS2; 28S rDNA-D3	Perennial foothill seepage water streams	Highly anthropophilic (01:00—04:00)	Human-dwellings indoors	Incriminated (3.0)	Highly susceptible to all residual insecticides	North-eastern of Arunachala Pradesh, Assam, Meghalaya, Manipur, Mizoram, Nagaland, Tripura, and Eastern State of Odisha
An. dirus s.l.	*An. baimaii* (8)	Karyotypic studies, polytene chromosome analysis, gene-enzyme variation, DNA probes, rDNA ITS2; SCAR-PCR	Jungle water pools, Elephant foot-prints	Highly anthropophilic (21:00—24:00)	Exophilic	Incriminated (1.9)	Highly susceptible to all residual insecticides	North-eastern of Arunachala Pradesh, Assam, Meghalaya, Manipur, Mizoram, Nagaland, Tripura
An. sundaicus s.l.	*An. sundaicus* cytotype D (4)	Mitochondrial DNA cytochrome oxidase 1 and cytochrome-b; rDNA ITS2; 28S rDNA-D3	Brackish water including swamps, salt water lagoons, creeks as well as fresh water	Predominantly zoophilic except indoor resting populations (21:00—04:00)	Both indoors and outdoors	Incriminated	Highly susceptible to all residual insecticides	Andaman & Nicobar Islands

Anopheles species/ taxa	Sibling species prevalent in India (total identified)	Diagnostic cytotaxonomic/ molecular tools	Breeding habitats	Feeding behavior (peak biting activity)	Resting habitats	Sporozoite infectivity (%)	Insecticide susceptibility status	Distribution range
An. stephensi	Not applicable		Domestic containers, building construction sites, overhead water storage tanks, underground cement tanks, desert coolers	Predominantly anthropophilic (22:00—24:00)	Endophilic	Incriminated	Resistant to DDT and Malathion	Urban metropolitan cities of India

[*]*Source*: Refs. [20, 23–25]; rDNA, ribosomal DNA; SCAR, sequence characterized amplified region; ITS2, internal transcribed spacer 2; PCR, polymerase chain reaction.

Table 2. Bionomics, distribution and sibling-species composition of the dominant mosquito vector taxa of human malaria in India[*].

studied for its sibling species composition (A, B, C, D and E), distribution range, seasonal prevalence, larval ecology, feeding and breeding behavior and disease transmission relationships [26]. Species E is the most efficient malaria vector of all having predilection for human host, while species B is a poor vector for its zoophilic characteristics. The other three species (A, C and D) are responsible for local transmission in areas of their predominance [27]. This taxon is the most abundant rural vector in plains of mainland India generating about 65% of cases annually and held responsible for focal disease outbreaks associated with build-up of vector density. It is regarded as highly adaptive species for its diverse breeding habitats and invading new territories in degraded forests of north-eastern India evidenced by records of rising density and incrimination [28–30]. Its control has become a formidable challenge for having grown multi-resistant virtually to all available insecticides including pyrethroids opening new vistas for research on newer interventions that are sustainable, cost-effective and community-based [31–33].

An. fluviatilis complex is just as widespread and have overlapping distribution with *An. culicifacies* throughout India [20]. Among its sibling species, that is, S, T, U and form 'V'; it is species S which is highly anthropophilic and responsible for maintaining hyperendemic malaria predominantly in foothills of eastern India contributing ~15% of reported cases [34]. It shares similar bionomical characteristics with yet another efficient malaria vector species *An. minimus s.s* for breeding in foothill seepage water streams and resting indoors in human dwellings [35]. Both are highly susceptible to residual insecticides. *An. minimus* instead is the most predominant vector species of north-eastern States of India and has long history of disappearance and re-appearance stymying the control authorities. It is reckoned as the most efficient vector species for its high anthropophily (human blood index > 90%) and fulminating focal disease outbreaks taking heavy toll of human lives [36]. It is a perennial species and widely incriminated practically all months of the year with average sporozoite infection rate of 3% [37]. This species exhibits high behavioral plasticity for avoiding sprayed surfaces for weeks and establishing extra-domiciliary transmission in response to indoor residual spraying (IRS). While this species has staged comeback in eastern State of Odisha after lapse of 45 years [38], the populations of *An. minimus* once again are reported diminishing in erstwhile domains of its distribution in northeast India corroborated by evidence of reducing disease transmission [35]. It presents an unprecedented opportunity to strengthen interventions to keep populations of this species at bay helping achieve malaria elimination specific to the region at sub-national level.

Within the *An. dirus* complex, *An. baimaii* is the only vector occurring in India with a wide prevalence in the north-eastern States and has been recorded in high densities and incriminated in range of its distribution [39]. It is just as efficient vector species with strong predilection for human host but distinct from *An. minimus* for its breeding and resting characteristics [40, 41]. It is a forest dweller affecting forest-fringe human settlements along inter-country and inter-state border areas causing devastating disease outbreaks often in conjunction with *An. minimus;* together they contribute 10% of reported cases in the country [42]. Its control has become difficult for peak biting activity during second quartile (21:00–00:00) of the night as well as exophilic resting behavior avoiding sprayed surfaces. Its populations along with that of *An. minimus* are also depleting owing to deforestation and urbanization [29, 30]. However, niche thus vacated by both these species is accessed by *An. culicifacies s.l.* and has established foothold erstwhile recorded in low-density [26, 28]. Among sibling species of the *An. sundaicus* complex, cytotype species D has been characterized with a regional importance presently confined to Andaman and Nicobar Islands [43]. It is a brackish water species, largely zoophilic and susceptible to residual insecticides.

An. stephensi is the only urban vector species breeding in domestic containers and often associated with tropical aggregation of labor at construction sites in metropolitan cities [44]. The species is resistant to multiple insecticides and its control focused on 'source reduction' to contain urban malaria. Due to continued urbanization and associated labor migration, urban malaria is viewed as a growing menace contributing about 10% of cases in the country [5–7].

Besides these dominant vectors, member species of *An. maculatus s.l.*, *An. annularis s.l.* and *An. subpictus s.l.* are also implicated; however, these species are considered of lesser significance for being predominantly zoophilic [45, 46]. Vector control is an integral part of the malaria control strategy in India and huge investment is made annually to contain build-up of disease vectors averting epidemic malaria. What is tantamount to vector control is the entomological surveillance for developing malaria-risk maps, judicious application of insecticides, monitoring insecticide-resistance and residual efficacy, universal coverage for population at risk and continued research for newer interventions, which are community-based and sustainable. We strongly believe that judicious mix of technologies that are situation-specific and doable would help save operational costs in resource-poor settings. The country is in dire need of skilled entomologist/taxonomists (an expertise that is getting scarce) to meet the human resource requirements for control of malaria, and other vector-borne diseases, as well as vector surveillance post-elimination to prevent re-establishment of local transmission in malaria-free territories.

4. Drug-resistant malaria

Of the two prevalent malaria parasite species, the rising proportions of *P. falciparum* is of grave concern for presently constituting >60% of total reported cases in the country [5, 7]. Rising trends of *P. falciparum* are largely attributed to fast emerging drug-resistance over space and time in parallel with phenomenon happening in countries of the Greater Mekong Subregion (GMS) of Southeast Asia [47]. Historically, chloroquine (CQ) was the most commonly used drug for treatment ever since inception of the control program in 1953 for its efficacy and affordability. It had become obsolete since its first report of treatment failure in Assam (northeast India) way back in 1973 [48]. Subsequently, drug-resistant foci had multiplied for which northeast is considered corridor for spread to rest of peninsular India resulting in steady rise in proportions of *P. falciparum* what was 13% in 1978 to 65% in present day malaria [49]. Northeast India shares wide border with Myanmar contiguous with GMS countries which is porous for cross-border migration, facilitating entry of drug-resistant strains enroute to the rest of India and beyond. Malaria transmission along this border is intense vectored by *An. minimus* and *An. baimaii* (the two most efficient vector species), and healthcare access is inadequate resulting in indiscriminate and sub-optimal doses *inter-alia*, poor vector control, illiteracy and treatment-seeking behavior; all contributing to propagation and spread of drug-resistant malaria strains [50]. Chloroquine therapy was subsequently upgraded to sulfadoxine-pyrimethamine (SP) in 2004 as first-line treatment in selected districts reporting CQ-resistant malaria [51]. The therapeutic efficacy of SP was short lived resulting in substantial rise in cases in the following years [52]. It was in 1990s that the development of artemisinin-derivatives raised new hopes for treatment of drug-resistant malaria for its fast acting schizontocidal properties. Initially, artemisinin was used as monotherapy for treatment of severe and complicated clinical malaria, discontinued in 2009 due to high recrudescence rate and risk of resistance for being commonly prescribed medicine by private practitioners and public sector alike [53]. In 2010, the program adopted ACT by combining it with SP, that is, artesunate + SP (AS + SP) for treatment of every single case of *P. falciparum* malaria in high-risk districts [54]. Mass scale introduction of this combination did result in appreciable transmission reduction in endemic communities formerly intractable. It continues to be in practice throughout India except in the northeast region where it has been replaced by yet another combination therapy, that is, artemether + lumefantrine (AL) in 2013 due to declining efficacy of AS + SP combination drug [55]. The emergence of artemisinin resistance in Southeast Asia [56]; however, is a matter of grave concern for its movement westwards to India for having it detected in Myanmar close to the Indian border in northeast [57]. Genomic studies have already detected mutations in the '*kelch 13*' propeller region (*Pfk 13*) linked to artemisinin resistance in north-eastern States, but to lesser frequency [58]. It is of utmost importance to periodically monitor the therapeutic efficacy of drug-regimen in force for radical cure and keep vigil on circulation of counterfeit drugs. The cost of spread of artemisinin-resistant malaria would be colossal, threatening the control and elimination efforts.

5. *Plasmodium vivax* malaria: the neglected parasite

The Southeast Asian countries contribute most of the vivax cases (58%) in the World of which India is the largest contributor [1]. Historically, much of the control efforts continue to be focused on control of falciparum malaria due to its associated severity and critical illness; the vivax malaria remained a neglected parasite [59]. Paradoxically, control of falciparum malaria is rather measurable in relation to interventions due to development of gametocytaemia 9–10 days post primary infection; instead the formation of gametocytes in vivax malaria is concurrent within few days of initial infection even before the patient seeks treatment permitting uninterrupted transmission. This biological characteristic of vivax malaria along with intrinsic ability of formation of latent hibernating 'hypnozoites' has made control efforts a difficult proposition. Nevertheless, the control of vivax malaria is gaining eminence in the context of malaria elimination across the continents [60].

The magnitude of vivax malaria is huge but grossly underestimated throughout India and continues to be neglected [61]. The transmission and distribution of vivax malaria varied across Indian States/UTs, but large concentrations of cases are occurring in urban metropolitan cities [7]. Although it remains highly susceptible to CQ therapy [62–66], its elimination is one difficult issue owing to latent stage 'hypnozoites' in the liver causing relapses amounting to extended morbidity over months/years. The only available anti-relapse drug 'primaquine (PQ)' does not guarantee radical cure much due to extended therapy over days coupled with poor compliance resulting in repeated episodes [67–69]. In addition, the administration of PQ is associated with several issues including contraindication in special groups, that is, infants, pregnant or lactating mothers, and inborn glucose-6-phosphate dehydrogenase (G6PD) deficiency syndromes due to associated hemolytic anemia; these population groups are excluded from primaquine therapy. There exists no diagnostics for detection of G6PD at point-of-care in the present surveillance system except few laboratories procedure for which it is time consuming and impractical in field conditions where the problem exists. Further, given the available technologies, the detection of latent hypnozoites and sub-patent parasitemia is presently not built in the disease surveillance.

The primary attack of vivax malaria is invariably associated with acute paroxysm presenting classical symptoms but treatable and rarely fatal [70–72]; although few sporadic cases of CQ-resistant cases have been reported in India and several other countries [73]. There is acute need of alternative 8-aminoquinolines, which are safe and universally applicable for radical cure across all population groups preventing relapses. As of today, we stand ill equipped to tackle this stubborn parasite calling for renewed attack both on parasite and disease vectors in reducing parasite reservoir which is likely to persist for long.

6. Asymptomatic malaria

India is historically endemic for malaria with record of devastating epidemics in the pre-DDT era and varied population groups have been subject to repeated attacks of malarial bouts, resulting in acquired immunity and consequent build-up of asymptomatic sub-patent parasitemia in the endemic communities, serving as infectious reservoir for continued transmission. In India, the surveillance program is aimed at taking blood-smears from those who are either febrile (active surveillance) or presenting themselves (passive surveillance) for malaria diagnosis or treatment. There is no built-in mechanism to detect asymptomatic cases or even low-density/sub-patent parasitemia in the endemic communities. These infections may go undetected with conventional diagnostic techniques leaving them untreated, except for mass-blood surveys/mass-drug administrations that are conducted only to contain epidemics. Asymptomatic malaria is more abundant than assumed and have been reported in different endemic States of India; however, the extent and distribution vary corresponding to transmission intensities [74–77]. Asymptomatic parasitemia is often associated with gametocyte carriage and may persist infectious throughout the year to mosquito vectors. These gametocytes are unable to cause clinical symptoms of malaria, rather ensure the uninterrupted transmission of malaria in the presence of efficient vectors. Asymptomatic cases remain undetected and not accounted for disease incidence amounting to gross underestimates.

Asymptomatic malaria in India remains entrenched in low-socioeconomic groupings living in forest-fringe communities, particularly along inter-border areas (both inter-province and international borders), which are largely inaccessible (marred with insurgent activities), wherein healthcare infrastructure is meager or even non-existent. Such areas are 'hot-spots' for explosive disease outbreaks due to mixing/importation of drug-resistant strains associated with illegal migration more so in the northeast (the gateway to India) that shares wide international border with Myanmar, a member country of GMS (an epicenter of multi-drug resistant malaria) and other WHO SEAR countries. Asymptomatic malaria has been documented for both *P. falciparum* and *P. vivax*, yet the magnitude was much higher for the former parasite species, more so in the winter months/dry-season, for example, in north-eastern State of Assam, for the high-risk districts surveyed, it varied from 7.1 to 31.1% in *P. falciparum* and 0.6–6.1% in *P. vivax* [78]. But on average, 12.8% of afebrile subjects were positive for malaria compared to 34.4% of those presenting with fever, and gametocyte carriage varied from 1.31 to 2.16%. Major bottleneck in eliminating asymptomatic malaria parasite is the absence of standard guidelines and diagnostic procedures aimed at targeting asymptomatic carriers. Malaria control program in practice is largely limited to the qualitative detection of parasite mostly in febrile human hosts and subsequently treating with suitable drugs; however, no attention is given on follow up for quantification of malaria parasite till radical cure. Moreover, a universally accepted parasite level for categorizing a patient as asymptomatic is also not available. Quantification and treating asymptomatic malaria has become increasingly important and relevant for disrupting transmission, requisite for achieving malaria elimination.

7. Cross-border malaria

India shares vast international border with Nepal, Bhutan and China to the North, Myanmar to the East, Bangladesh to the South and Pakistan to the West. Among these, borders with Myanmar and Bangladesh are of immediate concern for their high endemicity and common disease vectors and ecology in the adjoining vicinity on either side of the border [79, 80]. These border areas are porous for cross-migration and have high forest cover inhabited by indigenous tribes living in impoverished conditions. These communities have poor access to healthcare services and are at high-risk to disease outbreaks attributed to drug-resistant strains originating from the GMS countries. These populations are largely marginalized and just as reluctant to seek treatment amounting to unattended parasite reservoirs. Border with Myanmar in particular is believed to be the corridor for entry of drug-resistant strains to northeast India for onward spread. The detection of artemisinin-resistant malaria in closer proximity to Indian border is seen as threat for making its way to India and beyond, similar to the path that was followed by CQ-resistant malaria [48, 49]. Cross-border malaria transmission from neighboring endemic countries can be daunting task and has regional implications jeopardizing the elimination efforts [81, 82]. For example, most cases reported in Bhutan (a country that is heading for malaria elimination), are imported from adjoining districts of Assam seeking treatment on other side of the border. Labor migration across borders engaged in developmental projects is unstoppable for want of livelihood and there exists every possibility of re-entry of malaria given the similar vectors and ecology. It is important to characterize the imported malaria strains enabling interventions well in place and time to prevent re-establishment of local transmission in declared malaria-free territories [83]. Inter-country coordinated efforts are deemed essential to maintain vigil and strengthening border-posts (entry/exit doors) with capacity to detect and treat malaria in the migrant/itinerant labor force at the earliest available opportunity. In keeping the same mandate, India has joined hands with the Asia Pacific Malaria Elimination Network (APMEN) countries for shared experiences and coordinated action to achieve malaria elimination by 2030 [84]. Mitigating cross-border malaria should be accorded priority in context of malaria elimination.

8. Strengthening health systems

India has a well-structured vector-borne disease control program in place providing logistics support along with guidance and monitoring/evaluation services to malaria endemic States/

UTs [4, 7]. Utilizing the evidence-based intervention tools and large-scale implementation, India has registered notable decline in cases and malaria-attributable deaths in the preceding few years (**Figures 2** and **3**). Among these, roll-out of ACT for treatment of every single case of *P. falciparum* malaria, rapid diagnostics test (RDT) kits for on-the-spot diagnosis and large-scale provision of long-lasting insecticidal nets (LLINs) for vector control have resulted in rich dividends in reducing disease transmission in areas formerly intractable. Malaria threat is seen receding presenting an unprecedented opportunity for upscaling interventions in achieving universal coverage for populations at any risk making elimination an achievable target. However, the logistics requirement is huge for which increased funding from donors (both national and international agencies) and political commitment for sustained allocation of resources is of paramount importance for strengthening healthcare services reaching the outreach population groups for equitable access. A humble beginning has been made under National Health Mission (NHM), which envisages achievement of universal access to equitable, affordable and quality healthcare services both in urban and rural India [85]. Much needed disease surveillance in the country is further strengthened by Integrated Disease Surveillance Programme (IDSP) to detect early warning signals for impending disease outbreaks instituting interventions to thwart the disease onslaught and spread [86]. Both these establishments have helped the program immensely in strengthening laboratory services averting disease outbreaks, as well as human resource development in providing training to State surveillance officers, rapid response teams and other medical and paramedical staffs. However, continuing education program is need of the hour for upgrading skills to keep pace with the changing technologies as well as to fill the void due to attrition of skilled workforce. The induction of Accredited Social Health Activists (ASHA) have proven boon to the program ensuring door-to-door surveillance raising new levels of confidence in the poverty-stricken communities. Host of Non-Governmental Organizations (NGOs)/media coverage have increased the reach of services in remote/inaccessible areas helping combating illness and saving lives. Collectively, communities today stand better informed and clearly benefitted by increased awareness on disease prevention and control.

9. The way forward

In India, some States (Sikkim and Himachal Pradesh) and UTs (Lakshadweep, Daman & Diu and Puducherry) are already reporting <100 cases, while others recorded substantial decrease (>50%) in cases over past few years, for example, Assam and Karnataka (**Table 1**). Given the reducing transmission levels, malaria elimination at sub-national level is seemingly achievable. However, the emergence of artemisinin-resistant malaria and possible spread, coupled with multiple insecticide resistance in disease vectors (**Table 2**), could reverse the gains for which disease surveillance, monitoring and evaluation should be the corner-stone activity. *P. vivax* and asymptomatic malaria continue to be unattended and should be accorded priority for reducing parasite reservoir in the endemic communities. Priority should be accorded for strengthening healthcare services in high-risk States of eastern, central and north-eastern States helping mitigate disease onslaught and deter entry and spread of drug-resistant strains in India. Inter-sectoral linkages with research establishments and medical colleges for developing innovative newer interventions (possibly vaccines), assessing therapeutic efficacy of antimalarials and upgradation of drug-treatment policy, human resource development and field-evaluation of newer technologies, including innovative vector control approaches, are vital before these are incorporated in the control program. Disease epidemiology is rapidly changing in the face of fast urbanization, deforestation and anomalous weather conditions opening new vistas, which must be watched for targeting interventions in place and time. Mosquito vectors are invading new territories, and adapting to altered ecology establishing outdoor transmission in response to strengthening insecticide interventions, which are largely based on indoor residual applications. We strongly advocate the judicious mix of technologies used in an integrated manner to overcome the challenges of outdoor transmission and growing insecticide resistance threatening the efficacy of present day intervention tools. There remains of scope of newer interventions in Indian geo-epidemiological conditions, namely, eave tubes, attractive sugar baits, nano-synthesized pesticides loaded with microbial- and plant-borne compounds, for trapping adult mosquito vectors and population reduction presently being put to field evaluation in African countries (Beier, personal communication). It is the high time to strengthen the entomological component at the State/Zonal level for monitoring vector densities and insecticide resistance targeting interventions averting impending disease outbreaks. Above all, educating communities and stakeholders on disease prevention and control should be the guiding principle for increased compliance and harmonious action. Increased allocation of resources (both from State and Central assistance), for ensuring universal coverage of interventions, should be given utmost priority in reducing parasite reservoir much below threshold density disrupting transmission [87]. It is time accelerating towards elimination and let there be no complacency at various echelons of operation for keeping disease at bay. Outside Africa, Southeast Asia is the largest contributor of cases and source of spread of drug-resistant malaria for which it is strongly advocated that larger share of global investments in this part of the World would go a long way in alleviating poverty and malaria. In summary, given the enormity of disease burden and myriad of issues, odds are all against, yet concerted efforts should be made in rendering malaria a thing of the past; together we can beat malaria.

Acknowledgements

We are thankful to Professor S. Manguin (Montpellier, France) for inviting us to contribute this article for this compilation, and the Directorate of National Vector Borne Disease Control Programme, Directorate of Health Services, Government of India for grant of permission to data access.

Acronyms

ACT	artemisinin-based combination therapy
AIM	action and investment to defeat malaria

AL	artemether lumefantrine
API	annual parasite incidence
APLMA	Asia Pacific Leaders Malaria Alliance
APMEN	Asia-Pacific Malaria Elimination Network
ASHA	Accredited Social Health Activist
AS + SP	artesunate + sulfadoxine-pyrimethamine
CQ	chloroquine
DDT	dichloro-diphenyl-trichloroethane
G6PD	glucose-6-phosphate dehydrogenase
GMS	Greater Mekong Subregion
IDSP	Integrated Disease Surveillance Project
IRS	indoor residual spray
ITN	insecticide treated nets
ITS-2	internal transcribed spacer-2
LLIN	long-lasting insecticidal nets
NGO	Non-Governmental Organization
NHM	National Health Mission
NVBDCP	National Vector Borne Disease Control Programme
PCR	polymerase chain reaction
Pf	*Plasmodium falciparum*
Pfk 13	*Plasmodium falciparum kelch 13*
RBM	roll back malaria
RDT	rapid diagnostic test
r-DNA	ribosomal-DNA
SCAR	Sequence Characterized Amplified Region
SEAR	WHO Southeast Asia Region
SP	sulfadoxine-pyrimethamine
UT	Union Territory
WHO	World Health Organization

Author details

Sunil Dhiman[1]*, Vijay Veer[2] and Vas Dev[3]

*Address all correspondence to: sunildhiman81@gmail.com

1 Defence R&D Establishment (DRDE), Gwalior, Madhya Pradesh, India

2 Defence Research Laboratory, Tezpur, Assam, India

3 Senior Scientist (Retired), formerly with the National Institute of Malaria Research, New Delhi, India

References

[1] World Health Organization (WHO). World Malaria Report 2017. Geneva. Available from: http://www.who.int/malaria/world_malaria_report_2017 [Accessed: 20 February 2018]

[2] Newby G, Bennett A, Larson E, Cotter C, Shretta R, Phillips AA, Feachem RG. The path to eradication: A progress report on the malaria-eliminating countries. Lancet. 2016;**387**:1775-1784

[3] World Health Organization (WHO). Global Technical Strategy 2016-2030. Global Malaria Programme. Geneva: World Health Organization. 30 pp. Available from: http://www.who.int/malaria/areas/global_technical_strategy/en/ [Accessed: 20 February 2018]

[4] National Framework for Malaria Elimination in India 2016-2030. Directorate of National Vector Borne Disease Control Programme (NVBDCP). Ministry of Health & Family Welfare, Government of India. p. 43. Available from: http://www.nvbdcp.gov.in/malaria [Accessed: 20 February 2018]

[5] Sharma VP. Re-emergence of malaria in India. Indian Journal of Medical Research. 1996;**103**:26-45

[6] Sharma VP. Fighting malaria in India. Current Science. 1998;**75**:1127-1140

[7] National Vector Borne Disease Control Programme, Directorate General of Health Services, Ministry of Health & Family Welfare. Government of India. Malaria. Available from: http://www.nvbdcp.gov.in/malaria [Accessed: February 20, 2018]

[8] Das A, Anvikar AR, Cator LJ, Dhiman RC, Eapen A, Mishra N, Nagpal BN, Nanda N, Raghavendra K, Read AF, Sharma SK, Singh OP, Singh V, Sinnis P, Srivastava HC, Sullivan SA, Sutton PL, Thomas MB, Carlton JM, Valecha N. Malaria in India: The centre for the study of complex malaria in India. Acta Tropica. 2012;**121**:267-273

[9] Sharma VP. Continuing challenge of malaria in India. Current Science. 2012;**102**:678-682

[10] Yadav RS, Sharma VP, Ghosh SK, Kumar A. Quartan malaria—An investigation on the incidence of *Plasmodium malariae* in Bisra PHC, District Sundergarh, Orissa. Indian Journal of Malariology. 1990;**27**:85-94

[11] Dev V. *Plasmodium malariae*—A case of quartan malaria in Assam. Journal of Communicable Diseases. 2000;**32**:149-151

[12] Bharti PK, Chand SK, Singh MP, Mishra S, Shukla MM, Singh R, Singh N. Emergence of a new focus of *Plasmodium malariae* in forest villages of district Balaghat, Central India: Implications for the diagnosis of malaria and its control. Tropical Medicine & International Health. 2013;**18**:12-17

[13] Singh R, Jain V, Singh PP, Bharti PK, Thomas T, Basak S, Singh N. First report of detection and molecular confirmation of *Plasmodium ovale* from severe malaria cases in Central India. Tropical Medicine & International Health. 2013;**18**:1416-1420

[14] Prakash A, Mohapatra PK, Bhattacharya DR, Goswami BK, Mahanta J. *Plasmodium ovale:* First case report from Assam, India. Current Science. 2003;**84**:1187

[15] Jambulingam P, Mohapatra SS, Das LK, Das PK, Rajagopal PK. Detection of *Plasmodium ovale* in Koraput district of Orissa State. Indian Journal of Medical Research. 1989;**89**: 115-116

[16] Cox-Singh J. Zoonotic malaria: *Plasmodium knowlesi*, an emerging pathogen. Current Opinion in Infectious Diseases. 2012;**25**:530-536

[17] Dhingra N, Jha P, Sharma VP, Cohen AA, Jotker RM, Rodriguez PS, Bassani DG, Suraweera W, Laxminarayan R, Peto R. Adult and child mortality in India: A nationally representative mortality survey. Lancet. 2010;**376**:1768-1774

[18] Christopher SR. The fauna of British India, including Ceylon and Burma. Diptera, Vol. IV. Family Culicidae, Tribe Anophelini. London: Taylor and Francis; 1933. p. 371

[19] Das BP, Rajagopal R, Akiyama J. Pictorial key to the species of Indian anopheline mosquitoes. Journal of Pure and Applied Zoology. 1990;**2**:131-162

[20] Dev V, Sharma VP. The dominant mosquito vectors of human malaria in India. In: Manguin S, editor. *Anopheles* Mosquitoes: New Insights into Malaria Vectors. Croatia: InTech Open Access; 2013. pp. 239-271. DOI: 10.5772/55215

[21] Rao TR. The Anophelines of India. New Delhi: Indian Council of Medical Research; 1984. p. 596

[22] Nagpal BN, Sharma VP. Indian Anophelines. New Delhi: Oxford & IBH Publishing Co. Pvt. Ltd.; 1995. p. 416. ISBN: 81-204-0929-9

[23] Subbarao SK. Anopheline Species Complexes in South and South-East Asia. Geneva. World Health Organization (WHO); 2007. p. 102. ISBN: 978-92-9022-294-1

[24] Manguin S, Garros C, Dusfour I, Harbach RE, Coosemans M. Bionomics, taxonomy and distribution of the major vector taxa of *Anopheles* subgenus *Cellia* in Southeast Asia: An updated review. Infection, Genetics and Evolution. 2008;**8**:489-503

[25] Sinka ME, Bangs MJ, Manguin S, Chareonviriyaphap T, Patil AP, Temperley WH, Gething PW, Elyazar IRF, Kabaria CW, Harbach RE, Hay SI. The dominant *Anopheles* vectors of human malaria in the Asia-Pacific region: Occurrence data, distribution maps, and bionomics precis. Parasites & Vectors. 2011;**4**:89

[26] Sharma VP, Dev V. Biology and control of *Anopheles culicifacies* Giles 1901. Indian Journal of Medical Research. 2015;**141**:525-536

[27] Subbarao SK. The *Anopheles culicifacies* complex and control of malaria. Parasitology Today. 1988;**4**:72-75

[28] Bhuyan M, Das NG, Chakraborty BC, Talukdar PK, Sarkar PK, Das SC. Role of *Anopheles culicifacies* during an outbreak of malaria in Garubandha PHC, Assam. Journal of Communicable Diseases. 1997;**29**:243-246

[29] Saxena R, Nagpal BN, Singh VP, Srivastava A, Dev V, Sharma MC, Gupta HP, Tomar AS, Sharma S, Gupta SK. Impact of deforestation on known malaria vectors in Sonitpur district of Assam, India. Journal of Vector Borne Diseases. 2014;**51**:211-215

[30] Nasreen A, Nagpal BN, Kapoor N, Srivastava A, Gupta HP, Saxena R, Shamim A, Kumar V, Gupta SK, Singh VP, Dev V, Nanda N, Valecha N. Impact of ecological and climatic changes on vectors of malaria in four North-eastern States of India. Indian Journal of Ecology. 2016;**43**:1-15

[31] Singh OP, Raghavendra K, Nanda N, Mittal PK, Subbarao SK. Pyrethroid resistance in *Anopheles culicifacies* in Surat district Gujarat, West India. Current Science. 2002;**82**:547-550

[32] Raghavendra K, Verma V, Srivastava HC, Gunasekaran K, Sreehari U, Das AP. Persistence of DDT, malathion & deltamethrin resistance in *Anopheles culicifacies* after their sequential withdrawal from indoor residual spraying in Surat district, India. Indian Journal of Medical Research. 2010;**132**:260-264

[33] Sahu SS, Sahu K, Gunasekaran T, Vijayakumar JP. Triple insecticide resistance in *Anopheles culicifacies*: A practical impediment for malaria control in Odisha State, India. Indian Journal of Medical Research. 2015;**142**:59-63

[34] Nanda N, Yadav RS, Subbarao SK, Joshi H, Sharma VP. Studies on *Anopheles fluviatilis* and *Anopheles culicifacies* sibling species in relation to malaria in forested hilly and deforested riverine ecosystems in northern Orissa, India. Journal of American Mosquito Control Association. 2000;**16**:199-205

[35] Dev V, Manguin S. Biology, distribution and control of *Anopheles (Cellia) minimus* in the context of malaria transmission in northeastern India. Parasites & Vectors. 2016;**9**:585

[36] Dev V, Ansari MA, Hira CR, Barman K. An outbreak of *P. falciparum* malaria due to *Anopheles minimus* in Central Assam. Indian Journal of Malariology. 2001;**38**:32-38

[37] Dev V. *Anopheles minimus*: Its bionomics and role in the transmission of malaria in Assam, India. Bulletin of the World Health Organization. 1996;**74**:61-66

[38] Jambulingam P, Sahu SS, Manonmani A. Reappearance of *Anopheles minimus* in Singhbum hills of hills of East-Central India. Acta Tropica. 2005;**96**:31-35

[39] Prakash A, Walton C, Bhattacharyya DR, O'Loughlin SM, Mohapatra PK, Mahanta J. Molecular characterization and species identification of *Anopheles dirus* and *An. minimus* complexes in north-east India using r-DNA ITS-2. Acta Tropica. 2006;**100**:156-161

[40] Dutta P, Bhattacharyya DR, Khan SA, Sharma CK, Mahanta J. Feeding pattern of *Anopheles dirus*, the major vector of forest malaria in North-east India. Southeast Asian Journal of Tropical Medicine and Public Health. 1996;**27**:378-381

[41] Dutta P, Khan SA, Bhattacharyya DR, Khan AB, Sharma CK, Mahanta J. Studies on the breeding habitats of the vector mosquito *Anopheles baimaii* and its relationship to malaria incidence in Northeastern region of India. EcoHealth. 2010;**7**:498-506

[42] Prakash A, Mohapatra PK, Bhattacharyya DR, Sharma CK, Goswami BK, Hazarika NC, Mahanta J. Epidemiology of malaria outbreak (April/May 1999) in Titabor Primary Health Centre, district Jorhat (Assam). Indian Journal of Medical Research. 2000;**111**:121-126

[43] Das MK, Nagpal BN, Sharma VP. Mosquito fauna and breeding habitats of anophelines in Car Nicobar Island, India. Indian Journal of Malariology. 1998;**35**:197-205

[44] Sumodan PK, Kumar A, Yadav RS. Resting behaviour and malaria vector incrimination of *Anopheles stephensi* in Goa, India. Journal of the American Mosquito Control Association. 2004;**20**:317-318

[45] Prakash A, Bhattacharyya DR, Mohapatra PK, Mahanta J. Role of the prevalent *Anopheles* species in the transmission of *Plasmodium falciparum*, and *P. vivax* in Assam State and north-eastern India. Annals of Tropical Medicine & Parasitology. 2004;**98**:559-568

[46] Dhiman S, Bhola RK, Goswami D, Rabha B, Kumar D, Baruah I, Singh L. Polymerase chain reaction detection of human host preference and *Plasmodium* parasite infections in field collected potential malaria vector species. Pathogens and Global Health. 2012;**106**:177-180

[47] Shah NK, Dhillon GPS, Dash AP, Arora U, Meshnick SR, Valecha N. Antimalaria drug resistance of *Plasmodium falciparum* in India: Changes over space and time. Lancet Infectious Diseases. 2011;**11**:57-64

[48] Sehgal PN, Sharma MID, Sharma SL, Gogai S. Resistance to chloroquine in falciparum malaria in Assam State, India. Journal of Communicable Diseases. 1973;**5**:175-180

[49] Sharma VP. Status of drug-resistance in malaria in India. In: Mahajan RC, editor, Multi-drug Resistance in Emerging Re-emerging Diseases. Delhi: Narosa Publications. pp. 191-202

[50] Mohapatra PK, Namchoom NS, Prakash A, Bhattacharya DR, Goswami BK, Mahanta J. Therapeutic efficacy of anti-malarials in *Plasmodium falciparum* malaria in an Indo-Myanmar border area of Arunachal Pradesh. Indian Journal of Medical Research. 2003;**118**:71-76

[51] Dev V, Phookan S, Barman K. Therapeutic efficacies of antimalarial drugs in the treatment of uncomplicated *Plasmodium falciparum* malaria in Assam, north-eastern India. Annals of Tropical Medicine & Parasitology. 2003;**97**:783-791

[52] Dev V, Sharma VP. Hojai. Malaria transmission and disease burden in Assam: Challenges and opportunities. Journal of Parasitic Diseases. 2009;**33**:13-22

[53] Mishra N, Anvikar AR, K Shah NK, Kamal VK, Sharma SK, Srivastava HC, Das K, Pradhan K, Kumar H, Gupta YK, Gupta P, Dash AP, Valecha N. Prescription practices and availability of artemisinin monotherapy in India: Where do we stand? Malaria Journal. 2011;**10**:360

[54] Dev V, Biswas S, Joshi H, Prajapati SK, Valecha N, Dash AP. Safety and efficacy of aretsunate + sulfadoxine-pyrimethamine in the treatment of *Plasmodium falciparum* malaria in northeast India. Parassitologia. 2009;**51**:29-34

[55] Mishra N, Kaitholia K, Srivastava B, Shah NK, Narayan JP, Dev V, Phookan S, Anvikar AR, Rana R, Bharti RS, Sonal GS, Dhariwal AC, Valecha N. Declining efficacy of artesunate plus sulphadoxine-pyrimethamine in northeastern India. Malaria Journal. 2014;**13**:284

[56] Phyo AP, Nkhoma S, Stepniewska K, Ashley EA, Nair S, McGready R, ler Moo C, Al-Saai S, Dondorp AM, Lwin KM, Singhasivanon P, Day NP, White NJ, Anderson TJ, Nosten F. Emergence of artemisinin-resistant malaria on the western border of Thailand: A longitudinal study. Lancet. 2012;**379**:1960-1966

[57] Tun KM, Imwong M, Lwin KM, Win AA, Hlaing TM, Hlaing T, Lin K, Kyaw MP, Plewes K, Faiz MA, Dhorda M, Cheah PY, Pukrittayakamee S, Ashley EA, Anderson TJ, Nair S, McDew-White M, Flegg JA, Grist EP, Guerin P, Maude RJ, Smithuis F, Dondorp AM, Day NP, Nosten F, White NJ, Woodrow CJ. Spread of artemisinin-resistant *Plasmodium falciparum* in Myanmar: A cross-sectional survey of the *K13* molecular marker. Lancet Infectious Diseases. 2015;**15**(4):415-421

[58] Mishra N, Prajapati SK, Kaitholia K, Bharti RS, Srivastava B, Phookan S, Anvikar AR, Dev V, Sonal GS, Dhariwal AC, White NJ, Valecha N. Surveillance of artemisinin resistance in *Plasmodium falciparum* in India using the *kelch13* molecular marker. Antimicrobial Agents and Chemotherapy. 2015;**59**:2548-2553

[59] Joshi H, Prajapati SK, Verma A, Kang S, Carlton JM. *Plasmodium vivax* in India. Trends in Parasitology. 2008;**24**:228-235

[60] Shanks GD. Control and elimination of *Plasmodium vivax*. Advances in Parasitology. 2012;**80**:301-341

[61] Sharma VP, Dev V, Phookan S. Neglected *Plasmodium vivax* malaria in northeastern States of India. Indian Journal of Medical Research. 2015;**141**:546-555

[62] Srivastava HC, Yadav RS, Joshi H, Valecha N, Mallick PK, Prajapati SK, Dash AP. Therapeutic responses of *Plasmodium vivax* and *P. falciparum* to chloroquine, in an area of western India where *P. vivax* predominates. Annals of Tropical Medicine and Parasitology. 2008;**102**:471-480

[63] Rishikesh K, Kamath A, Hande MH, Vidyasagar S, Acharya RV, Acharya V, Belle J, Shastry AB, Saravu K. Therapeutic assessment of chloroquine-primaquine combined regimen in adult cohort of *Plasmodium vivax* malaria from a tertiary care hospital in southwestern India. Malaria Journal. 2015;**14**:310

[64] Nandy A, Addy M, Maji AK, Bandyopadhyay AK. Monitoring the chloroquine sensitivity of *Plasmodium vivax* from Calcutta and Orissa, India. Annals of Tropical Medicine and Parasitology. 2003;**97**:215-220

[65] Ganguly S, Saha P, Guha SK, Das S, Bera DK, Biswas A, Kundu PK, Saha B, Ray K, Maji AK. In vivo therapeutic efficacy of chloroquine alone or in combination with primaquine against *vivax* malaria in Kolkata, West Bengal, India, and polymorphism in *pvmdr1* and *pvcrt-o* genes. Antimicrobial Agents and Chemotherapy. 2013;**57**:1246-1251

[66] Valecha N, Joshi H, Eapen A, Ravinderan J, Kumar A, Prajapati SK, Ringwald P. Therapeutic efficacy of chloroquine in *Plasmodium vivax* from areas with different epidemiological patterns in India and their *Pvdhfr* gene mutation pattern. Transactions of the Royal Society of Tropical Medicine and Hygiene. 2006;**100**:831-837

[67] Adak T, Sharma VP, Orlov VS. Studies on the *Plasmodium vivax* relapse pattern in Delhi, India. American Journal of Tropical Medicine and Hygiene. 1998;**59**:175-179

[68] Yadav RS, Ghosh SK. Radical curative efficacy of five-day regimen of primaquine for treatment of *Plasmodium vivax* malaria in India. Journal of Parasitology. 2002;**88**:1042-1044

[69] Rajgor DD, Gogtay NJ, Kadam VS, Kamtekar KD, Dalvi SS, Chogle AR, Aigal U, Bichile LS, Kshirsagar KKC. Efficacy of 14-day primaquine regimen in preventing relapses in patients with *Plasmodium vivax* malaria in Mumbai, India. Transactions Royal Society Tropical Medicine & Hygiene. 2003;**97**:438-440

[70] Valecha N, Pinto RG, Turner GD, Kumar A, Rodrigues S, Dubhashi NG, Rodrigues E, Banaulikar SS, Singh R, Dash AP, Baird JK. Histopathology of fatal respiratory distress caused by *Plasmodium vivax* malaria. American Journal of Tropical Medicine and Hygiene. 2009;**81**:75-62

[71] Kochar DK, Das A, Kochar SK, Saxena V, Sirohi P, Garg S, Kochar A, Khatri MP, Gupta V. Severe *Plasmodium vivax* malaria: A report on serial cases from Bikaner in Northwestern India. American Journal of Tropical Medicine & Hygiene. 2009;**80**:194-198

[72] Mishra VN, Singh DJ. Cerebral malaria by *Plasmodium vivax*. Journal of Association of Physicians of India. 1989;**37**:411

[73] Dua VK, Kar PK, Sharma VP. Chloroquine resistant 7. *Plasmodium vivax* malaria in India. Tropical Medicine & International Health. 1996;**1**:816-819

[74] Das NG, Dhiman S, Talukdar PK, Goswami D, Rabha B, Baruah I, Veer V. Role of asymptomatic carriers and weather variables in persistent transmission of malaria in an endemic district of Assam, India. Infection Ecology and Epidemiology. 2015;**5**:25442

[75] Ganguly S, Saha P, Guha SK, Biswas A, Kundu PK, Mali AK. High prevalence of asymptomatic malaria in a tribal population of Eastern India. Journal of Clinical Microbiology. 2013;**51**(5):1439-1444

[76] Chourasia MK, Raghavendra K, Bhatt RM, Swain DK, Meshram HM, Meshram JK, Suman S, Dubey V, Singh G, Prasad KM, Kleinschmidt I. Additional burden of

asymptomatic and sub-patent malaria infections during low transmission season in forested tribal villages in Chhattisgarh, India. Malaria Journal. 2017;**16**:320

[77] Laishram DD, Sutton PL, Nanda N, Sharma VL, Sobti RC, Carlton JM, Joshi H. The complexities of malaria disease manifestations with a focus on asymptomatic malaria. Malaria Journal. 2012;**11**:29

[78] Dev V, Phookan S, Sharma VP, Dash AP, Anand SP. Malaria parasite burden and treatment seeking behavior in ethnic communities of Assam, Northeastern India. Journal of Infection. 2006;**52**:131-139

[79] Dev V, Sangma BM, Dash AP. Persistent transmission of malaria in Garo hills of Meghalaya bordering Bangladesh, north-east India. Malaria Journal. 2010;**9**:263

[80] Dhiman S, Goswami D, Rabha B, Gopalakrishnan R, Baruah I, Singh L. Malaria epidemiology along Indo-Bangladesh border in Tripura State, India. The Southeast Asian Journal of Tropical Medicine and Public Health. 2010;**41**(6):1279-1289

[81] Wangdi K, Gatton ML, Kelly GC, Banwell C, Dev V, Clements AC. Malaria elimination in India and regional implications. Lancet Infectious Diseases. 2016;**16**:e214-e224

[82] Wangdi K, Gatton ML, Kelly GC, Clements AC. Cross-border malaria: A major obstacle for malaria elimination. Advances in Parasitology. 2015;**89**:79-102

[83] Dharmawardena P, Premaratne RG, Gunasekera WM, Hewawitarane M, Mendis K, Fernando D. Characterization of imported malaria, the largest threat to sustained malaria elimination from Sri Lanka. Malaria Journal. 2015;**14**:177

[84] Asia Pacific Malaria Elimination Network (APMEN). Elimination 2030—Working Together for Malaria Free Asia Pacific. Available from: http://www.apmen.org [Accessed: 20 February 2018]

[85] National Health Mission. Ministry of Health & Family Welfare, Government of India. Available from: http://www.nhm.gov.in [Accessed: 28 February 2018]

[86] Integrated Disease Surveillance Programme, National Centre for Disease Control, Directorate General of Health Services, Ministry of Health & Family Welfare, Government of India. Available from: http://www.idsp.nic.in [Accessed: 28 February 2018]

[87] Sharma VP. Battling malaria iceberg incorporating strategic reforms in achieving Millennium Development Goals & malaria elimination in India. Indian Journal of Medical Research. 2012;**136**:907-925

6

New Approaches for an Old Disease: Studies on Avian Malaria Parasites for the Twenty-First Century Challenges

Luz García-Longoria, Sergio Magallanes, Manuel González-Blázquez, Yolanda Refollo, Florentino de Lope and Alfonso Marzal

Abstract

Emerging infectious diseases (EIDs) impose a burden on economies and public health. Because EIDs on wildlife are mainly affected by environmental and ecological factors, the study of EIDs in wildlife provides valuable insights to improve our understanding on their causes and their impact on global health. Malaria is an EID that has increased its prevalence in the last few decades at an alarming rate. Avian malaria parasites are abundant, widespread and diverse, which turn these parasites into an excellent model for the study of EIDs. In the face of new health and environmental challenges in the twenty- irst century, studies on avian malaria will provide new approaches for this old disease. The identfiication of essential genes for the malaria invasion, the study of modification of host behaviour by malaria parasites in order to promote the parasite transmission, and the knowledge of factors contributing to the emergence of infectious diseases in wildlife are essential for understanding parasite epidemiology, local patterns of virulence and evolution of host resistance. In this chapter, we will review the results of some recent investigations on these topics that will be useful for predicting and preventing EIDs in wildlife, livestock and humans.

Keywords: avian malaria, emerging infectious diseases, *Haemoproteus*, haemosporidians, *Plasmodium*

1. Introduction

Malaria is one of the world's deadliest diseases, with 214 million cases and an estimated 1 million malaria deaths every year. Although the first human recording of malaria was in China in 2700 B.C., most probably this disease is older than humans. Fossil evidence shows that modern malaria was transmitted by mosquitoes at least 20 million years ago, and the recent analysis of the pre-historic origin of malaria has suggested that earlier forms of the disease, carried by biting midges, are at least 100 million years old and probably much older [1]. Hence, malaria not only infects humans. In fact, systematic parasitologists have erected more than 500 described species belonging to 15 genera within the order Haemosporidia (phylum Apicomplexa) that infect reptiles, birds and mammals, and use at least seven families of dipteran vectors for transmission [2, 3]. These parasites are widely distributed in every terrestrial habitat on all the warm continents. Within these parasites, avian malaria is the largest group of haemosporidians by the number of species. They are widespread, abundant and diverse, and are easily sampled without disrupting the host populations. Although the term 'malaria parasites' has been a controversial issue among parasitologists, ecologists and evolutionary researchers [4, 5], authors usually include genera *Plasmodium*, *Haemoproteus* and *Leuocytozoon* among the malaria parasites [4].

Investigations on avian malaria have contributed significantly to the knowledge on biology and ecology of malaria parasites of other vertebrates, including human malaria [6]. Since the discovery of the mosquito transmission of malaria in birds by Sir Ronald Ross, studies on malaria parasites of birds have saved millions of human lives. For example, essential advances in medical parasitology such as the development of anti-malarial compounds (e.g. plasmochin, primaquine and atebrin), the study of the life cycle and cultivation in vitro were initially developed using bird haemosporidian models.

Also, during the 2000s, research on bird malaria was at the very peak because scientists recognised the benefits of using studies on avian malaria to answer ecological, behavioural and evolutionary questions. Nowadays, far to be outdated, investigations on avian malaria will be essential to face new health and environmental challenges in the twenty-first century. In this chapter, we will review the newest contributions on bird studies helping in the fight against malaria.

2. Emerging infectious diseases and wildlife studies

In the last century, advances in vaccines and antibiotics, as well as other improvements in food intake and sanitation, contributed to the fast development in demography and economic growth in many parts of the world [7]. These advances brought the erroneous idea of a possible world without the burden of pathogens, followed by a flawed policy of reducing investment in the research of infectious diseases [8]. Pathogenic microorganisms rapidly evolve using multiple genetic evolutionary mechanisms, thus steadily adapting to new environments and escaping host's defences. As a consequence, more than 300 events of emerging and re-emerging infectious diseases (EIDs) have killed millions of people since the 1940s and represent one of the major threats to human, livestock and wildlife in the twenty-first century [9]. These diseases are caused by pathogens from animals that now infect humans (HIV-1), or pathogens that have been probably presented in humans for centuries, but continue to appear in new locations (Lyme disease) or have evolved resistance to drugs (malaria resistance to chloroquine, mefloquine and artemisinin), or that reappear after apparent control or elimination (tuberculosis). Ironically, the health improvements and economic developments of the last century also contributed to the increase of these pathogenic diseases, as 'hidden costs' of this wellness. The economic and demographic growth led to millions of people live in crowded urban areas, thereby facilitating the spread of infections [10]. Also, the deforestation for logging and farming in tropical rainforests to meet the demands of growing population have provoked changes in the ecology and epidemiology of vector-borne diseases (e.g. malaria, leishmania and Chagas disease), thus favouring the spread of the disease [11].

Studies on wildlife may provide essential information in the fight against EIDs for several reasons. On the one hand, wildlife is an essential component in the epidemiology of many EIDs. In this sense, more than 60% of these diseases in humans are caused by pathogens spread from animals, and 71.8% of these zoonotic diseases events are provoked by pathogens with a wildlife origin [9]. On the other hand, socio-cultural and economic drivers (e.g. population density, economic growth), as well as ecological and environmental conditions (wildlife species richness, rainfall), may be major determinants of surge and spread of diseases in humans. In opposition to human studies on EIDs, wildlife studies are free of socio-economics and cultural confounding variables, thus providing reliable conclusions on the ecological drivers of the epidemiology.

2.1. Avian malaria and deforestation

Infections with vector-borne pathogens have become one of the main EIDs in the last years. Arthropods such as mosquitoes, ticks and bugs are responsible for transmission of viruses (dengue, chikungunya, Zika), bacteria (Lyme disease) and protozoans (malaria, Chagas). Anthropogenic deforestation and land use change have been proposed to cause the spread of vectors and the re-emergence of malaria in South America [12]. In this sense, it has been shown that the biting rate of *Anopheles darlingi* (primary human malaria vector in the Amazon) in deforested rainforest sites was more than 278 times higher than the rate determined for areas that were predominantly forested [13]. Also, it has been reported that deforestation can increase human malaria prevalence up to 50% [14]. However, as mentioned previously, the drivers favouring malaria outbreaks go beyond the basic biological elements and include ecological as well as socio-economic factors [15]. Because these puzzling effects are irrelevant in the context of wildlife malaria parasites, further studies (e.g. avian malaria studies) removing potential confounding variables are required to confirm whether anthropogenic land-use change is a key driver of disease emergence.

In recent years, several studies have analysed the effects of habitat fragmentation and deforestation on the prevalence of bird haemosporidian parasites in different continents. Bonneaud et al. [16] examined the prevalence of infection of bird malaria in both pristine and disturbed forests from Cameroon, showing a higher prevalence of *Plasmodium* lineages in pristine as compared with disturbed forest sites. Also, Chasar et al. [17] analysed the diversity, prevalence and distribution of avian haemosporidian parasites (*Plasmodium, Haemoproteus* and *Leucocytozoon*) from nine-paired sites (disturbed vs. undisturbed habitats) in Southern Cameroon in two widespread species of African rainforest birds. They found that the prevalence of *Haemoproteus* and *Leucocytozoon* infections was significantly higher in undisturbed than in deforested habitats. They also showed that the prevalence of *Plasmodium megaglobularis* was higher in undisturbed areas, whereas the prevalence of infection of *P. lucens* was higher in deforested areas. Furthermore, Loiseau et al. [18] reported the variation of parasitaemia intensity and co-infections of avian haemosporidian parasites in two common African bird species at three sites with distinct habitat characteristics in Ghana. They detected a variation in infection prevalence and intensity of parasitaemia that differ in environmental factors; thus suggesting that spatial heterogeneity can impact the prevalence, frequency of co-infections, and chronic parasitaemia intensity of haemosporidian parasites.

In Hawaiian Islands, malaria is thought to be responsible of the population decline and even extinctions of many native bird species [19]. In addition, deforestation could also have contributed to the population decimation by altering the patterns of malaria transmission [20, 21]. In this sense, it has been suggested that deforestation of the Alaka'i Wilderness Preserve on Kaua'i Island could have changed the pattern of seasonal transmission of avian malaria to a pattern of continuous transmission through all the year [20], which could enormously increase the prevalence and pathogenic effects of avian malaria.

Moreover, Laurance et al. [22] investigated the effects of habitat fragmentation and ecological parameters on the prevalence of malaria parasites (genera *Plasmodium* and *Haemoproteus*) in bird communities of Australia. They analysed the prevalence and genetic diversity of haemosporidians across six study sites including large sites and continuous-forest sites, finding that the prevalence of the dominant haemosporidian infection (*Haemoproteus*) was significantly higher in continuous forest than in habitat fragments.

In Brazil, Belo et al. [23] examined the presence and genetic diversity of haemosporidian parasites in 676 wild birds from three different environmental regions (intact cerrado, disturbed cerrado and transition area Amazonian rainforest-cerrado) with the aim to determine whether different habitats are associated with differences in the prevalence and diversity of malaria infection. Surprisingly, they found that neither the prevalence nor the diversity of infection of *Plasmodium* spp. or *Haemoproteus* spp. differed significantly among the three habitats studied. More recently, Ricopa and Villa-Galarce [24] have studied the prevalence and genetic characterisation of avian malaria lineages in one disturbed and one preserved area of National Reserve Allpahuayo-Mishana in Peruvian Amazon. They found a higher prevalence and a higher diversity of malaria infection in birds from the deforested area when compared to birds from pristine forest.

2.2. Avian malaria parasites as emerging infectious diseases: the role in biological invasions

Alien, also called non-indigenous, exotic or non-native species, are defined as those species that colonise an area beyond their natural range, where they reproduce and establish a population. In addition to urbanisation, demographic growth and land-use change, the introduction of domestic and wildlife alien species can also provoke emerging diseases with tremendous costs in terms of loss of biodiversity, mortality and economic expenses [25]. In this sense, several studies have shown zoonosis linked to birds spreading diseases to humans. For example, it is thought that the West Nile virus, a bird pathogen but also causing mortality to humans, was introduced to New York by migratory or invasive bird species [26]. Also, the bird flu virus (H5N1), which has been registered, was transported by invasive bird species [27]. But despite these negative impacts of invasive species and the efforts from scientists to understand biological invasions, the mechanisms that allow one species to become invasive are still poorly understood.

Since the eighteenth century, more than 1400 human attempts to introduce 400 bird species have been recorded worldwide [28]. But not all of these introduced birds have resulted in established populations of invasive birds in the new regions. In fact, only 10% of introduced species are able to colonise new environments and become successful invaders [29]. In consequence, some life history traits and ecological attributes could allow some alien species to maintain high survival and reproductive success in new locations and to become successful invaders [28]. It has been proposed that parasites may play this role facilitating the successful colonisation of their bird hosts [30]. Hence, parasitic infections (or sometimes, their absence) may facilitate or limit invasions impacting native species via both direct and indirect effects. Three hypotheses (novel weapon hypothesis, enemy release hypothesis and biotic resistance hypothesis) have been proposed to explain the role of parasites in invasions in bird- parasite systems (**Table 1**). On the one hand, exotic bird species can act as a 'Trojan horse' because they can bring alien parasites and pathogens inside them, which could favour the dissemination in the new areas of their avian host species. In the history, pathogens have played a role bringing diseases in humans that become epidemic in susceptible native populations [39]. As example, in European conquest in the Americas smallpox spread rapidly killing an estimated 95% of the indigenous population far in advance of the European themselves [39]. Following this idea, the novel weapon hypotheses (NWH) states that invasive species gain advantages over native species by bringing their own parasites to the new environments against which the introduced species but not the natives have evolved defences [40, 41]. These co-introduced parasites may switch to native bird hosts and spread in the new communities, hence becoming themselves invasive parasites provoking serious damages to indigenous bird species. But the role of parasites in invasions may extend well beyond such direct effects, and hence some indirect effects may also be expected. In this sense, the enemy release hypothesis (ERH) states that non-native bird species could become invaders because they have lost their co-evolved malaria parasites during the process of colonisation, and thus they may increase their competitive ability and displace native species in the new areas. Conversely, the biotic resistance hypothesis states that native parasites in the indigenous species may reduce the fitness of the potential bird invader and prevent its spread and establishment. Next, we will focus on the role of avian malaria parasites co-introduced with their bird hosts.

Avian malaria parasites are among the most pathogenic species of poultry and wildlife birds, being responsible for economic losses, mass mortality, population declines and even extinctions of many bird species worldwide after its introduction outside its native range [42]. For all these reasons, the International Union for Conservation of Nature (IUCN) classifies avian malaria to be among the 100 of the world's worst invasive alien species [43]. The spread of exotic avian malaria in Hawaiian Islands is the best documented example of the effects of invasive malaria on native bird communities. Since the discovery of Hawaiian Archipelago by the Captain Cook in 1774, more than a half of over 100 endemic bird taxa in Hawaii have been driven to extinction by a combination of habitat loss, introduced species and diseases [19, 44]. In 1826, the primary vector for avian malaria *Culex quinquesfasciatus* was accidentally introduced in Hawaii from shipping vessel HMS Wellington [19, 45]. The colonisation of this mosquito species, as well as the introduction of non-native bird species co-transporting avian malaria *Plasmodium relictum*, then provoked a wave of extinctions and endangerment among Hawaiian forest birds since the 1920s [21].

Novel weapon hypothesis (NWH)	**Reference**	**Observations**
Hawaii	van Ripper et al. [21]	
Hawaii	Atkinson et al. (2005) [46]	
Hawaii	Lapointe (2005) [47]	
Hawaii	Atkinson and Samuel (2010) [48]	
New Zealand	Doré (1920) [49]	
New Zealand	Tompkins and Gleeson [31]	
New Zealand	Barraclough et al. [32]	
New Zealand	Howe et al. [33]	
New Zealand	Ewen et al. (2012) [50]	
New Zealand	Schoener et al. (2014) [51]	
Galapagos Islands	Levin et al. [34]	
Galapagos Islands	Santiago-Alarcón et al. [35]	
Galapagos Islands	Levin et al. [36]	
Perú	Marzal et al. (2015) [52]	
Enemy release hypothesis (ERH)		
Southern Asia	Beadell et al. (2006) [53]	Mixed results with NWH
Seychelles Islands	Hutchings (2009) [54]	
Brazil	Lima et al. (2010) [55]	
6 continents (58 locations)	Marzal et al. [37]	
Biotic resistance hypothesis		
Lesser Antilles	Ricklefs et al. (2010) [56]	
sGarcía-Longoria et al. [38].		

Table 1. Main studies on the role of avian malaria parasites in the global spread of their bird hosts.

Similar to Hawaii, recent investigations have detected avian malaria *Plasmodium* spp. in New Zealand birds, thus suggesting that avian malaria could be an emerging threat to New Zealand avifauna [32, 33]. For example, an outbreak of malaria has killed more than 90% of the population of the endemic Yellowheads (*Mohoua ochrocephala*) [46]. Also, Howe et al. [33] have reported the death of native and exotic bird species due to acute *Plasmodium* spp. infection. In addition, Baillie et al. [46] have documented three exotic *Plasmodium* species infecting the endemic New Zealand passerine Bellbird *Anthornis melanura*. Finally, it is known that four alien species of mosquitoes have been established and rapidly spread in New Zealand [31, 47] and are likely to be the vectors responsible for some avian malaria outbreaks in the New Zealand [48].

Malaria parasites were historically considered to be absent in Galápagos Islands, because studies based on microscopic and molecular screening of parasites failed to detect malaria parasites in Galápagos birds [49, 50], most probably due to the absence of competent vectors. However, in the last decade, several studies have showed malaria-infected birds in several islands in the archipelago, thus suggesting recent arrival of avian malaria parasites. In this sense, the only known competent vector for *Plasmodium* parasites present in the archipelago is the mosquito *Culex quinquesfasciatus*, which was described for the first time in Galápagos in 1989 and it was well established by 2003 [51]. Following the mosquito introduction, the first report of malaria-infected birds in the Galápagos Archipelago come from Levin et al. [34], identifying penguins as positives for *Plasmodium*. Later, Santiago-Alarcon et al. [35] showed haemosporidian parasites infecting the endemic Galápagos dove (*Zenaida galapagoensis*). More recently, Levin et al. [35] have found different genetic lineages of *Plasmodium* parasites infecting Galápagos birds. Some of these lineages seem to be transient infections of parasites not established on the archipelago, whereas other parasite lineages are thought to be established and regularly transmitted in the archipelago.

P. relictum is an avian malaria parasite with highly virulence, genetic diversity and markedly invasive nature [19, 45, 52]. Recent molecular studies on partial sequences of the cytochrome oxidase b gene on this parasite have revealed different genetic diversity of this parasite, with two main parasite lineages: *P. relictum* GRW4 and *P. relictum* SGS1. *P. relictum* GRW4 is the parasite lineage responsible for devastating epizooties reported in Hawaii and New Zealand, and has a broad geographical range including Africa, Asia and the Americas [37, 45]. Its sister lineage, *P. relictum* SGS1 is widespread and actively transmitted in Europe, Africa and Asia [37], but until very recently, this invasive lineage had not been reported in the mainland Americas [37, 45, 53–55].

Marzal et al. [56] have recently showed the first report of this invasive pathogen in the mainland Americas. They analysed more than 100 blood samples from native bird species from South America, showing the presence of *P. relictum* SGS1 in neotropical birds from two different areas of Peru. In this study, *P. relictum* SGS1 was also geographically spread, and the most generalist and prevalent parasite lineage found in the study, infecting 13 individuals from eight host species (39.40% of the total infections). We must be particularly aware on the presence of this invasive parasite in birds of South America because it may represent a serious risk to this avifauna and a potential threat to over one-third of all bird species in the world.

Would it be possible to eliminate emerging infectious diseases? We do not think so. Indeed, it seems unlikely that most emerging infectious diseases will be eradicated in a close future [57]. In the fight against emerging infectious diseases, we have to follow the advice of the Red Queen to Lewis Carroll's Alice in Wonderland: '…it takes all the running you can do, to keep in the same place. If you want to get somewhere else, you must run at least twice as fast as that!' Therefore, this is a continuous process, where we have to keep on researching to avoid being out of step in the fight against malaria and other emerging infectious diseases. Studies on avian malaria research may play an essential role in these investigations to determine the key factors (e.g. deforestation and land-use change, biological invasions) contributing to the emergence of these diseases.

3. Identification of malaria genes

Approximately, 40% of the world population lives in areas where malaria is transmitted. In some areas, as sub-Saharan Africa, malaria may cause a rate of mortality in 5-year-old children around 90% [58]. An important tool in the fight against malaria parasites is the identification and sequencing of malaria genes that could give essential information about this harmful disease. Hence, in 1996, an international effort was launched to sequence the *Plasmodium falciparum* genome with the aim to open new paths for researching and for the development of new treatments and vaccines against malaria parasites. Some years later, the results were published showing that there was possible to sequence all the chromosomes of *P. falciparum* clone 3D7 [59–61]. The results showed that these chromosomes encode for 5300 genes and are the most (A + T)-rich genome sequence to date.

Moreover, these chromosomes possess a high number of genes related to immune evasion and host-parasite interactions and fewer enzymes and transporters. In the short term, however, it has been suggested that the genome sequence alone provides little information about malaria parasites. As Gardner et al. [59] claim 'much remains to be done'. These results might need to be accompanied by new methods of control, including new drugs and vaccines, improved diagnostics and effective vector control techniques. In this section, we will deal with some malaria genes that are essential for identification of malaria transmission areas and to develop strategies to avoid spread of the disease.

Also, we will show some recent studies on the identification of malaria genes that are crucial in the parasite life cycle, and could be used as a target for future vaccines or anti-malaria drugs.

3.1. Identification of merozoite surface protein gene 1 (MSP1) and malaria transmission areas

Malaria parasites have an important effect in populations where it is present affecting the survival of the community and laying out with facility [5]. Therefore, there is a general need to define populations at risk for appropriate resource allocation and to provide a robust framework for evaluation its global economic impact. The interest of mapping the global distribution of malaria parasite has increased in the last decade. Some authors have decided to identify some essential genes with an enormous variability in order to distinguish different location of the malaria parasites [62]. A commonly used good candidate gene is merozoite surface protein 1 (msp1). This gene is one of the most variable genes found in the human malaria parasite *P. falciparum* [63]. It encodes a protein involved in the attachment of the malaria parasite to the host red blood cell [64]. Within *P. falciparum,* the msp1 gene encodes for a 190 kDa protein that is separated in four different polypeptides (p83, p42, p38 and p30). During the erythrocyte invasion, the polypeptide p42 is split in two more polypeptides (p19 and p33). However, at the end of the process the only polypeptide that remains into the erythrocyte is p19 [65]. This gene has been analysed in a wide number of studies with the aim to determine whether it is a good candidate for developing vaccines or anti-malaria drugs. In this sense, [66] showed that antibodies to the p19 peptide are found in populations with high malaria prevalence and can be associated with immunity to the malaria parasite.

In 2013, Hellgren et al. [67] identified this gene in *P. relictum* SGS1, GRW11 and GRW4 lineages. They found that, within msp1 gene, there are nine different alleles split into the three

P. relictum lineages: SGS1 (alleles Pr1, Pr2, Pr3 and Pr7), GRW4 (alleles Pr4, Pr5, Pr6, Pr8 and Pr9) and GRW11 (alleles Pr2, Pr3 and Pr7). Theses alleles have a specific distribution around the world affecting areas as South America, Europe, Asia or Africa [68]. Moreover, they suggested that due to its high variability, this gene could be used as a candidate to investigate how different host species cope with the infection. In this sense, Hellgren et al. [68] confirmed some transmission events by the lineages analysing resident bird species or juvenile individuals before migration. Therefore, some alleles are restricted to a specific area. For instance, the allele Pr1 is, to date, only present in sub-Sahara areas, while the Pr2 allele has been mainly detected in European areas. This strict allocation may suggest the existence of transmission barriers (e.g. vector communities or abiotic factors) limiting transmission between regions.

By barcoding the msp1 gene in SGS1 and GRW4, a recent study has determined whether haemosporidian transmission in house martins occurs at European sites by sampling juvenile birds house martins (a migratory species with a high fidelity to its area of hatching and nesting) [30].

Moreover, they analysed the msp1 alleles in both adult and juvenile house martins in order to identify their potential areas of transmission. Surprisingly, their results showed that some juvenile and adult house martins were infected by Pr2 allele of *P. relictum* SGS1, an allele thought to be exclusively transmitted in Europe. These results showed, for the first time, that juvenile house martins may become infected with *Plasmodium* parasites already before their first migration to Africa, thus confirming that active transmission of *Plasmodium* spp. to house martins also occur in Europe. These findings emphasise not only the importance of using multiple independent loci of avian *Plasmodium* parasites to understand transmission areas of blood parasites but also the use of birds as study model in parasite analyses.

3.2. New target to avoid completion of malaria life cycle: the chitinase gene (CHT1)

Malaria parasites (including human malaria) show a complex life cycle that requires mechanisms adapted to enable the parasite invasion into the different tissues from the vertebrate host to the arthropod vector. Apparently, arthropods develop a protective peritrophic membrane (PM) against pathogens around their midgut after each blood meal. This PM blocks the penetration of blood parasites and avoids the spreading of the parasite to other organs. In turn, malaria parasites have developed a mechanism to overcome the PM barrier. Once the malaria parasite has complete its sexual stage in the mosquito stomach, the ookinete has the ability to cross the PM by secreting a chitinase that has catalytic and substrate-binding sites breaking down this layer. After crossing the PM, ookinetes finally transform into oocytes, which after maturing releases the sporozoites that move to the salivary glands where they are ready for infecting a new host [69]. Therefore, the role of the chitinase gene is essential in the life cycle of malaria parasites.

The chitinase gene has been study for years due to the variability of structures that it shows. In mammals, some *Plasmodium* parasites may present two different structures. For example, in human malaria (*Plasmodium vivax*), shared human and primate malaria (*Plasmodium knowlesi*) and in rodent malaria (*Plasmodium berghei, Plasmodium yoelii* and *Plasmodium chabaudi*) the chitinase gene presents a long structure and has a catalytic domain and a chitin-binding domain. However, the chitinase gene in human *P. falciparum* and in primate *Plasmodium reichenowi* presents a short structure and lacks the chitin-binding domain [70]. Concerning birds, it has been shown that *Plasmodium gallinaceum* has functional copies of both the long (PgCHT1) and the short (PgCHT2) chitinase gene suggesting that *P. gallinaceum* could be a common ancestor of the mammalian *Plasmodium* parasites that subsequently lost either the short or the long copy of this gene. However, the phylogenetic relationship among *Plasmodium* parasites infecting mammals and birds has been intensively debated over the past decades. On the one hand, some authors suggest that *P. falciparum* is closer phylogenetically to bird parasites than other mammalian malaria parasites [71]. On the other hand, several authors claim that mammalian parasites form a monophyletic clade [72]. Additionally, it has been suggested that *P. gallinaceum* is not the most prevalence parasite in birds and new studies would be needed in order to clarify this relationship. In this sense, Garcia-Longoria et al. [73] identified the chitinase gene in one of the most harmfulness and widespread avian malaria parasites, *P. relictum*. They demonstrated that *P. relictum* presents both copies encoding for chitinase (PrCHT1 and PrCHT2), thus supporting the hypothesis that avian malaria parasites could be the ancestor for the chitinase gene in malaria parasites of primates and rodents. Therefore, given the current phylogenetic hypothesis, it could be assumed that mammalian parasites evolved from an avian parasite that carried two copies of the chitinase gene. These findings are quite remarkable if we take into account that the evolutionary pathway of the malaria parasites is being decoded day-by-day, and the ancestors of human malaria parasites may give essential gene information that could be used for development of new anti-malaria treatment.

4. Malaria parasites and escape behaviour

Behavioural traits are an important factor in the life cycle of all live organisms. Behaviour may determine whether an individual ends up as a survivor or as a prey [74] or it can even acts as a defence against some parasites. For example, some organisms modified their behaviour by plastically changing their life history in order to evade parasite or to minimise the impact of infection [75]. A good example of behaviour as a defence mechanism to avoid is displayed in *Drosophila melanogaster*. Since small larvae are better protected from parasites, this fly can reduce the size of their larvae in habitats with high concentration of pathogens [76]. Ants also can modify their behaviour as a defence against parasites, as they reallocate their nests more often in areas where parasites are common [77]. All these examples suggest that behaviour is an essential key in the survival of individuals.

Anti-predator behaviour is a specific kind of behaviour that is consistent in the presence of a predator across time and contexts [78] and imposes an important selection pressure on preys [79]. Thus, when a predator stalks a prey, the first mean of avoidance of predation is escaping from the predator. However, when the prey is already captured by the predator, the behaviour displayed by the prey can be much more specific: the escape behaviour. Among others, escape behaviour includes several behavioural traits such as (i) the intensity with which a captured individual wriggles to escape, (ii) biting or attacking the predator,(iii) whether it loses feathers, limbs, or a tail and thereby manages to escape, (iv) fear screaming and (v) akin behaviour to feigning death [80]. These variables are closely related to the probabilities that one individual has to escape; thus, the more intense this escape behaviour in one individual is, the more probabilities would have this individual to escape from the predator. For example, a prey individual may emit a loud fear scream that can either warn co-specifics or to attract secondary predators, thus facilitating the escape [81]. Additionally, in 2011, Møller et al. [82] showed that birds with high levels of predation wriggled more when captured by a human, hence increasing their probabilities to escape from the predator, showing that intense escape behaviour is related with high levels of predation.

In addition to predation, parasite represents another major cause of mortality in birds. Some studies demonstrated that the presence of parasites and predators may provoke stress to animals and reduce the immune function in one individual suggesting a relationship between malaria parasites and predation [83]. Later, Møller and Nielsen [81] showed that individuals infected with blood parasites showed lower intense of escape behaviour. Both studies reveal an underlying mechanism that links predation to prevalence of blood parasites. Recently, this underlying mechanism has been analysing. In this sense, Garcia-Longoria et al. [84] tested whether species with higher prevalence of *Haemoproteus*, *Plasmodium* or *Leucocytozoon* infection differed in escape behaviour from species with lower prevalence. They found that some escape behaviours are positively related with the prevalence of these blood parasites, where bird species with an intense escape behaviour showed higher parasitaemia of blood parasites. The observed correlation between blood parasite infections and escape behaviour may suggest a correlation between host behaviour and parasite infection, where individuals showing brave behaviours (e.g. exploratory behaviours or escape behaviours) could increase their likelihood of become infected by increasing the chances of co-specific encounters, injuries or vector bites. Alternatively, this correlation may also show a possible manipulation by the parasite of the behaviour of its host to enhance its chances of transmission.

Regarding to this latter hypothesis, the behavioural manipulation hypothesis posits that manipulation of host behaviour by parasites may confer fitness benefits to the parasite, usually increasing transmission success to the parasite [85]. There are some studies supporting this hypothesis. One of the most well-known examples is the manipulation displayed by *Toxoplasma gondii*, a blood parasite that may infect rodent and other mammals. A mice infected with *T. gondii* lose its fear against feline predators (the definitive host of *T. gondii*), thus increasing the likelihoods of transmission of the parasite to its final host [86]. Concerning malaria parasites, little is known about whether malaria parasites can manipulate the behaviour of their avian host. Malaria parasites show a complex life cycle with both vertebrate (e.g. birds, reptiles and mammals) and invertebrate host (e.g. mosquitoes). In 2013, Cornet et al. [87] demonstrated that infected birds attract more vectors than uninfected ones suggesting that malaria parasites may modify the behaviour of their vector in order to increase their own transmission. However, whether malaria parasites may manipulate escape behaviour of their vertebrate host has been poorly analysed. To date, only one study has explored the association between avian malaria parasites and behaviour in the vertebrate host [88]. Garcia-Longoria et al. [88] experimentally tested whether malaria parasites could manipulate the escape behaviour of their bird hosts. They experimentally infected house sparrows with *P. relictum* and measured the escape behaviour of sparrows before and after the malaria infection. They showed that experimentally infected individuals increased the intensity of their escape behaviour after the parasite inoculation, hence demonstrating that *P. relictum* may modify the escape behaviour of their avian hosts. These results agree with the behavioural manipulation hypothesis, because the facility to escape from predators would indirectly increase the transmission of the parasite, as well as enhance the survival of the hosts. One remaining question concerns the identification of the mechanisms that malaria parasites may use to boost the escape behaviour of their avian hosts. In this sense, some parasites are known to modify the behaviour of their host by secreting substances capable of altering the neuronal activity of the host. For example, the trematode *Schistosoma mansoni* secretes opioid peptides that change the function in the brain of its hosts by producing cystic fibrosis causing the necrosis of some brain areas. Other parasites, like helminths, can alter the concentration of serotonin or dopamine in the host, thus altering some neurological mechanism in their host. Hence, the mechanisms that *P. relictum* might use in order to modify the escape behaviour of its avian host it remains unknown. Future studies on avian malaria research should go deeper with the aim to identifying the mechanisms underlying the behaviour alterations of their bird hosts after malaria infection.

5. Conclusions

Malaria parasites and other emerging infectious diseases are one of the major challenges for global health in the twenty-first century. Despite the efforts made by scientist and health care providers, malaria parasites are becoming drug-resistant, as well as they are boosting their mortality rate in some regions and increasing their areas of transmission. These risings can be provoked by some anthropogenic alterations as deforestation or biological invasions, thus provoking changes in the ecology and epidemiology of vector-borne diseases and outbreaks in human, livestock and wildlife emerging infectious diseases. Moreover, in human malaria studies, it is very difficult to assess if the changes in parasite prevalence are due to socio-ecological factors or to the effects of environmental alterations. These facts emphasise the importance of the study of malaria parasites in wild animals, free from social and economic factors, to fight against this pathogen. Here, we have also focused our attention in the identification of new avian malaria genes that could help in the detection of malaria transmission areas around the world. In addition, the identification of malaria genes with high genetic variability will supply essential information in the evolution of both human and avian malaria pathogens and would provide scientists with new tools for the development of anti-malaria drugs. Our current knowledge about malaria and EIDs is still limited. Further investigation and exploration are needed in order to gain a better understanding of the malaria distribution and the global economic and health impact of malaria. Moreover, it is important to increase awareness of the consequences of introducing non-native species in different habitats and to increase the control in biosecurity borders for avoiding the introduction of alien pathogens such as malaria parasites. Finally, we should be fully aware that there is no ending in the fight against EIDs, where 'it will take all the running (*researching*) you can do, to keep in the same place'.

Acknowledgements

This study was funded by research projects of the Spanish Ministry of Economy and Competitiveness (CGL2015-64650P) and Junta de Extremadura (GRU15117). Sergio Magallanes was supported by a PhD grant from Ministry of Economy and Competition of Spain.

Author details

Luz García-Longoria*, Sergio Magallanes, Manuel González-Blázquez, Yolanda Refollo, Florentino de Lope and Alfonso Marzal

*Address all correspondence to: luzlongoria@unex.es

Department of Anatomy, Cellular Biology and Zoology, University of Extremadura, Badajoz, Spain

References

[1] Poinar G. What fossils reveal about the protozoa progenitors, geographic provinces, and early hosts of malarial organisms. American Entomologist. 2016;62:22-25. DOI org/ 10.1093/ ae/tmw006

[2] Vittor A, Gilman R, Tielsch T, Glass G, Shields T, Sánches W, et al. The effect of deforestation on the human-biting rate of *Anopheles darlingi*, the primary vector of

falciparum malaria in the Peruvian Amazon. American Journal of Tropical Medicine and Hygyene. 2006;74:3–11.

[3] Martinsen ES, Perkins SL, Schall JJ. A three-genome phylogeny of malaria parasites (*Plasmodium* and closely related genera): Evolution of life-history traits and host switches. Molecular Phylogenetics and Evolution. 2008;47:261–73. DOI: 10.1016/j.ympev.2007.11.012

[4] Pérez-Tris J, Bensch S. Diagnosing genetically diverse avian malarial infections using mixed-sequence analysis and TA-cloning. Parasitology. 2005;131:15–23. DOI: 10.1017/S003118200500733X

[5] Valkiunas G, Anwar AM, Atkinson C, Greiner E, Paperna I, Peirce M. What distinguishes malaria parasites from other pigmented haemosporidians? Trends in Parasitology. 2005;21:357–8. DOI: 10.1016/j.pt.2005.06.005

[6] Marzal A. Recent advances in studies on avian malaria parasites. Malaria Parasites. 2012. InTech. Rijeka, Croatia. pp. 135–58. DOI: 10.5772/33730

[7] Preston SH, Keyfitz N, Schoen R. Causes of death: Life tables for national populations. The World Health Report New York 1999. pp. 13–28.

[8] Berkelman RL, Bryan RT. Infectious disease surveillance: A crumbling foundation. Science. 1994;264:368.

[9] Jones KE, Patel NG, Levy MA, Storeygard A, Balk D, Gittleman JL, et al. Global trends in emerging infectious diseases. Nature. 2008;451:990–3. DOI: 10.1038/nature06536

[10] Neiderud CJ. How urbanization affects the epidemiology of emerging infectious diseases. Infection Ecology and Epidemiology. 2015;5:27060. DOI: 10.3402/iee.v5.27060

[11] Sehgal RNM. Deforestation and avian infectious diseases. Journal of Experimental Biology. 2010;213:955–60. DOI: 10.1242/jeb.037663

[12] Daszak P, Cunningham AA, Hyatt AD. Emerging infectious diseases of wildlife threats to biodiversity and human health. Science. 2000;287:443–9.

[13] Vittor A, Gilman Y, Tielsch RH, Glass J, Shields GT, Lozano S, et al. The effect of deforestation on the human-biting rate of *Anopheles darlingi*, the primary vector of *falciparum* malaria in the Peruvian Amazon. Brazilian Journal of Biological Science. 2006;68:949–56.

[14] Olson SH, Gangnon R, Silveira GA, Patz JA. Deforestation and malaria in Mancio Lima country, Brazil. Emerging Infectious Diseases. 2010;16:1108–15. DOI: 10.3201/eid1607.091785

[15] Wilson ML. Ecology and infectious disease. In: Aron J, Patz JA, editors. Ecosystem Change and Public Health Baltimore, USA; 2001. pp. 283–324.

[16] Bonneaud C, Sepila I, Miláa B, Buermanna W, Pollingera J, Sehgal RNM, et al. The prevalence of avian *Plasmodium* is higher in undisturbed tropical forests of Cameroon. Journal of Tropical Ecology. 2009;25:439–47. DOI: 10.1017/S0266467409006178

[17] Chasar A, Loiseau C, Valkiunas G, Iezhova T, Smith TB, Sehgal RNM. Prevalence and diversity patterns of avian blood parasites in degraded African rainforest habitats. Molecular Ecology. 2009;18:4121–33. DOI: 10.1111/j.1365-294X.2009.04346.x

[18] Loiseau C, Iezhova T, Valkiūnas G, Chasar A, Hutchinson A, Buermann W, et al. Spatial variation of haemosporidian parasite infection in African rainforest bird species. Journal of Parasitology. 2010;96:21–9. DOI: 10.1645/GE-2123.1

[19] LaPointe DA, Goff ML, Atkinson CT. Comparative susceptibility of introduced forest-dwelling mosquitoes in Hawai'i to avian malaria, *Plasmodium relictum*. Journal of Parasitology. 2005;91:843–9. DOI: 10.1645/GE-3431.1

[20] Atkinson CT, Lapointe DA. Introduced avian diseases, climate change, and the future of Hawaiian honeycreepers. Journal of Avian Medicine and Surgery. 2009;23:53–63. DOI: 10.2307/1942550

[21] Van Riper III C, Van Riper SG, Goff ML, Laird M. The epizootiology and ecological significance of malaria in Hawaiian land birds. Ecological Monographs. 1986;56:327–44. DOI: 10.2307/1942550

[22] 22. Laurance SGW, Jones D, Westcott D, Mckeown A, Harrington G, Hilbert DW. Habitat fragmentation and ecological traits influence the prevalence of avian blood parasites in a tropical rainforest landscape. PLoS One. 2013;8. DOI: 10.1371/journal.pone.0076227

[23] Belo NO, Pinheiro RT, Reis ES, Ricklefs RE, Braga ÉM. Prevalence and lineage diversity of avian haemosporidians from three distinct cerrado habitats in Brazil. PLoS One. 2011;6. DOI: 10.1371/journal.pone.0017654

[24] Ricopa L, Villa-Galarce ZH. HAemosporidians prevalence and diversity in birds from the National Reserve of Allpahuayo Mishana, Iquitos-Perú. MS thesis. Iquitos, Universidad Nacional de la Amazonía Peruana. 2014.

[25] Waterman SH, Margolis HS, Sejvar JJ. Surveillance for dengue and dengue-associated neurologic syndromes in the United States. American Journal of Tropical Medicine Hygiene. 2015;92:996–8. DOI: 10.4269/ajtmh.14-0016

[26] Calisher CHC. West Nile virus in the New World: Appearance, persistence, and adaptation to a new econiche—an opportunity taken. Viral Immunology. 2000;13:411–4.

[27] Webster RG, Govorkova EA. H5N1 influenza—Continuing evolution and spread. The New England Journal of Medicine. 2006;2174–7.

[28] Sodhi N. Birds. In: Encyclopedia of Invasive Introduced Species. Simberloff D. & Rejmanek M., editors. University of California Press. California , USA; 2010

[29] Williamson MH, Fitter A. The characters of successful invaders. Biological Conservation. 1996;78:163–70. DOI: 10.1016/0006-3207(96)00025-0

[30] Garcia-Longoria L, Hellgren O, Bensch S, De Lope F, Marzal A. Detecting transmission areas of malaria parasites in a migratory bird species. Parasitology. 2015;1–6. DOI: 10.1017/S0031182015000487

[31] Tompkins DM, Gleeson DM. Relationship between avian malaria distribution and an exotic invasive mosquito in New Zealand. Journal of Royal Society of New Zealand. 2006;36:51–62. DOI: 10.1080/03014223.2006.9517799

[32] Barraclough TG, Balbi KJ, Ellis RJ. Evolving concepts of bacterial species. Evolutionary Biology. 2012;39:148–57. DOI: 10.1007/s11692-012-9181-8

[33] Howe L, Castro IC, Schoener ER, Hunter S, Barraclough RK, Alley MR. Malaria parasites (*Plasmodium* spp.) infecting introduced, native and endemic New Zealand birds. Parasitology Research. 2012;110:913–23. DOI: 10.1007/s00436-011-2577-z

[34] Levin II, Outlaw DC, Vargas FH, Parker PG. Plasmodium blood parasite found in endangered Galapagos penguins (*Spheniscus mendiculus*). Biological Conservation. 2009;142:3191–5. DOI: 10.1016/j.biocon.2009.06.017

[35] Santiago-Alarcon D, Outlaw DC, Ricklefs RE, Parker PG. Phylogenetic relationships of haemosporidian parasites in New World Columbiformes, with emphasis on the endemic Galapagos dove. International Journal of Parasitology. 2010;40:463–70. DOI: 10.1016/j.ijpara.2009.10.003

[36] Levin II, Zwiers P, Deem SL, Geest EA, Higashiguchi JM, Iezhova TA, et al. Multiple lineages of avian malaria parasites (*Plasmodium*) in the Galapagos Islands and evidence for arrival via migratory birds. Conservation Biology. 2013;27:1366–77. DOI: 10.1111/cobi.12127

[37] Marzal A, Ricklefs RE, Valkiūnas G, Albayrak T, Arriero E, Bonneaud C, et al. Diversity, loss, and gain of malariap in a globally invasive bird. PLoS One. 2011;6:8. DOI: 10.1371/journal.pone.0021905

[38] García-Longoria L, Magallanes S, de Lope F, Marzal A (2015). Biological invasions of malaria parasites and their bird hosts. in Waterman R (Ed.) Biological invasions. Patterns, Management and Economic Impact. Nova-Publisher, New York.

[39] Diamond J. Guns, germs, and steel: The fates of human societies. Revision of Mexican Sociology. New York, USA: Random House; 1997.

[40] Callaway RM, Ridenour WM. Novel weapons: Invasive success and the evolution of increased competitive ability. Frontiers in Ecology and Environment. 2004;436–43.

[41] Prenter J, MacNeil C, Dick JTA, Dunn AM. Roles of parasites in animal invasions. Trends in Ecology and Evolution. 2004;385–90.

[42] Valkiūnas G. Avian malaria parasites and other haemosporidia. Boca Raton. 2005.

[43] Lowe S, Browne M, Boudjelas S, De Poorter M. 100 of the World's Worst Invasive Alien Species. A selection from the Global Invasive Species Database. Invasive Species Spec. Gr. a Spec. Gr. Species Surviv. Comm. World Conservation Union. 2000;12:12.

[44] Olson SL, James HF. Fossil birds from the Hawaiian Islands: Evidence for wholesale extinction by man before western contact. Science. 1982;217:633–638. DOI: 10.1126/science.217.4560.633

[45] Beadell JS, Ishtiaq F, Covas R, Melo M, Warren BH, Atkinson CT, et al. Global phylogeographic limits of Hawaii's avian malaria. Proceeding of the Royal Society B: Biological Science. 2006;273:2935–44. DOI: 10.1098/rspb.2006.3671

[46] Derraik JGB. Bitten birds. Piecing together the avian malaria puzzle. Biosecurity New Zeal. 2006;16–7.

[47] Derraik JGB. A survey of the mosquito (Diptera :Culicidae) fauna of the Auckland Zoological park. New Zealand Entomology. 2004;27:51–5. DOI: 10.1080/00779962.2004.9722124

[48] Derraik JGB. Exotic mosquitoes in New Zealand: A review of species intercepted, their pathways and ports of entry. Australian and New Zealand Journal of Public Health. 2004;433–44. DOI: 10.1111/j.1467- 842X.2004.tb00025.x

[49] Miller GD, Hofkin BV, Snell H, Hahn A, Miller RD. Avian malaria and Marek's disease: Potential threats to Galapagos penguins *Spheniscus mendiculus*. Marine Ornithology. 2001;29:43–6.

[50] Travis EK, Vargas FH, Merkel J, Gottdenker N, Miller RE, Parker PG. Hematology, serum chemistry, and serology of Galapagos penguins (*Spheniscus mendiculus*) in the Galapagos Islands, Ecuador. Journal of Wildlife Diseases. 2006;42:14–20. DOI: 10.7589/0090-3558- 42.3.625

[51] Whiteman NK, Goodman SJ, Sinclair BJ, Walsh T, Cunningham AA, Kramer LD, et al. Establishment of the avian disease vector *Culex quinquefa*sciatus Say, 1823 (Diptera:Culicidae) on the Galapagos Islands, Ecuador. Ibis (Lond. 1859). 2005;147:843–7. DOI: 10.1111/j.1474- 919X.2005.00468.x

[52] Palinauskas V, Valkiūnas G, Bolshakov C V, Bensch S. *Plasmodium relictu*m (lineage P-SGS1): Effects on experimentally infected passerine birds. Experimental Parasitology. 2008;120:372–80. DOI: 10.1016/j.exppara.2008.09.001

[53] Durrant KL, Beadell JS, Ishtiaq F, Graves GR, Olson SL, Gering E, et al. Avian Haematozoa in South America: A comparison of temperate and tropical zones. Ornithological Monographs. 2006;60:98.

[54] Merino S, Moreno J, Vásquez RA, Martínez J, Sánchez-Monsálvez I, Estades CF, et al. Haematozoa in forest birds from Southern Chile: Latitudinal gradients in prevalence and parasite lineage richness. Australian Ecology. 2008;33:329–40. DOI: 10.1111/j. 1442-9993.2008.01820.x

[55] 56. Lacorte GA, Flix GMF, Pinheiro RRB, Chaves AV, Almeida-Neto G, Neves FS, et al. Exploring the diversity and distribution of neotropical avian malaria parasites—A molecular survey from Southeast Brazil. PLoS One. 2013;8:e1003456. DOI: 10.1371/ journal.pone.0057770

[56] Marzal A, García-Longoria L, Cárdenas Callirgos JM, Sehgal RN. Invasive avian malaria as an emerging parasitic disease in native birds of Peru. Biological Invasions. 2014;17:39–45. DOI: 10.1007/s10530-014-0718-x

[57] Morens DM, Fauci AS. Emerging infectious diseases: Threats to human health and global stability. PLoS Pathogenic. 2013;9:e1003467. DOI: 10.1371/journal.ppat.1003467

[58] Breman JG. The ears of the hippopotamus: Manifestations, determinants, and estimates of the malaria burden. American Journal of Tropical Medicine and Hygiene. 2001;64:1–11.

[59] Gardner MJ, Shallom SJ, Carlton JM, Salzberg SL, Nene V, Shoaibi A, et al. Sequence of *Plasmodium falciparum* chromosomes 2, 10, 11 and 14. Nature. 2002;419:531–4. DOI: 10.1038/nature01094

[60] Hall N, Pain A, Berriman M, Churcher C, Harris B, Harris D, et al. Sequence of *Plasmodium falciparum* chromosomes 1, 3–9 and 13. Nature. 2002;419:527–31. DOI: 10.1038/nature01095

[61] Hyman RW, Fung E, Conway A, Kurdi O, Mao J, Miranda M, et al. Sequence of *Plasmodium falciparum* chromosome 12. Nature. 2002;419:534–7. DOI: 10.1038/ nature01102

[62] Snow RW, Guerra CA, Noor AM, Myint HY, Hay SI. The global distribution of clinical episodes of Plasmodium falciparum malaria. Nature. 2005;434:214–7 DOI: 10.1038/ nature03342

[63] Barry AE, Schultz L, Buckee CO, Reeder JC. Contrasting population structures of the genes encoding ten leading vaccine-candidate antigens of the human malaria parasite, *Plasmodium falciparum*. PLoS One. 2009;4:e849. DOI: 10.1371/journal.pone.0008497

[64] Gerold P, Schofieldb L, Blackman MJ, Holder AA, Schwarz RT. Structural analysis of the glycosyl-phosphatidylinositol membrane anchor of the merozoite surface proteins-1 and -2 of *Plasmodium falciparum*. Molecular and Biochemical Parasitology. 1996;75:131–43.

[65] Blackman MJ, Heidrich HG, Donachie S, McBride JS, Holder AA. A single fragment of a malaria merozoite surface protein remains on the parasite during red cell invasion

and is the target of invasion-inhibiting antibodies. The Journal of Experimental Medicine. 1990;172:379–82.

[66] Hui G, Hashimoto C. *Plasmodium falciparum* anti-MSP1-19 antibodies induced by MSP1-42 and MSP1-19 based vaccines differed in specificity and parasite growth inhibition in terms of recognition of conserved versus variant epitopes. Vaccine. 2007;25:948–56. DOI: 10.1016/j.vaccine.2006.08.041

[67] Hellgren O, Kutzer M, Bensch S, Valki Nas G, Palinauskas V. Identification and characterization of the merozoite surface protein 1 (msp1) gene in a host-generalist avian malaria parasite, *Plasmodium relict*um (lineages SGS1 and GRW4) with the use of blood transcriptome. Malaria Journal. 2013;12:381. DOI: 10.1186/1475-2875-12-381

[68] Hellgren O, Atkinson CT, Bensch S, Albayrak T, Dimitrov D, Ewen JG, et al. Global phylogeography of the avian malaria pathogen *Plasmodium relictum* based on MSP1 allelic diversity. Ecography. 2015;38:842–50.

[69] Vinetz JM, Valenzuela JG, Specht CA, Aravind L, Langer RC, Ribeiro JM, et al. Chitinases of the avian malaria parasite *Plasmodium gallinaceum*, a class of enzymes necessary for parasite invasion of the mosquito midgut. Journal of Biological Chemistry. 2000;275:10331–41. DOI: 10.1074/jbc.275.14.10331

[70] Li F, Patra KP, Vinetz JM. An anti-chitinase malaria transmission-blocking single-chain antibody as an effector molecule for creating a *Plasmodium falciparum*-refractory mosquito. The Journal of Infectious Diseases. 2005;192:878–87. DOI: 10.1086/432552

[71] Waters AP, Higgins DG, McCutchan TF. *Plasmodium falciparum* appears to have arisen as a result of lateral transfer between avian and human hosts. Proceedings of the National Academy of Sciences.1991;88:3140–4.

[72] Perkins SL, Schall JJ. A molecular phylogeny of malarial parasites recovered from cytochrome b gene sequences. Journal of Parasitology. 2002;88:972–8. DOI: 10.1645/0022-3395(2002)088[0972:AMPOMP]2.0.CO;2)

[73] Garcia-Longoria L, Hellgren O, Bensch S. Molecular identification of the chitinase genes in *Plasmodium relictum*. Malaria Journal. 2014;13:239. DOI: 10.1186/1475-2875-13-239

[74] Bell AM, Hankison SJ, Laskowski KL. The repeatability of behaviour: A meta-analysis. Animal Behaviour. 2009;77:771–83. DOI: 10.1016/j.anbehav.2008.12.022

[75] Sorensen RE, Minchella DJ. Snail-trematode life history interactions: Past trends and future directions. Parasitology. 2001;123:3–18.

[76] Kraaijeveld AR, Godfray HCJ. Potential life-history costs of parasitoid avoidance in *Drosophila melanogaster*. Evolutionary Ecology Research. 2003;5:1251–61.

[77] Schmid-Hempel P. Evolutionary parasitology: The integrated study of infections, immunology, ecology and genetics. Trends Parasitology. 2011. ISBN: 9780199229482

[78] Hellgren O, Kutzer M, Bensch S, Valki Nas G, Palinauskas V. Identification and characterization of the merozoite surface protein 1 (msp1) gene in a host-generalist avian malaria parasite, *Plasmodium* relictum (lineages SGS1 and GRW4) with the use of blood transcriptome. Malaria Journal. 2013;12:381. DOI: 10.1186/1475-2875-12-381

[79] Roulin A, Wink M. Predator-prey relationships and the evolution of colour polymorphism: A comparative analysis in diurnal raptors. Biological Journal of the Linnean Society. 2004;81:565–78. DOI: 10.1111/j.1095-8312.2004.00308.x

[80] Møller AP, Nielsen JT, Erritzøe J. Losing the last feather: Feather loss as an antipredator adaptation in birds. Behaviour Ecology. 2006;17:1046–56. DOI: 10.1093/beheco/arl044

[81] Møller AP, Nielsen JT. Fear screams and adaptation to avoid imminent death: Effects of genetic variation and predation. Ethology Ecology & Evolution. 2010;22:183–202. DOI: 10.1080/03949371003707968

[82] Møller A, Christiansen S, Mousseau T. Sexual signals, risk of predation and escape behavior. Behaviour Ecology. 2011;22:800–7. DOI: 10.1093/beheco/arr046

[83] Navarro C, de Lope F, Marzal A, Møller AP. Predation risk, host immune response, and parasitism. Behaviour Ecology. 2004;15:629–35. DOI: 10.1093/beheco/arh054.

[84] Garcia-Longoria L, Garamszegi LZ, Møller AP. Host escape behaviour and blood parasite infections in birds. Behaviour Ecology. 2014;25:890–900. DOI: 10.1093/beheco/aru066

[85] Bell AM, Hankison SJ, Laskowski KL. The repeatability of behaviour: A meta-analysis. Animal Behaviour. 2009;77:771&83. DOI: 10.1016/j.anbehav.2008.12.022.

[86] Sorensen RE, Minchella DJ. Snail-trematode life history interactions: Past trends and future directions. Parasitology. 2001;123:3–18.

[87] Kraaijeveld AR, Godfray HCJ. Potential life-history costs of parasitoid avoidance in *Drosophila melanogaster*. Evolutionary Ecology Research. 2003;5:1251–61.

[88] Schmid-Hempel P. Evolutionary parasitology: The integrated study of infections, immunology, ecology and genetics. Trends Parasitology. 2011. ISBN: 9780199229482

[89] Dammhahn M, Almeling L. Is risk taking during foraging a personality trait ? A field test for cross-context consistency in boldness. Animal Behaviour. 2012;84:1131–1139. DOI: 10.1016/j.anbehav.2012.08.014

[90] Roulin A, Wink M. Predator-prey relationships and the evolution of colour polymorphism: A comparative analysis in diurnal raptors. Biological Journal of the Linnean Society. 2004;81:565–78. DOI: 10.1111/j.1095-8312.2004.00308.x

[91] Møller AP, Nielsen JT, Erritzøe J. Losing the last feather: Feather loss as an antipredator adaptation in birds. Behaviour Ecology. 2006;17:1046–56. DOI: 10.1093/beheco/arl044

[92] Møller AP, Nielsen JT. Fear screams and adaptation to avoid imminent death: Effects of genetic variation and predation. Ethology Ecology & Evolution. 2010;22:183–202. DOI: 10.1080/03949371003707968

[93] Møller A, Christiansen S, Mousseau T. Sexual signals, risk of predation and escape behavior. Behaviour Ecology. 2011;22:800–7. DOI: 10.1093/beheco/arr046

[94] Navarro C, de Lope F, Marzal A, Møller AP. Predation risk, host immune response, and parasitism. Behaviour Ecology. 2004;15:629–35. DOI: 10.1093/beheco/arh054.

[95] Garcia-Longoria L, Garamszegi LZ, Møller AP. Host escape behaviour and blood parasite infections in birds. Behaviour Ecology. 2014;25:890–900. DOI: 10.1093/beheco/aru066

[96] Poulin R. Parasite Manipulation of Host Behavior: An Update and Frequently Asked Questions. 1st ed. Adv. Study Behavior. Elsevier; 2010.

[97] Webster JP, McConkey GA. *Toxoplasma gondii*-altered host behaviour: Clues as to mechanism of action. Folia Parasitol. 2010;57:95–104. DOI: 10.1016/S0924-9338(11)73825-1

[98] Cornet S, Nicot A, Rivero A, Gandon S. Malaria infection increases bird attractiveness to uninfected mosquitoes. Ecology Letters. 2013;16:323–9. DOI: 10.1111/ele.12041

[99] Garcia-Longoria L, Møller AP, Balbontín J, de Lope F, Marzal A. Do malaria parasites manipulate the escape behaviour of their avian hosts? An experimental study. Parasitology Research. 2015;114:4493–4501. DOI: 10.1007/s00436-015-4693-7

7

Enabling Vaccine Delivery Platforms and Adjuvants for Malaria

Amy R. Noe, Vinayaka Kotraiah and
Gabriel M. Gutierrez

Abstract

Enabling vaccine delivery platforms and adjuvants with promising attributes for malaria vaccine development are reviewed within the framework of accessibility, efficacy, clinical status, cost, and cold-chain considerations. An emphasis is placed on commercially available platforms and adjuvants including virus-like particle, nanoparticle, microneedle, and mRNA vaccine delivery platforms as well as lipid vesicle, microparticle, and emulsion-based adjuvants. Strategies for addressing complications of vaccine delivery in endemic regions due to concatenate vaccination and infection, and parasite immune avoidance mechanisms are presented. Additionally, recent findings regarding how malaria infection triggers inflammatory pathways and T cell exhaustion along with negative impacts to the development of effective memory responses are described in a context relevant to vaccine development.

Keywords: *Plasmodium falciparum*, malaria, adjuvant, vaccine, delivery platform, VLP, virus-like particle, microneedle, mRNA, nanoparticle, microparticle, liposome, emulsion, nanoemulsion, TLR agonist, T cell exhaustion, PD-1, immune response, CSP

1. Introduction

Efforts to develop an effective malaria vaccine have been ongoing for decades. In order to promote better coordination and acceleration of malaria vaccine development, the World Health Organization (WHO) initiated a process that resulted in the Malaria Vaccine Technology Roadmap, which was first published in 2006 [1] and updated in 2013 [2]. The vision in the roadmap includes development of vaccines for *Plasmodium falciparum* and *P. vivax* to prevent disease, death, and malaria transmission as part of enabling malaria eradication efforts. As per the updated Malaria Vaccine Technology Roadmap, the goal of a successful vaccine candidate is ≥75% protective efficacy over 2 years with no more than one annual booster that can be administered to all age groups. Transmission-blocking vaccines were also included in this development effort. Importantly, the Roadmap prioritized access to low cost GMP vaccine manufacture for commercial production, which encompasses a direct pathway to licensure, ability to manufacture at a large scale, as well as vaccine availability and ease of access, inclusive of delivery platforms and adjuvants. With these considerations in mind, we review enabling vaccine delivery platforms and adjuvants with favorable attributes, to both facilitate the fusion of promising malaria targets with novel technology platforms and meet Roadmap vaccine development, efficacy, and accessibility goals.

A brief overview of recent findings regarding development of immune responses during and after malaria infection is relevant to vaccine development (particularly regarding parasite immune evasion mechanisms that engage inflammatory pathways, promote T cell exhaustion, and stimulate regulatory T cell expansion), as vaccination and malaria infection occur concatenately in endemic regions. Traditionally, the intended outcome of any combination of malaria vaccine target and adjuvant/delivery platform would be to elicit as strong of an immunostimulatory response as possible to the Th1 and/or Th2 immune compartments. However, studies of chronic disease in humans and mice, in the cancer and infectious disease fields, have shown that magnitude of the immune stimulus may not be as important as the balance of immune presentation to immune overreaction (e.g., regulatory T cell stimulation and T cell exhaustion/ablation) [3–5]. Recent studies in rodent malaria models have significantly increased our understanding regarding how chronic malaria infection can hamper development of effective Th1 and Th2 immune responses as well as development of B and T cell memory. For example, in a mouse model of severe malaria infection, it has been shown that proinflammatory cytokines (IFN-γ and TNF) and pathways mediating the disease are detrimental to development of humoral response by inhibiting/exhausting T helper cells [6]. That these cytokines are the same as those monitored in regards to enhanced cellular response to many adjuvanted vaccines is of particular concern. Furthermore, in mouse malaria models, chronic malaria infection triggers CD8+ T cell exhaustion (loss of T cell effector function) through a programmed cell death-1 (PD-1) pathway [7, 8]. In humans, the state of T cell exhaustion has been documented following numerous infections, during chronic infection, as well as in cancer patients, with expression of PD-1 as a hallmark exhaustion [9]. Taken together, these phenomena suggest an explanation for some of the difficulties encountered during malaria vaccine development as well as provide insight into why vaccine-induced protective immunity quickly wanes. A knowledge base on preventing T cell exhaustion has been developed in the therapeutic cancer vaccine field, which can be used as a launching point for how to address this issue in malaria vaccine development. One of the key areas of interest is the use of adjuvants to downregulate pathways leading to T cell exhaustion (e.g., PD-1 and LAG-3 inhibitors) [10–12]. Therefore, we suggest that the information presented herein be considered in the context of careful characterization of the mode of action for the combined antigen and adjuvant/delivery technology to overcome the evolving hallmarks of malaria immune evasion.

1.1. Enabling vaccine delivery platforms

A range of novel vaccine delivery platforms are described herein, including those that can accommodate different antigen/immunogen formats such as recombinant proteins, peptides, epitopes, and/or nuclei acids. Many of these platforms can deliver multiple antigens and in different formats, simultaneously. In describing these platforms, we included state-of-the-art technologies with the potential for major impacts to vaccine delivery where the regulatory and/ or licensure pathways may not yet be defined. As there are a significant number of published preclinical and clinical studies on different viral vectored malaria antigens (e.g., adenovirus and modified vaccinia Ankara (MVA) vectors), these platforms have not been detailed herein, but have been recently reviewed elsewhere [13–15]. In addition, several particulate-based platforms that have been used in combination with malaria candidate vaccines, but not described here, have been recently reviewed [16].

1.2. Virus-like particles

The ability of viral capsid proteins to self-assemble and incorporate foreign antigens has been exploited in the development of virus-like particles (VLPs) as a vaccine delivery platform [17, 18]. While many VLP platforms for human pathogens have been developed and utilized to deliver native epitopes of the subject virus, other VLP platforms can be used to deliver foreign epitopes; only the latter is discussed herein. Platforms capable of integrating foreign epitopes include human pathogens (e.g., hepatitis B virus (HBV) and human papillomavirus) and many nonhuman pathogens (e.g., bacteriophages, plant viruses, and animal viruses). Foreign antigens can be incorporated into VLPs by genetic modification of the capsid protein at one or more sites or by chemical conjugation of antigen to the capsid protein. Immunogens can also be encapsidated within the VLP lumen. Even with these modifications, capsid proteins can retain the structure and morphology of the originating virus. VLPs are known to induce strong humoral and cellular immune responses as foreign antigens are displayed in a repetitive manner on VLPs, which boost immune responses by facilitating cross-linking of immunoglobulin receptors and B cell activation; VLPs are easily taken up by antigen-presenting cells that ultimately lead to cytokine production, stimulation of CD4+ T helper cells, and induction of potent cytotoxic immune responses through cross-presentation to cytotoxic CD8+ T cells [18–24]. For most VLPs, single-stranded RNA (ssRNA) is packaged within the particles during assembly. The presence of ssRNA is thought to enhance immunity, as this is a natural ligand for Toll-like receptor (TLR) 7 and TLR8 [25]. Of note is that the described plant-based VLP platforms do not meet a strict definition of VLP as they are infectious to and propagate in the organism in which they are grown (but not in humans). For simplicity, and as these platforms are often identified as VLPs in the literature, they are presented together in a single section.

The main drawback of VLP-based vaccines is size constraints of the foreign antigen incorporated or fused to capsid protein, which is dependent on the specific VLP platform. Note that larger antigens can be chemically conjugated to some capsid proteins; however, this is also a drawback as the antigen and capsid must be expressed and purified separately for conjugation, which can elevate cost. Currently, three VLP-based malaria vaccine candidates have been evaluated in the clinic, and one of these was recently approved for use in humans. These are RTS,S (tradename Mosquirix when in combination with AS01), ICC-1132, and Pfs25 VLP-FhCMB, which are each described below. A recent review of the different GlaskoSmithKline (GSK) adjuvants (AS01, AS02, etc.) can be found elsewhere [26].

1.2.1. Hepatitis virus VLPs

Viruses of the family *Hepadnaviridae*, including the human pathogen HBV, can be utilized as vaccine delivery platforms. These viral particles have both an outer lipid envelope containing a surface antigen (e.g., HBsAg) as well as a nucleocapsid composed of a core protein (e.g., HBcAg). Both the surface protein and core protein can accept foreign peptides and thus be utilized as VLP-based vaccine delivery platforms. RTS,S is composed of the repeat and C-terminal regions of *P. falciparum* circumsporozoite protein (PfCSP) fused to hepatitis B virus surface antigen (HBsAg) and has been licensed in combination with AS01 by the European Medicines Agency (EMA). The vaccine candidate ICC-1132 is comprised of the hepatitis B virus core protein (HBcAg) with PfCSP T cell and B cell epitope insertions. ICC-1132 has been tested in multiple clinical studies [27–30]; however, upon controlled human malaria challenge (CHMI) of vaccinees administered with ICC-1132 formulated in Montanide, no sterile protection was seen [30].

Core protein-based VLPs possess a number of favorable characteristics for vaccine development as compared to surface protein-based VLPs. These include the ability of the recombinant core protein to self-assemble into VLPs, flexibility of the expression system, and increased immunogenicity of the core protein as compared to the surface protein [31–34]. Considerations of immune tolerance issues when using VLPs based on the human pathogen HBV are also important given the number of chronic HBV carriers worldwide. Additionally, as antibodies to the HBcAg serve as the basis for HBV diagnostics, widespread use of HBcAg-based VLPs may compromise use of anti-HBc antibodies to diagnose infection. These concerns have been addressed through use of nonhuman pathogenic hepadnaviruses in VLP platform development, including viruses that infect rodents and ducks [35–37]. In addition to RTS,S and ICC-1132, which are VLPs based on the human hepatitis B virus, a woodchuck hepatitis B virus VLP platform (WHcAg) containing PfCSP T cell and B cell epitopes (developed by VLP Biotech) has shown promise in challenge studies with a rodent malaria model where 80–100% protection was seen with different formulations [38]. In this same study, a WHcAg VLP carrying *P. vivax* circumsporozoite protein (PvCSP) repeat epitopes was used for challenge with a rodent malaria model and 100% protection was seen. A comparative study of antigenicity and immunogenicity of different rodent hepatitis virus core proteins (woodchuck, ground squirrel, and artic squirrel) and HBcAg demonstrated that rodent core proteins are (1) equal in immunogenicity to, or more immunogenic than HBcAg for both B cell and T cell responses, (2) not significantly cross-reactive with the HBcAg for B cell responses and only partially cross-reactive with HBcAg for T cell (CD4) responses, and (3) competent to function as vaccine carrier platforms for heterologous, B cell epitopes [36, 39]. In consideration of cost, WHcAg VLPs can be easily expressed at high levels in *E. coli*. In addition, this platform can accommodate insertion of foreign sequences at multiple sites within the coat protein and large inserts at both the N- and C-termini. Note that this platform has not yet been tested in the clinic.

1.2.2. Bacteriophage VLPs

VLPs based on ssRNA bacteriophages can be used as vaccine delivery platforms through conjugation of foreign antigens to the coat protein, encapsidation of foreign antigens within the VLP, or genetic insertion of foreign sequences into the coat protein. One application of the last is creation of VLP-based peptide display libraries by the University of New Mexico (based on MS2, PP7, and AP205 bacteriophage VLP platforms) using a series of plasmid vectors that allow insertion of high complexity random sequence peptides into the coat protein enabling construction of libraries with up to 10^{10} to 10^{11} unique random sequence peptide VLP clones with inserts from 6 to 20 base pairs in length [40, 41]. Biopanning can be performed on these libraries using neutralizing or inhibitory antibodies to affinity select VLPs containing mimotopes—peptide sequences that mimics the structure of epitopes. As opposed to traditional peptide display technologies, affinity selected bacteriophage VLPs can be used directly as immunogen without modification. For example, a VLP mimotope to reticulocyte-binding protein homologue 5 (RH5) found through affinity selection of MS2 libraries using a monoclonal antibody able to block parasite invasion of erythrocytes (*in vitro* via growth inhibition assay) was shown to elicit inhibitory antibodies when administered to mice as an immunogen [42]. In addition, MS2 VLP library affinity selection has also been performed with two anti-AMA-1 monoclonal antibodies [42, 43]. Of note is that Agilvax LLC (a startup that was spun out of the Science & Technology Corporation at the University of New Mexico) holds an exclusive license to commercialize this technology for vaccines and immunotherapies based on the MS2 and AP205 VLP platforms. The MS2 VLP platform can also be used to encapsidate RNA and RNA-modified cargo [44]. Similar to the Qbeta VLPs, foreign antigen can be conjugated to AP205 VLPs [45]. Additionally, while most bacteriophage VLPs can only tolerate small foreign insertions, relatively large insertions are tolerated by the AP205 platform [46]. This has been exploited to create a platform whereby antigens can be irreversibly bound to and displayed on AP205 VLPs by simple mixing using SpyCatcher and SpyTag; further, AP205 VLPs utilizing the SpyCatcher/SpyTag system and displaying Pfs25 (a transmission-blocking vaccine target) are immunogenic in mice [47, 48]. Note that use of the SpyCatcher/SpyTag technology might easily be extended to several other platforms included here, in particular to nanoparticles and lipid vesicle-based platforms; however, it will be important to understand if this technology can meet regulatory requirements for clinical use.

1.2.3. Plant-based virus VLPs

A number of plant viruses have been developed into replication-competent platforms whereby VLPs can infect and replicate in plants (generally tobacco or spinach), but not in humans. Two of the more advanced platforms include alfalfa mosaic virus (AlMV) and tobacco mosaic virus (TVM), both of which can be produced at high levels in plants [49]. While the benefits of biologics production in plants include the ability to produce large quantities of material with relatively low cost starting materials, there are logistical challenges in housing and transfecting plants on a large-scale under conditions that meet GMP requirements as well as development of downstream purification processes to recover VLPs from fibrous plant material [50]. Of note is that significant improvements have been made in plant cell culture for expression of pharmaceutical products (conducted in bioreactors), which has the potential to alleviate some of these challenges and increase the feasibility of using plant VLPs platforms for large-scale vaccine production [50, 51]. Malaria vaccine research efforts have included development of a AlMV VLP containing Pfs25 by Fraunhofer USA Center for Molecular Biotechnology [52], which has been tested in a phase I clinical trial (ClinicalTrials.gov Identifier: NCT02013687); however, results of the trial have not yet been published.

1.3. Polymeric nanoparticle delivery platforms

Polymeric nanoparticles share many of the immunological advantages of VLPs in that their size and structure are similar to that of a pathogen, which leads to interaction with antigen presenting cells [53]. An additional attribute of polymeric nanoparticles is that these can be tailored to a specific purpose through adjusting physical attributes such as size, shape, and charge as well as customizing the type and concentration of polymer [54]. A number of different nanoparticle-based vaccine delivery platforms are available, some of which have been used in the clinic and some of which have thus far only been assessed in animals. The main components of these platforms are biodegradable polymers/composites that function to create a depot for antigen presentation. Immunostimulators can also be incorporated into these delivery platforms. Antigens may be encapsulated or bounded by covalent or noncovalent bonds.

1.3.1. PLGA nanoparticle delivery platforms

Poly-DL-lactide-co-glycolide acid (PLGA) is a biodegradable polymer approved for human use by FDA for several indications. Published applications of PLGA nanoparticles in regards to malaria vaccine development include the targets Pfs25 and PvCSP [55, 56]. PLGA nanoparticle delivery platforms of interest for malaria vaccine development include Selecta Biosciences' synthetic vaccine particle (SVP™) platform and Orbis Biosciences Stratum™ platform. The SVP™ platform in combination with TLR7/8 and TLR9 agonists can enable robust cellular and humoral immune responses, and is flexible regarding how antigens are incorporated [57]. The Stratum™ technology is based on PLGA microspheres that encapsulate aqueous material (including antigens) and degrades in a controlled manner to permit delayed release of encapsulated material [58, 59]. For example, this platform can enable provision of both prime and booster antigen within a single administration with the booster contained in extended release microspheres that degrade 30 days after administration. Clinical studies have been conducted on PLGA-based platforms from both Selecta and Orbis.

1.3.2. Multilayer nanofilm-based nanoparticles

Artificial Cell Technologies, Inc. (ACT) has developed an innovative method for producing nanoparticle vaccines utilizing artificial biofilms comprised of oppositely charged polymers and target antigens constructed on solid $CaCO_3$ cores (nonimmunogenic carrier) using layer-by-layer (LbL) fabrication. This platform can accommodate multiple target antigens applied at different layers (depths) within the biofilms as well as immunostimulators, as needed for optimizing the immune response. Additionally, the biolayers can include innate immune stimulants to increase vaccine potency. Biofilm generation and LbL fabrication of nanoparticles have been previously described [60–62]. Of note is that experimental studies have shown that proteins/polypeptides are stabilized in nanofilms by noncovalent interactions, and secondary structure is maintained during the manufacturing process [62]. Additionally, disulfide bonds between cysteine-containing peptides increase nanofilm stability, mimicking the stabilization of the native protein structure [62]. Several ACT nanoparticle constructs, including different B and T cell epitopes of PfCSP, have been developed and tested in mice with encouraging results [63]. While this platform has not yet been assessed in the clinic, ACT is fast approaching intuition of a phase I study with this platform.

1.4. Microneedle platforms

Recent advances have increased interest in intradermal/transdermal vaccine delivery due to an improved understanding of the high immune response achievable within the skin, based on plasticity and high numbers of antigen-presenting cells (APCs) within this tissue, including Langerhans cells, dendritic cells, and macrophages [64–66]. Traditional intradermal vaccine delivery, using the Mantoux or skin scarification methods, requires special training to perform correctly and can be inaccurate regarding the dose of vaccine that is delivered or difficult to achieve based on volume limitations (skin scarification). Therefore, platforms that provide easy and accurate transdermal delivery of vaccines are of high interest [67, 68]. Microneedle arrays described herein are solid-state platforms that either integrate vaccine components into a biodegradable polymer, which is subsequently formed into an array, or are manufactured from nonbiodegradable materials into an array and then coated with vaccine components. In either case, size and length of the microneedle array is controlled so that temporary pores are created in the stratum corneum (the protective outer layer of the skin), and the vaccine is administered to the desired depth. In addition to the benefit of "needleless" administration, the depth at which microneedles penetrate does not reach underlying blood vessels or pain receptors. Stabilization of antigens and adjuvants on or within the microneedle array is also of benefit, particularly in regards to cold-chain requirements. One potential drawback of these platforms is that relatively high concentrations of antigen and adjuvant must be possible in order to achieve a relevant dosing range for most vaccines. Also of note is that development costs for microneedle platforms that incorporate antigens are higher than those where antigens are coated on the microarrays. In addition, consideration must be given to the administration device used to place the array regarding cost and ease of use. However, cost savings are achieved with these platforms because a needle and syringe is not required for administration.

Viral vectored ME-TRAP, PbCSP, and PyMSP-1 have been assessed with silicone microneedle arrays in mice where increased immune response to the target antigen (compared to the vector) and protective efficacy were found [69–71]. However, better responses were found using a mixed administration regimen where antigen(s) were first given via the microneedle platform and then boosted via the intradermal route. For these studies, antigen was applied to the skin just prior to application of the microarray rather than being incorporated into or coated on to the microneedle array itself.

1.4.1. Natural polymeric microneedles

Silk fibroin is a biocompatible, biodegradable block copolymer that self-assembles into β-sheets separated by flexible hydrophilic spacers. This natural polymer is approved by FDA for human use in medical devices such as wound dressings and sutures, and GMP grade silk fibroin is available from Vaxess Technologies. Significant progress has been made by Vaxess in developing a consistent, repeatable manufacturing process for silk fibroin microneedles [72]. Additionally, several protein immobilization strategies can be used with this polymer including adsorption, covalent bonding, entrapment, and encapsulation [73]. One attribute of this platform that is highly attractive for malaria vaccine development is that silk fibroin microneedles can be designed such that an initial bolus of vaccine is delivered upon administration followed by low-level sustained release of vaccine over a period of several weeks or longer [74]. Note that this microneedle platform has not yet been tested in the clinic.

1.4.2. Synthetic polymeric microneedles

Microneedle arrays can also be constructed from synthetic biodegradable polymeric materials such as PLGA. Corium International has a vaccine-in-tip platform where antigen and adjuvant are combined with MicroCor excipients and then the solution is cast into molds to create the microstructure array (MSA) [75]. A PLGA backing layer is applied and the patch integrated into an applicator. The MicroCor platform is designed such that the needles fully dissolve over a period of several minutes after which the backing is removed. Arrays can also be constructed from nonbiodegradable polymers, which are then coated with antigen and adjuvant. Such a platform is available from 3M's drug delivery systems division whereby arrays are molded from medical grade liquid crystalline polymer and substances (antigens, adjuvants, etc.) are coated on the microneedles using a dip coating process [76]. This type of array is designed to be left *in situ* for a short period of time and then removed once the coating has dissolved. Note that liquid crystalline polymer is not biodegradable. Microneedle platforms from both Corium and 3M have been tested in the clinic.

1.5. mRNA-based vaccine delivery platforms

Recent advances in mRNA vaccine delivery have elevated these platforms to the point at which feasibility of mRNA-based vaccines has been demonstrated in the clinic. The CureVac RNActive platform uses mRNA for vaccine delivery and relies on sequence modifications at the 5′ and 3′ ends to enhance protein expression and inclusion of a protamine sequence to increase immunogenicity [77]. An RNActive prostate cancer vaccine has been tested in the clinic with encouraging results regarding safety and immunogenicity, where induction of both Th1 and Th2 responses was seen [78]. There are significant advantages in using a nucleic acid-based platform including (1) the cost benefits of neither having to manufacture/purify antigen nor formulate with adjuvant, (2) the possibility for development of multivalent vaccines without concerns regarding formulation, and (3) quick manufacturing speeds where gene synthesis to completion of GMP production can take less than 2 months. A parallel mRNA-based delivery platform has been developed by Moderna; however, relatively limited information is available regarding Moderna's mRNA Therapeutics™ platform with the published studies relating to injection of mRNA into the heart (in a mouse model) to treat myocardial infarction [79, 80].

1.6. Densigen™ platform

The Densigen™ platform (available from Altimmune) is based on rationally designed long, fully synthetic peptides (30–40mers) containing natural clusters of CD4+ and CD8+ T cell epitopes (termed densigens). A proprietary bioinformatics approach is applied to select the most immunogenic and conserved domains. Densigens are conjugated to a fluorocarbon moiety, which allows the densigens to self-assemble into micelle-based nanoparticles. The self-adjuvanting properties of densigens are thought to be attributed to persistence of the nanoparticles at the administration site (depot effect) and resistance of the nanoparticles to proteolytic degradation [81]. Multiple densigens can be incorporated into a single formulation. A Phase I clinical study with a densigen-based influenza vaccine demonstrated good immunogenicity to all six peptides contained in the vaccine (across divergent influenza strains) [82]. In addition, a Phase 1 study of an HBV therapeutic densigen vaccine (HepTcell, which is composed of nine densigens) is ongoing (clinicaltrials.gov identifier: NCT02496897).

2. Enabling vaccine adjuvant platforms

Malaria vaccine enabling adjuvant platforms and immunostimulators are detailed in this section. Many of these can be combined with different immunogen formats and vaccine delivery platforms. We describe novel adjuvants as well as those where studies have been performed with malaria vaccine candidates. Also noted is if an adjuvant has been or can be combined with additional immunostimulators. Similar to the vaccine delivery platforms, we included state-of-the-art technologies where the regulatory and/or licensure pathways may not yet be defined.

2.1. Lipid vesicle-based platforms

Several different classes of lipids can be incorporated into vesicle-based vaccine adjuvant and delivery platforms. These include traditional liposomes (phospholipids as well as anionic, neutral, and cationic lipids from bacteria and eukaryotes), lipids derived from viral envelopes (virosomes), and lipids from Archaea (archaeosomes). The versatility and plasticity of lipid vesicle-based platforms are a major advantage as liposomal compositions can be customized to achieve desired characteristics including lipid type(s), charge, size, antigen association type, and inclusion of adjuvants and immunostimulators [83, 84]. Depending on the chemical properties of the liposomes, antigens may be entrapped in the aqueous core, intercalated into the lipid bilayer, and/or attached to the liposome surface by adsorption or conjugation. Additionally, different antigens/adjuvants can be combined to tailor liposomal vaccines for specific applications [85, 86]. In general, these systems provide adjuvant activity by enhancing antigen delivery to effector cells and/or by potentiating immune responses. Of note is that some of the platforms in this section can serve as both adjuvants as well as delivery platforms, depending on how antigen is incorporated. A comprehensive review of liposome vaccine delivery platforms is provided in [87].

2.1.1. Aqueous liposomal platforms

Several aqueous liposomal platforms have been built around the capabilities of cholesterol to stabilize lipid bilayers and QS-21 to create pores in lipid bilayers through association with cholesterol. In addition to these properties, QS-21 has also been shown to stimulate Th1-type responses and production of antigen-specific cytotoxic T lymphocytes (CTLs) [88]. The molecular stability of QS-21 is increased when incorporated into liposomes [86], as free molecules undergo deacylation above pH 6 and at temperatures problematic for vaccine administration in warm climates where cold-chain may not be maintained [88]. Aqueous liposomal formulations containing QS-21 provided in a format that can be directly mixed with antigen include AS01 from GSK (which also contains monophosphoryl lipid A – MPLA), GLA-LSQ developed by IDRI (which contains a synthetic form of MPLA known as GLA), ALF-Q developed by WRAIR (which contains MPLA), and Matrix-M from Novavax, previously known as AbISCO-100 (which is a unique 40-nm-sized complex and can be combined with immunostimulators such as TLR agonists [89]). These adjuvants are known to promote elicitation of both Th1 and Th2 immune responses [86, 90, 91]. One of the biggest drawbacks for several of these adjuvants is limited access/availability. However, GMP grade MPLA and QS-21 are available from Avanti Polar Lipids, Inc. and Agenus Inc., respectively. In addition, GMP grade lipids suitable for liposomal preparations are available from Avanti Polar Lipids.

Multiple clinical studies combining malaria vaccines/candidates (RTS,S, LSA-1, AMA-1, MSP-1, and CelTOS) with this class of adjuvants have been performed [16]. The different levels of protection seen with RTS,S/AS01 are well documented in the literature, and therefore not reviewed here. A high level of protective efficacy has not been found with any of the other malaria antigens combined with AS01, which has been recently reviewed in Ref. [16]. Preclinical studies have been conducted with full length PfCSP recombinant protein adjuvanted with GLA-LSQ where 40% sterile protection was seen upon challenge in a mouse malaria model [92]. This adjuvant has also been used in combination with PfCelTOS recombinant protein where a statistically significant reduction in liver load was found in challenged mice [93]. In addition, a clinical study with GLA-LSQ and the placental malaria vaccine candidate PAMVAC (VAR2CSA) has been registered on clinicaltrials.gov (identifier: NCT02647489); however, no published information is available. ALF-Q is a relative newcomer, and there are currently no published studies using ALF-Q in combination with malaria vaccine candidates. Matrix-M has been tested in preclinical studies with a variety of antigens including viral-vectored Pv Duffy binding protein (DBP) vaccine candidates. High levels of *in vitro* erythrocyte binding inhibition (>90%) were achieved with Matrix-M formulations in this study [94]. Additionally, Matrix-M has been assessed in a Phase I clinical study in combination with chimpanzee adenovirus 63

(ChAd63) ME-TRAP and MVA ME-TRAP (ClinicalTrials.gov identifier: NCT01669512); however, study results have not yet been published.

A platform related to Matrix-M and also comprised of lipids, cholesterol, and QS21 is immune stimulating complex (ISCOM) technology. ISCOMs are spherical open cage-like structures formed by cholesterol binding QS-21 and then stabilized with phospholipids [95]. Similar to Matrix-M, ISCOMs have a mean diameter of ~40 nm; however, this technology incorporates antigens into the ISCOM such that they are displayed in a multimeric fashion on the particles. ISCOMs are known to traffic antigen into the cytosol of dendritic cells, stimulate both Th1 and Th2 immune responses, and link innate and adaptive immune responses *in vivo* in a MyD88-dependent manner [96, 97]. The major drawback of this platform is that the type and amount of antigen displayed can be limiting; however, researchers have developed additional methods for incorporating antigen into ISCOMs, including using cationic ISCOMATRIX particles to attract anionic proteins, adding a lipid tail to the antigen, or using a fusion protein strategy to add hydrophobic peptide tags to the antigen [98]. Although modification of a vaccine candidate for inclusion in such a platform can add a layer of complexity and additional expense to the development process, ISCOMs might be of interest to adjuvant malaria immunogens containing a GPI-anchor. No studies with ISCOMs and GPI-anchored proteins were found in the literature. ISCOMs are commercially available from CSL Behring as ISCOMATRIX.

Another aqueous liposomal platform of potential interest is the adjuvant CAF01, developed by Statens Serum Institute. A clinical study conducted with this adjuvant demonstrated long-lived Th1 responses over a 3-year monitoring period (ClinicalTrials.gov identifier: NCT00922363) [99]. This adjuvant is comprised of two synthetic components, cationic liposomes and a glycolipid immunomodulator (synthetic mycobacterial cell wall cord factor). In a recent preclinical mouse study, five approved or clinically tested adjuvants (Alum, MF59®, GLA-SE, IC31®, and CAF01) were each combined with antigens from *M. tuberculosis*, influenza, and chlamydia and compared head-to-head [100]. Of the five adjuvants tested, CAF01 was the only adjuvant to elicit a Th1 immune response when formulated with each of the three antigens. In addition, the CAF01 formulation demonstrated the highest reduction of *M. tuberculosis* and *Chlamydia trachomatis* in challenge models. However, in most cases, the humoral response elicited was similar to the no adjuvant and/or alum formulations. Note that MF59®, GLA-SE, and IC31® are discussed in subsequent sections.

2.1.2. Lipid-in-oil platforms

The DepoVax™ platform, developed by ImmunoVaccine Inc., contains lipids, cholesterol, oil, emulsifier, and an immunostimulant (e.g., polyIC or Pam_3Cys) [101]. This unique lipid-in-oil platform is designed to present antigen(s) and adjuvant(s) at a long lasting depot that effectively attracts APCs and from which antigen is released over an extended period of time, from weeks to months [102]. Based on this long lasting depot, a single dose of vaccine formulated in DepoVax has been shown to be superior to multiple doses of the same vaccine formulated in traditional adjuvants [103, 104]. In addition, DepoVax has been shown to not only promote Th2 responses, but also enhance Th1 immune responses without triggering regulatory T cell [101]. DepoVax has been used in the clinic as part of a Phase I/II study for a cancer vaccine (ClinicalTrials.gov identifier: NCT01095848) [105]. Of note is that there are no aqueous components in this formulation; therefore, antigen is lyophilized for use with DepoVax and components are mixed and emulsified prior to administration using materials provided as part of an administration kit.

2.1.3. *Virosomes*

Virosomes are liposomes prepared by reconstituting virus envelope phospholipids. Those from influenza virus are the most common with the virosome physicochemical properties modulated by the amount and type of lipids used [106]. In contrast to liposomes, virosomes can contain functional viral glycoproteins (i.e., influenza virus hemagglutinin and neuraminidase) within the phospholipid bilayer membrane, which enhance immunogenicity. Additionally, virosomes can induce both B and T cell responses through antigen presentation in the context of both MHC-I and MHC-II [87, 106, 107]. Antigen can be encapsulated within the virosomes, conjugated to phospholipids, or adsorbed to the virosome surface [108]. Malaria antigens have been incorporated into influenza virosomes including epitopes from AMA-1, CSP, MSP-3, and GLURP [109–111]. Clinical studies were performed with virosomes containing an AMA-1 peptide from domain 3 (PEV301) and a CSP repeat region peptide constituting constrained NPNA units (PEV302). In a Phase 1a trial, volunteers immunized with PEV301, PEV302, or a combination of the two (PEV301 + PEV 302) had good seroconversion and long-lived humoral responses when assessed at a 1-year follow-up [112–114]. A Phase 1b trial was conducted in a malaria-endemic area where adults and children were immunized with PEV3B (a formulation including both the subject AMA-1 and CSP epitopes) or a comparator virosome-based vaccine to influenza, Inflexal®V [115]. While not statistically significant, the malaria incidence rate in children administered PEV3B was lower than children given Inflexal®V (67% versus 80%, respectively) over the 1-year follow-up period.

2.1.4. *Archaeosomes*

Species of the domain *Archaea* contain unique polar lipids that have adjuvanting properties when used as liposomes (archaeosomes) containing encapsulated antigens. The lipid backbones found in *Archaea* have a higher resistance to acid hydrolysis compared to those from *Eukarya* and *Bacteria*, and surface tension and permeability characteristics of archaeosomes differ in comparison to traditional liposomes; these properties are also thought to increase adjuvanting potential of archaeosomes [116]. The type of immune response generated with archaeosomes can be manipulated by changing composition of the head groups attached to archaeol, and lipids from some *Archaea* have been used to chemically synthesize additional lipid types with interesting characteristics [117, 118]. Several studies with archaeosomes and encapsulated ovalbumin (for cancer applications) have shown elicitation of both Th1 and Th2 immune responses as well as the ability to modulate the immune response by varying the types of polar lipids within the archaeosomes [117–119]. As this is a relatively new platform, a pathway to regulatory approval for clinical testing and licensure is needed.

2.2. Polymeric microparticle-based adjuvants

Advax^{TM} (developed by Vaxine) is a microparticle-based adjuvant comprised of microcrystalline delta inulin, a plant-derived polysaccharide. Of note is that delta inulin is insoluble at body temperature. This adjuvant generates Th1 and Th2 immune responses and activates the alternative compliment pathway [120]. However, Advax^{TM} does not activate nuclear factor-kappa B (NFkB) so an inflammatory response is not seen with this adjuvant [121]. Given the mounting data regarding the ability of malaria to hinder development of effective immune responses, adjuvants that do not trigger inflammatory responses are of interest, particularly for use in malaria-endemic regions. Although there are no published studies with Advax^{TM} and malaria antigens, preclinical assessments have been conducted with a variety vaccine candidates formulated in this adjuvant [121]. In addition, this adjuvant has been assessed in multiple clinical studies [122, 123].

2.3. Emulsion-based adjuvants

All of the adjuvants described in this section are oil-in-water emulsions. Those that include solvents and surfactants form nanoemulsions, which facilitate antigen uptake by dendritic cells [124]. Formulation of malaria vaccines with emulsion-based adjuvants is of interest in part because there are examples of a high level of sterile protection in clinical studies with CHMI challenge when RTS,S was combined with an oil-in-water emulsion-based adjuvant [125, 126]. The GSK adjuvants AS02 and AS03 are both oil-in-water emulsions. AS03 contains squalene, vitamin E, and Tween 80, while AS02 contains these components plus MPLA and QS21. In a clinical study with CHMI where RTS,S was combined with either AS02 or AS03, sterile protection was seen in 6/7 (86%) volunteers given RTS,S/AS02, and 2/7 (29%) volunteers given RTS,S/AS03 [126]. However, 6 months after the last vaccination only 1/5 (20%) of the volunteers given RTS,S/AS02 showed sterile protection upon a second CHMI [125]. For these volunteers, the factors contributing to loss of protective efficacy in such a short period of time is unclear but may relate to challenge and the ability of malaria parasites to compromise development of long-term immunity. In light of these and similar results, improvements in sustaining established immunity must be made regarding development of an effective malaria vaccine.

2.3.1. MF59

MF59 is an oil-in-water nanoemulsion that consists of squalene oil, Tween 80, and sorbitan trioleate (Span 85). MF59 (available from Novartis) is licensed in Europe as a clinical vaccine adjuvant for influenza and has been intramuscularly administered to millions of people ranging in age from children to elderly adults. This adjuvant has been assessed in animal studies with MSP-1 and PvDBP malaria antigens; however, immunogenicity and binding assay (PvDBP) results were poor in comparison to other adjuvants [127–129]. While these results were discouraging, using MF59 in combination with small molecule immunostimulators, particularly those known to induce a Th1 response such as CpG (which has been previously used MF59 with encouraging results [130]), may improve efficacy with malaria antigens. In a recent study, five approved or clinically tested adjuvants

(Alum, MF59®, GLA-SE, IC31®, and CAF01) were each combined with antigens from *M. tuberculosis*, influenza, and chlamydia and compared in head-to-head mouse studies [100]. Of the five adjuvants tested, only MF59 and GLA-SE were able to induce inhibitory titers to influenza; however, inhibitory titers with MF59 were >60% higher than with GLA-SE. Note that MF59 formulations did not induce a Th1 immune response for any of the antigens.

2.3.2. NanoStat™ platform

NanoStat™ (available from NanoBio Corporation) is an oil-in-water nanoemulsion composed of soybean oil, ethanol, Tween 80, cetylpyridinium chloride, and water. Note that these components are quite inexpensive as compared to those of some of the other adjuvants described herein. The adjuvant activity of this nanoemulsion is dependent on the nanodroplet structure and positive charge, which enables the penetration of the mucous layer, binding to cell membranes, and cellular uptake [124, 131]. In mice, NanoStat™ has been shown to produce systemic and mucosal immune responses including MyD88-independent Ab responses and MyD88-dependent Th-1 and Th-17 cell-mediated responses [132]. While most of the published research (including a Phase I clinical [133]) is with NanoStat™ formulated for intranasal delivery, a formulation that contains the same components in proportions tailored for intramuscular administration is also available. These adjuvants can be combined with small molecule immunostimulators. Currently, there are no published studies of NanoStat™ used in combination with malaria antigens.

2.3.3. GLA-SE

GLA-SE (developed by IDRI) is an oil-in-water emulsion containing squalene and glucopyranosyl lipid A (GLA), a synthetic Toll-like receptor 4 (TLR4) agonist that is similar to MPLA. This adjuvant is known to generate both Th1 and Th2 immune responses. Multiple clinical studies have been conducted with GLA-SE formulated vaccines [134–136] including several with malaria antigens; however, results from the latter have not yet been published. Preclinical studies with GLA-SE have been conducted with a number of malaria vaccine candidates. As an example, in a study conducted with a full length PfCSP recombinant protein (produced by Pfenex) adjuvanted with GLA-SE, 50% sterile protection was seen upon challenge in a mouse malaria model (Pb/PfCSP repeats and C-terminal region replacement) [92]. With a different full length PfCSP recombinant protein (produced by WRAIR), 60% protection was seen upon challenge in a different mouse malaria model (Pb/PfCSP full-length replacement) [137]. This adjuvant has also been used in combination with PfCelTOS recombinant protein in preclinical studies, where a statistically significant reduction in liver load was found in challenged mice [93]. A clinical study with PfCelTOS formulated in GLA-SE has been conducted, but data have not yet been published (ClinicalTrials.gov identifier: NCT01540474). Additionally, in a preclinical study with PvRII (region II of PvDBP) where moderate levels of in vitro erythrocyte binding inhibition (>50%) was achieved with GLA-SE, slightly higher levels (>60%) were seen when GLA-SE was combined with the TLR 7/8 agonist R848 [138].

In a recent study, five approved or clinically tested adjuvants (Alum, MF59®, GLA-SE, IC31®, and CAF01) were each combined with antigens from *M. tuberculosis*, influenza, and chlamydia and compared in head-to-head mouse studies [100]. Of the five adjuvants tested, only GLA-SE demonstrated statistically significant inhibition in all three challenge models. However, it was not the best performer in any of the models.

2.3.4. Nutritive immune-enhancing delivery system (NIDS)

NIDS (developed by Epitogenesis, Inc.) is an oil-in-water nanoemulsion containing vitamin A, a polyphenol-flavonoid, catechin hydrate, Tween 80, and mustard oil that were originally developed to boost mucosal immune responses to a variety of antigens without triggering inflammatory responses [139]. All the adjuvant components are generally regarded as safe (GRAS) by the FDA and are available at GMP-grade. Note that these components are quite inexpensive as compared to those of some of the other adjuvants described herein. The NIDS platform allows modification of the NIDS components toward more Th1 or Th2 responses [140]. In addition, this adjuvant can be administered systemically (e.g., IM injection) or delivered via a mucosal route. Although this adjuvant has not yet be assessed in the clinic and no preclinical studies have been published that use NIDS in combination with malaria antigens, it is worth consideration regarding both its low cost and ability to adjuvant in the absence of triggering an inflammatory response.

2.4. Small molecule adjuvants and immunostimulants

Several small molecule-based adjuvants and immunostimulators relevant to malaria vaccine development are described herein. Note that although a number of TLR agonists have been used in preclinical (and in some cases clinical) assessments of malaria vaccine candidates, these have been thoroughly reviewed elsewhere [141, 142]. Such TLR agonists include MPLA/GLA (TLR4 agonists), CpG oligodeoxynucleotides (ssDNA containing cytosines and guanines, which are TLR9 agonists), Poly:IC (dsRNA, which is a TLR3 agonist), Pam3Cys (lipopeptide and TLR1/2 agonist), as well as imiquimod and resiquimod (TLR 7/8 agonists), none of which are detailed herein.

2.4.1. IC31® adjuvant platform

IC31® (developed by Valneva) is a two-component adjuvant comprised of a polycationic peptide (poly-L-arginine) and ODN1a (a TLR9 agonist). Activity of this adjuvant includes recruitment of MHC class II at the injection site as well as migration of antigen to the draining lymph node [26]. The poly-L-arginine contributes to development of humoral and Th2 immune responses [143], while ODN1a is a single-stranded DNA oligonucleotide that stimulates Th1 responses [144]. No studies of malaria vaccine candidates formulated IC31® have been published. In a recent study, five approved or clinically tested adjuvants (Alum, MF59®, GLA-SE, IC31®, and CAF01) were each combined with antigens from *M. tuberculosis*, influenza, and chlamydia and compared in head-to-head mouse studies [100]. Of the five adjuvants tested, IC31® elicited Th1 and Th2 immune responses and demonstrated a statistically significant reduction (but not the biggest reduction) of *M. tuberculosis* and *C. trachomatis* in challenge models. This adjuvant has been assessed in the clinic [145–149].

2.4.2. 7DW8-5

7DW8-5 (developed by ADARC) is a glycolipid α-galactosylceramide (α-GalCer) analog identified as part of structure-activity relationship (SAR) screening of α-GalCer analogs for increased adjuvant activity as compared to the parent molecule [150]. 7DW8-5 induces Th1 immune responses by binding CD1d (nonclassical MHC proteins expressed on APCs that present lipid antigens), stimulating natural killer cells, and inducing dendritic cell activation/ maturation as well as dendritic cell trafficking to the draining lymph node [150, 151]. This adjuvant has been assessed in preclinical studies with several malaria vaccine candidates including CSP, AMA-1, and irradiated sporozoites [151–153]. In formulations with 7DW8-5, enhanced Th1 responses were found as well significantly reduced liver load [153] and a high level of sterile protection (90%) upon challenge [151].

2.4.3. Saponins (QS-21)

Saponins (particularly QS-21), which can be extracted from the bark the *Quillaja saponaria* Molina tree or be semisynthetic, are of interest because they have been shown to stimulate Th1-type responses and production of antigen-specific cytotoxic T lymphocytes (CTLs) [88]. However, a major concern regarding use of QS-21 in malaria vaccines is instability at pH above six and at elevated temperatures [88]. While it is possible to stabilize QS-21 (e.g., in lipids with cholesterol), this small molecule is not recommended for malaria vaccines formulations (intended for use in endemic regions) without assessments of stability at elevated temperatures in the selected formulation.

3. Conclusions

In recent years, there has been a proliferation of novel and promising adjuvant and vaccine delivery systems that together cast a wide net over the effector targets offered by our current understanding of immune system's pathways. Accordingly, this review surveys the field of vaccine delivery platforms and adjuvants in the context of their potential utility for improving the sterile or protective immunity conferred by malaria vaccine candidates. These technologies have the potential to positively affect the induction of immune response elicited by a vaccine candidate through more effective antigen delivery and presentation, ability to present multiple epitopes/copies of epitopes, and mobilizing different components of the immune system appropriate to the antigen and the malarial life-cycle stage being targeted.

Indeed, the judicious selection of vaccine delivery platforms and adjuvants is a necessary part of the malaria vaccine development process. For example, RTS,S was tested with a range of different adjuvants in both preclinical and clinical studies prior to section of AS01 for the commercial formulation. Additionally, while many other malaria vaccine targets have since been tested with AS01, none of these has achieved the same level of protective efficacy seen with RTS,S/AS01 [16]. These data demonstrate the necessity of evaluating malaria vaccine targets with a range of delivery platforms and adjuvants prior to selection of the platform(s)/adjuvant(s) for clinical testing. In addition, testing multiple formulations will likely be necessary to sufficiently evaluate efficacy. In endemic regions, this process is compounded by the parasite's ability to hamper development of effective, long-lived immune responses as the intersection of vaccination and infection varies greatly depending on the level of malaria transmission. Several strategies for addressing these complications have been presented including, (1) platforms capable of sustained antigen release, (2) adjuvants that function without triggering inflammatory immune responses, and (3) use of blockage inhibitors to reduce T cell exhaustion.

Additional considerations include affordability and cold-chain requirements. As the principal target populations for vaccination against malaria are individuals residing in endemic regions, primarily Africa and other developing countries, an effective vaccine must be relatively inexpensive to manufacture, store, and deliver. Several of the enabling technologies presented are relatively inexpensive. Additionally, some have the potential to stabilize the vaccine formulation for room temperature storage and transport. However, accessibility is problematic for several of these technologies, and there is a significant cost component regarding the development process, particularly for the vaccine delivery platforms. Due to the complex nature of malaria vaccine development, it is clear that a team approach capable of tapping into expertise in the commercial, academic, government, and nonprofit sectors to efficiently assemble the right combination of vaccine development and delivery technologies is critical to success of malaria vaccine development strategies.

Acknowledgements

This publication was made possible through support provided by the Office of Health, Infectious Diseases, and Nutrition; Bureau for Global Health, U.S. Agency for International Development, under the terms of the Malaria Vaccine Development Program (MVDP) Contract AID-OAA-C-15-00071, for which Leidos, Inc. is the prime contractor. The opinions expressed herein are those of the author(s) and do not necessarily reflect the views of the U.S. Agency for International Development. The authors would like to thank Carter Diggs and Lorraine Soisson for helpful discussions regarding the adjuvants and vaccine delivery platforms described herein.

Author details

Amy R. Noe, Vinayaka Kotraiah and Gabriel M. Gutierrez*

*Address all correspondence to: gabriel.m.gutierrez@leidos.com

Leidos Life Sciences, Leidos Inc., Frederick, MD, USA

References

[1] Malaria Vaccine Funders Group. Malaria Vaccine Technology Roadmap. 2006. Available from: http://www.who.int/immunization/sage/meetings/2013/april/7_Malaria_Vaccine_TRM_Final.pdf. [Accessed: 2016-05-10]

[2] Malaria Vaccine Funders Group. Malaria Vaccine Technology Roadmap. 2013. Available from: http://www.who.int/immunization/topics/malaria/vaccine_roadmap/TRM_update_nov13.pdf?ua=1. [Accessed: 2016-05-10]

[3] Callendret B, Eccleston HB, Satterfield W, Capone S, Folgori A, Cortese R, et al. Persistent hepatitis C viral replication despite priming of functional CD8(+) T cells by combined therapy with a vaccine and a direct-acting antiviral. Hepatology. 2016;63:1442–54. DOI: 10.1002/hep.28309

[4] Rodrigues V, Cordeiro-da-Silva A, Laforge M, Silvestre R, Estaquier J. Regulation of immunity during visceral leishmania infection. Parasit Vectors. 2016;9:118. DOI: 10.1186/s13071-016-1412-x

[5] Wherry EJ, Kurachi M. Molecular and cellular insights into T cell exhaustion. Nat Rev Immunol. 2015;15:486–99. DOI: 10.1038/nri3862

[6] Ryg-Cornejo V, Ioannidis LJ, Ly A, Chiu CY, Tellier J, Hill DL, et al. Severe malaria infections impair germinal center responses by inhibiting T follicular helper cell differentiation. Cell Rep. 2016;14:68–81. DOI: 10.1016/j.celrep.2015.12.006

[7] Horne-Debets JM, Faleiro R, Karunarathne DS, Liu XQ, Lineburg KE, Poh CM, et al. PD-1 dependent exhaustion of CD8+ T cells drives chronic malaria. Cell Rep. 2013;5:1204–13. DOI: 10.1016/j.celrep.2013.11.002

[8] Wykes MN, Horne-Debets JM, Leow CY, Karunarathne DS. Malaria drives T cells to exhaustion. Front Microbiol. 2014;5:249. DOI: 10.3389/fmicb.2014.00249

[9] Yi JS, Cox MA, Zajac AJ. T-cell exhaustion: characteristics, causes and conversion. Immunology. 2010;129:474–81. DOI: 10.1111/j.1365-2567.2010.03255.x

[10] Kano Y, Iguchi T, Matsui H, Adachi K, Sakoda Y, Miyakawa T, et al. Combined adjuvants of poly(I:C) plus LAG-3-Ig improve antitumor effects of tumor-specific T cells, preventing their exhaustion. Cancer Sci. 2016;107:398–406. DOI: 10.1111/cas.12861

[11] Nagato T, Lee YR, Harabuchi Y, Celis E. Combinatorial immunotherapy of polyinosinic-polycytidylic acid and blockade of programmed death-ligand 1 induce effective CD8 T-cell responses against established tumors. Clin Cancer Res. 2014;20:1223–34. DOI: 10.1158/1078-0432.ccr-13-2781

[12] Pulko V, Liu X, Krco CJ, Harris KJ, Frigola X, Kwon ED, et al. TLR3-stimulated dendritic cells up-regulate B7-H1 expression and influence the magnitude of CD8 T cell responses to tumor vaccination. J Immunol. 2009;183:3634–41. DOI: 10.4049/jimmunol.0900974

[13] Capone S, D'Alise AM, Ammendola V, Colloca S, Cortese R, Nicosia A, et al. Development of chimpanzee adenoviruses as vaccine vectors: challenges and successes emerging from clinical trials. Expert Rev Vaccines. 2013;12:379–93. DOI: 10.1586/erv.13.15

[14] Gilbert SC. Clinical development of modified vaccinia virus Ankara vaccines. Vaccine. 2013;31:4241–6. DOI: 10.1016/j.vaccine.2013.03.020

[15] Schuldt NJ, Amalfitano A. Malaria vaccines: focus on adenovirus based vectors. Vaccine. 2012;30:5191–8. DOI: 10.1016/j.vaccine.2012.05.048

[16] Wu Y, Narum DL, Fleury S, Jennings G, Yadava A. Particle-based platforms for malaria vaccines. Vaccine. 2015;33:7518–24. DOI: 10.1016/j.vaccine.2015.09.097

[17] Pushko P, Pumpens P, Grens E. Development of virus-like particle technology from small highly symmetric to large complex virus-like particle structures. Intervirology. 2013;56:141–65. DOI: 10.1159/000346773

[18] Chackerian B. Virus-like particles: flexible platforms for vaccine development. Expert Rev Vaccines. 2007;6:381–90. DOI: 10.1586/14760584.6.3.381

[19] Deml L, Speth C, Dierich MP, Wolf H, Wagner R. Recombinant HIV-1 Pr55gag virus-like particles: potent stimulators of innate and acquired immune responses. Mol Immunol. 2005;42:259–77. DOI: 10.1016/j.molimm.2004.06.028

[20] Grgacic EV, Anderson DA. Virus-like particles: passport to immune recognition. Methods. 2006;40:60–5. DOI: 10.1016/j.ymeth.2006.07.018

[21] Murata K, Lechmann M, Qiao M, Gunji T, Alter HJ, Liang TJ. Immunization with hepatitis C virus-like particles protects mice from recombinant hepatitis C virus-vaccinia infection. Proc Natl Acad Sci U S A. 2003;100:6753–8. DOI: 10.1073/pnas.1131929100

[22] Paliard X, Liu Y, Wagner R, Wolf H, Baenziger J, Walker CM. Priming of strong, broad, and long-lived HIV type 1 p55gag-specific CD8+ cytotoxic T cells after administration of a virus-like particle vaccine in rhesus macaques. AIDS Res Hum Retroviruses. 2000;16:273–82. DOI: 10.1089/088922200309368

[23] Schirmbeck R, Bohm W, Reimann J. Virus-like particles induce MHC class I-restricted T-cell responses. Lessons learned from the hepatitis B small surface antigen. Intervirology. 1996;39:111–9.

[24] Win SJ, Ward VK, Dunbar PR, Young SL, Baird MA. Cross-presentation of epitopes on virus-like particles via the MHC I receptor recycling pathway. Immunol Cell Biol. 2011;89:681–8. DOI: 10.1038/icb.2010.161

[25] Heil F, Hemmi H, Hochrein H, Ampenberger F, Kirschning C, Akira S, et al. Species-specific recognition of single-stranded RNA via toll-like receptor 7 and 8. Science. 2004;303:1526–9. DOI: 10.1126/science.1093620

[26] Levast B, Awate S, Babiuk L, Mutwiri G, Gerdts V, van Drunen Littel-van den Hurk S. Vaccine potentiation by combination adjuvants. Vaccines (Basel). 2014;2:297–322. DOI: 10.3390/vaccines2020297

[27] Nardin EH, Oliveira GA, Calvo-Calle JM, Wetzel K, Maier C, Birkett AJ, et al. Phase I testing of a malaria vaccine composed of hepatitis B virus core particles expressing *Plasmodium falciparum* circumsporozoite epitopes. Infect Immun. 2004;72:6519–27. DOI: 10.1128/IAI.72.11.6519-6527.2004

[28] Oliveira GA, Wetzel K, Calvo-Calle JM, Nussenzweig R, Schmidt A, Birkett A, et al. Safety and enhanced immunogenicity of a hepatitis B core particle *Plasmodium falciparum* malaria vaccine formulated in adjuvant Montanide ISA 720 in a phase I trial. Infect Immun. 2005;73:3587–97. DOI: 10.1128/IAI.73.6.3587-3597.2005

[29] Walther M, Dunachie S, Keating S, Vuola JM, Berthoud T, Schmidt A, et al. Safety, immunogenicity and efficacy of a pre-erythrocytic malaria candidate vaccine, ICC-1132 formulated in Seppic ISA 720. Vaccine. 2005;23:857–64. DOI: 10.1016/j.vaccine.2004.08.020

[30] Gregson AL, Oliveira G, Othoro C, Calvo-Calle JM, Thorton GB, Nardin E, et al. Phase I trial of an alhydrogel adjuvanted hepatitis B core virus-like particle containing epitopes of *Plasmodium falciparum* circumsporozoite protein. PLoS One. 2008;3:e1556. DOI: 10.1371/journal.pone.0001556

[31] Hoofnagle JH, Gerety RJ, Barker LF. Antibody to hepatitis-B-virus core in man. Lancet. 1973;2:869–73.

[32] Milich DR, McLachlan A, Thornton GB, Hughes JL. Antibody production to the nucleocapsid and envelope of the hepatitis B virus primed by a single synthetic T cell site. Nature. 1987;329:547–9. DOI: 10.1038/329547a0

[33] Pumpens P, Grens E. Hepatitis B core particles as a universal display model: a structure-function basis for development. FEBS Lett. 1999;442:1–6.

[34] Whitacre DC, Lee BO, Milich DR. Use of hepadnavirus core proteins as vaccine platforms. Expert Rev Vaccines. 2009;8:1565–73. DOI: 10.1586/erv.09.121

[35] Billaud JN, Peterson D, Lee BO, Maruyama T, Chen A, Sallberg M, et al. Advantages to the use of rodent hepadnavirus core proteins as vaccine platforms. Vaccine. 2007;25:1593–606. DOI: 10.1016/j.vaccine.2006.11.013

[36] Billaud JN, Peterson D, Schodel F, Chen A, Sallberg M, Garduno F, et al. Comparative antigenicity and immunogenicity of hepadnavirus core proteins. J Virol. 2005;79:13641–55. DOI: 10.1128/JVI.79.21.13641-13655.2005

[37] Paoletti LC, Peterson DL, Legmann R, Collier RJ. Preclinical evaluation of group B streptococcal polysaccharide conjugate vaccines prepared with a modified diphtheria toxin and a recombinant duck hepatitis B core antigen. Vaccine. 2001;20:370–6.

[38] Whitacre DC, Espinosa DA, Peters CJ, Jones JE, Tucker AE, Peterson DL, et al. P. falciparum and P. vivax epitope-focused VLPs elicit sterile jmmunity to blood stage infections. PLoS One. 2015;10:e0124856. DOI: 10.1371/journal.pone.0124856

[39] Billaud JN, Peterson D, Barr M, Chen A, Sallberg M, Garduno F, et al. Combinatorial approach to hepadnavirus-like particle vaccine design. J Virol. 2005;79:13656–66. DOI: 10.1128/JVI.79.21.13656-13666.2005

[40] Peabody DS, Manifold-Wheeler B, Medford A, Jordan SK, do Carmo Caldeira J, Chackerian B. Immunogenic display of diverse peptides on virus-like particles of RNA phage MS2. J Mol Biol. 2008;380:252–63. DOI: 10.1016/j.jmb.2008.04.049

[41] Tumban E, Peabody J, Tyler M, Peabody DS, Chackerian B. VLPs displaying a single L2 epitope induce broadly cross-neutralizing antibodies against human papillomavirus. PLoS One. 2012;7:e49751. DOI: 10.1371/journal.pone.0049751

[42] Ord RL, Caldeira JC, Rodriguez M, Noe A, Chackerian B, Peabody DS, et al. A malaria vaccine candidate based on an epitope of the *Plasmodium falciparum* RH5 protein. Malar J. 2014;13:326. DOI: 10.1186/1475-2875-13-326

[43] Crossey E, Frietze K, Narum DL, Peabody DS, Chackerian B. Identification of an immunogenic mimic of a conserved epitope on the *Plasmodium falciparum* blood stage antigen AMA1 using virus-like particle (VLP) peptide display. PLoS One. 2015;10:e0132560. DOI: 10.1371/journal.pone.0132560 [doi] PONE-D-15-07386 [pii]

[44] Ashley CE, Carnes EC, Phillips GK, Durfee PN, Buley MD, Lino CA, et al. Cell-specific delivery of diverse cargos by bacteriophage MS2 virus-like particles. ACS Nano. 2011;5:5729–45. DOI: 10.1021/nn201397z

[45] Spohn G, Jennings GT, Martina BE, Keller I, Beck M, Pumpens P, et al. A VLP-based vaccine targeting domain III of the West Nile virus E protein protects from lethal infection in mice. Virol J. 2010;7:146. DOI: 10.1186/1743-422X-7-146

[46] Tissot AC, Renhofa R, Schmitz N, Cielens I, Meijerink E, Ose V, et al. Versatile virus-like particle carrier for epitope based vaccines. PLoS One. 2010;5:e9809. DOI: 10.1371/journal.pone.0009809

[47] Brune KD, Leneghan DB, Brian IJ, Ishizuka AS, Bachmann MF, Draper SJ, et al. Plug-and-display: decoration of virus-like particles via isopeptide bonds for modular immunization. Sci Rep. 2016;6:19234. DOI: 10.1038/srep19234

[48] Thrane S, Janitzek CM, Matondo S, Resende M, Gustavsson T, de Jongh WA, et al. Bacterial superglue enables easy development of efficient virus-like particle based vaccines. J Nanobiotechnol. 2016;14:30. DOI: 10.1186/s12951-016-0181-1

[49] Chen Q, Lai H. Plant-derived virus-like particles as vaccines. Hum Vaccin Immunother. 2013;9:26–49. DOI: 10.4161/hv.22218

[50] Yao J, Weng Y, Dickey A, Wang KY. Plants as factories for human pharmaceuticals: applications and challenges. Int J Mol Sci. 2015;16:28549–65. DOI: 10.3390/ijms161226122

[51] Tekoah Y, Shulman A, Kizhner T, Ruderfer I, Fux L, Nataf Y, et al. Large-scale production of pharmaceutical proteins in plant cell culture-the protalix experience. Plant Biotechnol J. 2015;13:1199–208. DOI: 10.1111/pbi.12428

[52] Jones RM, Chichester JA, Mett V, Jaje J, Tottey S, Manceva S, et al. A plant-produced Pfs25 VLP malaria vaccine candidate induces persistent transmission blocking antibodies against *Plasmodium falciparum* in immunized mice. PLoS One. 2013;8:e79538. DOI: 10.1371/journal.pone.0079538

[53] Yue H, Ma G. Polymeric micro/nanoparticles: particle design and potential vaccine delivery applications. Vaccine. 2015;33:5927–36. DOI: 10.1016/j.vaccine.2015.07.100

[54] Vartak A, Sucheck SJ. Recent advances in subunit vaccine carriers. Vaccines (Basel). 2016;4. DOI: 10.3390/vaccines4020012

[55] Kumar R, Ledet G, Graves R, Datta D, Robinson S, Bansal GP, et al. Potent functional immunogenicity of Plasmodium falciparum transmission-blocking antigen (Pfs25) delivered with nanoemulsion and porous polymeric nanoparticles. Pharm Res. 2015;32:3827–36. DOI: 10.1007/s11095-015-1743-x

[56] Moon JJ, Suh H, Polhemus ME, Ockenhouse CF, Yadava A, Irvine DJ. Antigen-displaying lipid-enveloped PLGA nanoparticles as delivery agents for a *Plasmodium vivax* malaria vaccine. PLoS One. 2012;7:e31472. DOI: 10.1371/journal.pone.0031472

[57] Ilyinskii PO, Roy CJ, O'Neil CP, Browning EA, Pittet LA, Altreuter DH, et al. Adjuvant-carrying synthetic vaccine particles augment the immune response to encapsulated antigen and exhibit strong local immune activation without inducing systemic cytokine release. Vaccine. 2014;32:2882–95. DOI: 10.1016/j.vaccine.2014.02.027

[58] Berkland C, Pollauf E, Pack DW, Kim K. Uniform double-walled polymer microspheres of controllable shell thickness. J Control Release. 2004;96:101–11. DOI: 10.1016/j.jconrel.2004.01.018

[59] Berkland C, Pollauf E, Varde N, Pack DW, Kim KK. Monodisperse liquid-filled biodegradable microcapsules. Pharm Res. 2007;24:1007–13. DOI: 10.1007/s11095-006-9197-9

[60] Powell TJ, Palath N, DeRome ME, Tang J, Jacobs A, Boyd JG. Synthetic nanoparticle vaccines produced by layer-by-layer assembly of artificial biofilms induce potent protective T-cell and antibody responses in vivo. Vaccine. 2011;29:558–69. DOI: 10.1016/j.vaccine.2010.10.001

[61] Zhang L, Haynie DT. Reversibility of structural changes of polypeptides in multilayer nanofilms. Biomacromolecules. 2008;9:185–91. DOI: 10.1021/bm700967k

[62] Zhang L, Zhao W, Rudra JS, Haynie DT. Context dependence of the assembly, structure, and stability of polypeptide multilayer nanofilms. ACS Nano. 2007;1:476–86. DOI: 10.1021/nn700267g

[63] Powell TJ, Tang J, Derome ME, Mitchell RA, Jacobs A, Deng Y, et al. *Plasmodium falciparum* synthetic LbL microparticle vaccine elicits protective neutralizing antibody and parasite-specific cellular immune responses. Vaccine. 2013;31:1898–904. DOI: 10.1016/j.vaccine.2013.02.027

[64] Combadiere B, Liard C. Transcutaneous and intradermal vaccination. Hum Vaccin. 2011;7:811–27. DOI: 10.4161/hv.7.8.16274

[65] Nicolas JF, Guy B. Intradermal, epidermal and transcutaneous vaccination: from immunology to clinical practice. Expert Rev Vaccines. 2008;7:1201–14. DOI: 10.1586/14760584.7.8.1201

[66] Hegde NR, Kaveri SV, Bayry J. Recent advances in the administration of vaccines for infectious diseases: microneedles as painless delivery devices for mass vaccination. Drug Discov Today. 2011;16:1061–8. DOI: 10.1016/j.drudis.2011.07.004

[67] Marshall S, Sahm LJ, Moore AC. Microneedle technology for immunisation: perception, acceptability and suitability for paediatric use. Vaccine. 2016;34:723–34. DOI: 10.1016/j.vaccine.2015.12.002

[68] Suh H, Shin J, Kim YC. Microneedle patches for vaccine delivery. Clin Exp Vaccine Res. 2014;3:42–9. DOI: 10.7774/cevr.2014.3.1.42

[69] Carey JB, Pearson FE, Vrdoljak A, McGrath MG, Crean AM, Walsh PT, et al. Microneedle array design determines the induction of protective memory CD8+ T cell responses induced by a recombinant live malaria vaccine in mice. PLoS One. 2011;6:e22442. DOI: 10.1371/journal.pone.0022442

[70] Carey JB, Vrdoljak A, O'Mahony C, Hill AV, Draper SJ, Moore AC. Microneedle-mediated immunization of an adenovirus-based malaria vaccine enhances antigen-specific antibody immunity and reduces anti-vector responses compared to the intradermal route. Sci Rep. 2014;4:6154. DOI: 10.1038/srep06154

[71] Pearson FE, O'Mahony C, Moore AC, Hill AV. Induction of CD8(+) T cell responses and protective efficacy following microneedle-mediated delivery of a live adenovirus-vectored malaria vaccine. Vaccine. 2015;33:3248–55. DOI: 10.1016/j.vaccine.2015.03.039

[72] Lee J, Park SH, Seo IH, Lee KJ, Ryu W. Rapid and repeatable fabrication of high A/R silk fibroin microneedles using thermally-drawn micromolds. Eur J Pharm Biopharm. 2015;94:11–9. DOI: 10.1016/j.ejpb.2015.04.024

[73] Pritchard EM, Dennis PB, Omenetto F, Naik RR, Kaplan DL. Review physical and chemical aspects of stabilization of compounds in silk. Biopolymers. 2012;97:479–98. DOI: 10.1002/bip.22026

[74] DeMuth PC, Min Y, Irvine DJ, Hammond PT. Implantable silk composite microneedles for programmable vaccine release kinetics and enhanced immunogenicity in transcutaneous immunization. Adv Healthc Mater. 2014;3:47–58. DOI: 10.1002/adhm.201300139

[75] Bonificio A, Ghartey-Tagoe E, Gallorini S, Baudner B, Chen G, Singh P, et al. Fabrication of cell culture-derived influenza vaccine dissolvable microstructures and evaluation of immunogenicity in guinea pigs. Vaccine. 2015;33:2930–8. DOI: 10.1016/j.vaccine.2015.04.059

[76] Zhang Y, Brown K, Siebenaler K, Determan A, Dohmeier D, Hansen K. Development of lidocaine-coated microneedle product for rapid, safe, and prolonged local analgesic action. Pharm Res. 2012;29:170–7. DOI: 10.1007/s11095-011-0524-4

[77] Kallen KJ, Thess A. A development that may evolve into a revolution in medicine: mRNA as the basis for novel, nucleotide-based vaccines and drugs. Ther Adv Vaccines. 2014;2:10–31. DOI: 10.1177/2051013613508729

[78] Kubler H, Scheel B, Gnad-Vogt U, Miller K, Schultze-Seemann W, Vom Dorp F, et al. Self-adjuvanted mRNA vaccination in advanced prostate cancer patients: a first-in-man phase I/IIa study. J Immunother Cancer. 2015;3:26. DOI: 10.1186/s40425-015-0068-y

[79] Huang CL, Leblond AL, Turner EC, Kumar AH, Martin K, Whelan D, et al. Synthetic chemically modified mrna-based delivery of cytoprotective factor promotes early cardiomyocyte survival post-acute myocardial infarction. Mol Pharm. 2015;12:991–6. DOI: 10.1021/mp5006239

[80] Zangi L, Lui KO, von Gise A, Ma Q, Ebina W, Ptaszek LM, et al. Modified mRNA directs the fate of heart progenitor cells and induces vascular regeneration after myocardial infarction. Nat Biotechnol. 2013;31:898–907. DOI: 10.1038/nbt.2682

[81] Francis JN, Thaburet JF, Bonnet D, Sizer PJ, Brown CB, Georges B. Increasing cellular immunogenicity to peptide-based vaccine candidates using a fluorocarbon antigen delivery system. Vaccine. 2015;33:1071–6. DOI: 10.1016/j.vaccine.2014.12.061

[82] Francis JN, Bunce CJ, Horlock C, Watson JM, Warrington SJ, Georges B, et al. A novel peptide-based pan-influenza A vaccine: a double blind, randomised clinical trial of immunogenicity and safety. Vaccine. 2015;33:396–402. DOI: 10.1016/j.vaccine.2014.06.006

[83] Kersten GF, Crommelin DJ. Liposomes and ISCOMs. Vaccine. 2003;21:915–20.

[84] Watson DS, Endsley AN, Huang L. Design considerations for liposomal vaccines: influence of formulation parameters on antibody and cell-mediated immune responses to liposome associated antigens. Vaccine. 2012;30:2256–72. DOI: 10.1016/j.vaccine.2012.01.070

[85] Apellaniz B, Nieva JL. The use of liposomes to shape epitope structure and modulate immunogenic responses of peptide vaccines against HIV MPER. Adv Protein Chem Struct Biol. 2015;99:15–54. DOI: 10.1016/bs.apcsb.2015.03.002

[86] Alving CR, Rao M, Steers NJ, Matyas GR, Mayorov AV. Liposomes containing lipid A: an effective, safe, generic adjuvant system for synthetic vaccines. Expert Rev Vaccines. 2012;11:733–44. DOI: 10.1586/erv.12.35

[87] Schwendener RA. Liposomes as vaccine delivery systems: a review of the recent advances. Ther Adv Vaccines. 2014;2:159–82. DOI: 10.1177/2051013614541440

[88] Marciani DJ, Press JB, Reynolds RC, Pathak AK, Pathak V, Gundy LE, et al. Development of semisynthetic triterpenoid saponin derivatives with immune stimulating activity. Vaccine. 2000;18:3141–51.

[89] Dasari V, Smith C, Zhong J, Scott G, Rawlinson W, Khanna R. Recombinant glycoprotein B vaccine formulation with Toll-like receptor 9 agonist and immune-stimulating complex induces specific immunity against multiple strains of cytomegalovirus. J Gen Virol. 2011;92:1021–31. DOI: 10.1099/vir.0.029413-0

[90] Reimer JM, Karlsson KH, Lovgren-Bengtsson K, Magnusson SE, Fuentes A, Stertman L. Matrix-M adjuvant induces local recruitment, activation and maturation of central immune cells in absence of antigen. PLoS One. 2012;7:e41451. DOI: 10.1371/journal.pone.004145

[91] Beck Z, Matyas GR, Jalah R, Rao M, Polonis VR, Alving CR. Differential immune responses to HIV-1 envelope protein induced by liposomal adjuvant formulations containing monophosphoryl lipid A with or without QS21. Vaccine. 2015;33:5578–87. DOI: 10.1016/j.vaccine.2015.09.001

[92] Noe AR, Espinosa D, Li X, Coelho-Dos-Reis JG, Funakoshi R, Giardina S, et al. A full-length Plasmodium falciparum recombinant circumsporozoite protein expressed by *Pseudomonas fluorescens* platform as a malaria vaccine candidate. PLoS One. 2014;9:e107764. DOI: 10.1371/journal.pone.0107764

[93] Espinosa D, Vega-Rodriguez J, Flores-Garcia Y, Noe AR, Salman AM, Janse CJ, et al. The *P. falciparum* cell-traversal protein for ookinetes and sporozoites as a candidate for pre-erythrocytic and transmission-blocking vaccines. Submitted for publication. 2016.

[94] de Cassan SC, Shakri AR, Llewellyn D, Elias SC, Cho JS, Goodman AL, et al. Preclinical assessment of viral vectored and protein vaccines targeting the duffy-binding protein region II of *Plasmodium vivax*. Front Immunol. 2015;6:348. DOI: 10.3389/fimmu.2015.00348

[95] Cox RJ, Major D, Pedersen G, Pathirana RD, Hoschler K, Guilfoyle K, et al. Matrix M H5N1 vaccine induces cross-H5 clade humoral immune responses in a randomized clinical trial and provides protection from highly pathogenic influenza challenge in ferrets. PLoS One. 2015;10:e0131652. DOI: 10.1371/journal.pone.0131652

[96] Wilson NS, Yang B, Morelli AB, Koernig S, Yang A, Loeser S, et al. ISCOMATRIX vaccines mediate CD8+ T-cell cross-priming by a MyD88-dependent signaling pathway. Immunol Cell Biol. 2012;90:540–52. DOI: 10.1038/icb.2011.71

[97] Morelli AB, Becher D, Koernig S, Silva A, Drane D, Maraskovsky E. ISCOMATRIX: a novel adjuvant for use in prophylactic and therapeutic vaccines against infectious diseases. J Med Microbiol. 2012;61:935–43. DOI: 10.1099/jmm.0.040857-0

[98] Sun HX, Xie Y, Ye YP. ISCOMs and ISCOMATRIX. Vaccine. 2009;27:4388–401. DOI: 10.1016/j.vaccine.2009.05.032

[99] van Dissel JT, Joosten SA, Hoff ST, Soonawala D, Prins C, Hokey DA, et al. A novel liposomal adjuvant system, CAF01, promotes long-lived Mycobacterium tuberculosis-specific T-cell responses in human. Vaccine. 2014;32:7098–107. DOI: 10.1016/j.vaccine.2014.10.036

[100] Knudsen NP, Olsen A, Buonsanti C, Follmann F, Zhang Y, Coler RN, et al. Different human vaccine adjuvants promote distinct antigen-independent immunological signatures tailored to different pathogens. Sci Rep. 2016;6:19570. DOI: 10.1038/srep19570

[101] Karkada M, Weir GM, Quinton T, Sammatur L, MacDonald LD, Grant A, et al. A novel breast/ovarian cancer peptide vaccine platform that promotes specific type-1 but not Treg/Tr1-type responses. J Immunother. 2010;33:250–61. DOI: 10.1097/CJI.0b013e3181c1f1e9

[102] Brewer KD, Lake K, Pelot N, Stanford MM, DeBay DR, Penwell A, et al. Clearance of depot vaccine SPIO-labeled antigen and substrate visualized using MRI. Vaccine. 2014;32:6956–62. DOI: 10.1016/j.vaccine.2014.10.058

[103] MacDonald LD, Fuentes-Ortega A, Sammatur L, Mansour M. Efficacy of a single dose hepatitis B depot vaccine. Vaccine. 2010;28:7143–5. DOI: 10.1016/j.vaccine.2010.08.084

[104] Mansour M, Brown RG, Morris A, Smith B, Halperin SA. Improved efficacy of a licensed acellular pertussis vaccine, reformulated in an adjuvant emulsion of liposomes in oil, in a murine model. Clin Vaccine Immunol. 2007;14:1381–3. DOI: 10.1128/cvi.00143-07

[105] Berinstein NL, Karkada M, Morse MA, Nemunaitis JJ, Chatta G, Kaufman H, et al. First-in-man application of a novel therapeutic cancer vaccine formulation with the capacity to induce multi-functional T cell responses in ovarian, breast and prostate cancer patients. J Transl Med. 2012;10:156. DOI: 10.1186/1479-5876-10-156

[106] Moser C, Muller M, Kaeser MD, Weydemann U, Amacker M. Influenza virosomes as vaccine adjuvant and carrier system. Expert Rev Vaccines. 2013;12:779–91. DOI: 10.1586/14760584.2013.811195

[107] Gluck R. Immunopotentiating reconstituted influenza virosomes (IRIVs) and other adjuvants for improved presentation of small antigens. Vaccine. 1992;10:915–9.

[108] Trovato M, De Berardinis P. Novel antigen delivery systems. World J Virol. 2015;4:156–68. DOI: 10.5501/wjv.v4.i3.156

[109] Mueller MS, Renard A, Boato F, Vogel D, Naegeli M, Zurbriggen R, et al. Induction of parasite growth-inhibitory antibodies by a virosomal formulation of a peptidomimetic

of loop I from domain III of Plasmodium falciparum apical membrane antigen 1. Infect Immun. 2003;71:4749–58.

[110] Okitsu SL, Kienzl U, Moehle K, Silvie O, Peduzzi E, Mueller MS, et al. Structure-activity-based design of a synthetic malaria peptide eliciting sporozoite inhibitory antibodies in a virosomal formulation. Chem Biol. 2007;14:577–87. DOI: 10.1016/j.chembiol.2007.04.008

[111] Tamborrini M, Mueller MS, Stoffel SA, Westerfeld N, Vogel D, Boato F, et al. Design and pre-clinical profiling of a *Plasmodium falciparum* MSP-3 derived component for a multi-valent virosomal malaria vaccine. Malar J. 2009;8:314. DOI: 10.1186/1475-2875-8-314

[112] Genton B, Pluschke G, Degen L, Kammer AR, Westerfeld N, Okitsu SL, et al. A randomized placebo-controlled phase Ia malaria vaccine trial of two virosome-formulated synthetic peptides in healthy adult volunteers. PLoS One. 2007;2:e1018. DOI: 10.1371/journal.pone.0001018

[113] Okitsu SL, Silvie O, Westerfeld N, Curcic M, Kammer AR, Mueller MS, et al. A virosomal malaria peptide vaccine elicits a long-lasting sporozoite-inhibitory antibody response in a phase 1a clinical trial. PLoS One. 2007;2:e1278. DOI: 10.1371/journal.pone.0001278

[114] Peduzzi E, Westerfeld N, Zurbriggen R, Pluschke G, Daubenberger CA. Contribution of influenza immunity and virosomal-formulated synthetic peptide to cellular immune responses in a phase I subunit malaria vaccine trial. Clin Immunol. 2008;127:188–97. DOI: 10.1016/j.clim.2008.01.012

[115] Cech PG, Aebi T, Abdallah MS, Mpina M, Machunda EB, Westerfeld N, et al. Virosome-formulated *Plasmodium falciparum* AMA-1 & CSP derived peptides as malaria vaccine: randomized phase 1b trial in semi-immune adults & children. PLoS One. 2011;6:e22273. DOI: 10.1371/journal.pone.0022273

[116] Gonzalez RO, Higa LH, Cutrullis RA, Bilen M, Morelli I, Roncaglia DI, et al. Archaeosomes made of Halorubrum tebenquichense total polar lipids: a new source of adjuvancy. BMC Biotechnol. 2009;9:71. DOI: 10.1186/1472-6750-9-71

[117] Sprott GD, Yeung A, Dicaire CJ, Yu SH, Whitfield DM. Synthetic archaeosome vaccines containing triglycosylarchaeols can provide additive and long-lasting immune responses that are enhanced by archaetidylserine. Archaea. 2012;2012:513231. DOI: 10.1155/2012/513231

[118] Whitfield DM, Yu SH, Dicaire CJ, Sprott GD. Development of new glycosylation methodologies for the synthesis of archaeal-derived glycolipid adjuvants. Carbohydr Res. 2010;345:214–29. DOI: 10.1016/j.carres.2009.10.011

[119] Sprott GD, Dicaire CJ, Cote JP, Whitfield DM. Adjuvant potential of archaeal synthetic glycolipid mimetics critically depends on the glyco head group structure. Glycobiology. 2008;18:559–65. DOI: 10.1093/glycob/cwn038

[120] Silva DG, Cooper PD, Petrovsky N. Inulin-derived adjuvants efficiently promote both Th1 and Th2 immune responses. Immunol Cell Biol. 2004;82:611–6. DOI: 10.1111/j.1440-1711.2004.01290.x

[121] Petrovsky N, Cooper PD. Advax, a novel microcrystalline polysaccharide particle engineered from delta inulin, provides robust adjuvant potency together with tolerability and safety. Vaccine. 2015;33:5920–6. DOI: 10.1016/j.vaccine.2015.09.030

[122] Gordon D, Kelley P, Heinzel S, Cooper P, Petrovsky N. Immunogenicity and safety of Advax, a novel polysaccharide adjuvant based on delta inulin, when formulated with hepatitis B surface antigen: a randomized controlled Phase 1 study. Vaccine. 2014;32:6469–77. DOI: 10.1016/j.vaccine.2014.09.034

[123] Gordon DL, Sajkov D, Woodman RJ, Honda-Okubo Y, Cox MM, Heinzel S, et al. Randomized clinical trial of immunogenicity and safety of a recombinant H1N1/2009 pandemic influenza vaccine containing Advax polysaccharide adjuvant. Vaccine. 2012;30:5407–16. DOI: 10.1016/j.vaccine.2012.06.009

[124] Smith DM, Simon JK, Baker JR, Jr. Applications of nanotechnology for immunology. Nat Rev Immunol. 2013;13:592–605. DOI: 10.1038/nri3488

[125] Stoute JA, Kester KE, Krzych U, Wellde BT, Hall T, White K, et al. Long-term efficacy and immune responses following immunization with the RTS,S malaria vaccine. J Infect Dis. 1998;178:1139–44.

[126] Stoute JA, Slaoui M, Heppner DG, Momin P, Kester KE, Desmons P, et al. A preliminary evaluation of a recombinant circumsporozoite protein vaccine against Plasmodium falciparum malaria. RTS,S Malaria Vaccine Evaluation Group. N Engl J Med. 1997;336:86–91. DOI: 10.1056/NEJM199701093360202

[127] Sachdeva S, Mohmmed A, Dasaradhi PV, Crabb BS, Katyal A, Malhotra P, et al. Immunogenicity and protective efficacy of Escherichia coli expressed Plasmodium falciparum merozoite surface protein-1(42) using human compatible adjuvants. Vaccine. 2006;24:2007–16. DOI: 10.1016/j.vaccine.2005.11.041

[128] Stowers AW, Cioce V, Shimp RL, Lawson M, Hui G, Muratova O, et al. Efficacy of two alternate vaccines based on Plasmodium falciparum merozoite surface protein 1 in an Aotus challenge trial. Infect Immun. 2001;69:1536–46. DOI: 10.1128/IAI.69.3.1536-1546.2001

[129] Yazdani SS, Shakri AR, Mukherjee P, Baniwal SK, Chitnis CE. Evaluation of immune responses elicited in mice against a recombinant malaria vaccine based on *Plasmodium vivax* Duffy binding protein. Vaccine. 2004;22:3727–37. DOI: 10.1016/j.vaccine.2004.03.030

[130] Baudner BC, Ronconi V, Casini D, Tortoli M, Kazzaz J, Singh M, et al. MF59 emulsion is an effective delivery system for a synthetic TLR4 agonist (E6020). Pharm Res. 2009;26:1477–85. DOI: 10.1007/s11095-009-9859-5

[131] Makidon PE, Bielinska AU, Nigavekar SS, Janczak KW, Knowlton J, Scott AJ, et al. Pre-clinical evaluation of a novel nanoemulsion-based hepatitis B mucosal vaccine. PLoS One. 2008;3:e2954. DOI: 10.1371/journal.pone.0002954

[132] Beletskii A, Galloway A, Rele S, Stone M, Malinoski F. Engineered PRINT((R)) nanoparticles for controlled delivery of antigens and immunostimulants. Hum Vaccin Immunother. 2014;10:1908–13. DOI: 10.4161/hv.28817

[133] Stanberry LR, Simon JK, Johnson C, Robinson PL, Morry J, Flack MR, et al. Safety and immunogenicity of a novel nanoemulsion mucosal adjuvant W805EC combined with approved seasonal influenza antigens. Vaccine. 2012;30:307–16. DOI: 10.1016/j.vaccine.2011.10.094

[134] Falloon J, Ji F, Curtis C, Bart S, Sheldon E, Krieger D, et al. A phase 1a, first-in-human, randomized study of a respiratory syncytial virus F protein vaccine with and without a toll-like receptor-4 agonist and stable emulsion adjuvant. Vaccine. 2016. DOI: 10.1016/j.vaccine.2016.04.002

[135] Santini-Oliveira M, Coler RN, Parra J, Veloso V, Jayashankar L, Pinto PM, et al. Schistosomiasis vaccine candidate Sm14/GLA-SE: Phase 1 safety and immunogenicity clinical trial in healthy, male adults. Vaccine. 2016;34:586–94. DOI: 10.1016/j.vaccine.2015.10.027

[136] Treanor JJ, Essink B, Hull S, Reed S, Izikson R, Patriarca P, et al. Evaluation of safety and immunogenicity of recombinant influenza hemagglutinin (H5/Indonesia/05/2005) formulated with and without a stable oil-in-water emulsion containing glucopyranosyl-lipid A (SE+GLA) adjuvant. Vaccine. 2013;31:5760–5. DOI: 10.1016/j.vaccine.2013.08.064

[137] Schwenk R, DeBot M, Porter M, Nikki J, Rein L, Spaccapelo R, et al. IgG2 antibodies against a clinical grade Plasmodium falciparum CSP vaccine antigen associate with protection against transgenic sporozoite challenge in mice. PLoS One. 2014;9:e111020. DOI: 10.1371/journal.pone.0111020

[138] Wiley SR, Raman VS, Desbien A, Bailor HR, Bhardwaj R, Shakri AR, et al. Targeting TLRs expands the antibody repertoire in response to a malaria vaccine. Sci Transl Med. 2011;3:93ra69. DOI: 10.1126/scitranslmed.3002135

[139] Yu M, Vajdy M. A novel retinoic acid, catechin hydrate and mustard oil-based emulsion for enhanced cytokine and antibody responses against multiple strains of HIV-1 following mucosal and systemic vaccinations. Vaccine. 2011;29:2429–36. DOI: 10.1016/j.vaccine.2011.01.024

[140] Patel S, Vajdy M. Induction of cellular and molecular immunomodulatory pathways by vitamin A and flavonoids. Expert Opin Biol Ther. 2015;15:1411–28. DOI: 10.1517/14712598.2015.1066331

[141] Baxevanis CN, Voutsas IF, Tsitsilonis OE. Toll-like receptor agonists: current status and future perspective on their utility as adjuvants in improving anticancer vaccination strategies. Immunotherapy. 2013;5:497–511. DOI: 10.2217/imt.13.24

[142] Lahiri A, Das P, Chakravortty D. Engagement of TLR signaling as adjuvant: towards smarter vaccine and beyond. Vaccine. 2008;26:6777–83. DOI: 10.1016/j.vaccine.2008.09.045

[143] Fritz JH, Brunner S, Birnstiel ML, Buschle M, Gabain A, Mattner F, et al. The artificial antimicrobial peptide KLKLLLLLKLK induces predominantly a TH2-type immune response to co-injected antigens. Vaccine. 2004;22:3274–84. DOI: 10.1016/j.vaccine.2004.03.007

[144] Lingnau K, Riedl K, von Gabain A. IC31 and IC30, novel types of vaccine adjuvant based on peptide delivery systems. Expert Rev Vaccines. 2007;6:741–6. DOI: 10.1586/14760584.6.5.741

[145] van Dissel JT, Arend SM, Prins C, Bang P, Tingskov PN, Lingnau K, et al. Ag85B-ESAT-6 adjuvanted with IC31 promotes strong and long-lived Mycobacterium tuberculosis specific T cell responses in naive human volunteers. Vaccine. 2010;28:3571–81. DOI: 10.1016/j.vaccine.2010.02.094

[146] van Dissel JT, Soonawala D, Joosten SA, Prins C, Arend SM, Bang P, et al. Ag85B-ESAT-6 adjuvanted with IC31(R) promotes strong and long-lived Mycobacterium tuberculosis specific T cell responses in volunteers with previous BCG vaccination or tuberculosis infection. Vaccine. 2011;29:2100–9. DOI: 10.1016/j.vaccine.2010.12.135

[147] Geldenhuys H, Mearns H, Miles DJ, Tameris M, Hokey D, Shi Z, et al. The tuberculosis vaccine H4:IC31 is safe and induces a persistent polyfunctional CD4 T cell response in South African adults: a randomized controlled trial. Vaccine. 2015;33:3592–9. DOI: 10.1016/j.vaccine.2015.05.036

[148] Luabeya AK, Kagina BM, Tameris MD, Geldenhuys H, Hoff ST, Shi Z, et al. First-in-human trial of the post-exposure tuberculosis vaccine H56:IC31 in Mycobacterium tuberculosis infected and non-infected healthy adults. Vaccine. 2015;33:4130–40. DOI: 10.1016/j.vaccine.2015.06.051

[149] Reither K, Katsoulis L, Beattie T, Gardiner N, Lenz N, Said K, et al. Safety and immunogenicity of H1/IC31(R), an adjuvanted TB subunit vaccine, in HIV-infected adults with CD4+ lymphocyte counts greater than 350 cells/mm3: a phase II, multi-centre, double-blind, randomized, placebo-controlled trial. PLoS One. 2014;9:e114602. DOI: 10.1371/journal.pone.0114602

[150] Li X, Fujio M, Imamura M, Wu D, Vasan S, Wong CH, et al. Design of a potent CD1d-binding NKT cell ligand as a vaccine adjuvant. Proc Natl Acad Sci U S A. 2010;107:13010–5. DOI: 10.1073/pnas.1006662107

[151] Li X, Kawamura A, Andrews CD, Miller JL, Wu D, Tsao T, et al. Colocalization of a CD1d-binding Glycolipid with a radiation-attenuated sporozoite vaccine in lymph

node-resident dendritic cells for a robust adjuvant effect. J Immunol. 2015;195:2710–21. DOI: 10.4049/jimmunol.1403017

[152] Padte NN, Boente-Carrera M, Andrews CD, McManus J, Grasperge BF, Gettie A, et al. A glycolipid adjuvant, 7DW8-5, enhances CD8+ T cell responses induced by an adenovirus-vectored malaria vaccine in non-human primates. PLoS One. 2013;8:e78407. DOI: 10.1371/journal.pone.0078407

[153] Coelho-Dos-Reis JG, Huang J, Tsao T, Pereira FV, Funakoshi R, Nakajima H, et al. Co-administration of alpha-GalCer analog and TLR4 agonist induces robust CD8 T-cell responses to PyCS protein and WT-1 antigen and activates memory-like effector NKT cells. Clin Immunol. 2016;168:6–15. DOI: 10.1016/j.clim.2016.04.014

8

The Biology of Malaria Gametocytes

Che Julius Ngwa, Thiago F. de A. Rosa and Gabriele Pradel

Abstract

Gametocytes are sexual precursor cells of the malaria parasite that mediate the transmission of the parasite from its mammalian host to the *Anopheles* mosquito. Unlike the asexual blood stages, which are responsible for the clinical outcome of malaria, gametocytes cause no clinical manifestations. However, they are very crucial for the transmission of the disease thus represent key targets for transmission-blocking interventions. Despite their essential role in malaria transmission, only in the last decade gametocytes became a hot topic of research and their biology is not well understood. This chapter provides a detailed review on the biology of the human malaria gametocytes with emphasis on aspects such as gametocyte commitment, gametocyte maturation (gametocytogenesis), gametocyte metabolism and gametogenesis. Proper understanding of these processes will deepen our knowledge on the gametocyte biology and therefore open up more avenues for the development of malaria transmission-blocking intervention strategies.

Keywords: gametocyte, gametocytogenesis, transmission, gametogenesis, sexual reproduction, mosquito

1. Introduction

Gametocytes are specialized sexual precursor cells that mediate the transmission of the malaria parasite from the mammalian host to the mosquito. Once these cells have gained maturity, they are picked up by an *Anopheles* mosquito during a blood meal. In the midgut of the mosquito, they become activated and differentiate into male and female gametes. The male gamete then fertilizes the female gamete resulting in the formation of a zygote. The zygote further develops into a motile ookinete, which penetrates the gut epithelium and subsequently develops into an oocyst. The oocyst then matures releasing sporozoites, which migrate to the salivary gland of the mosquito. The parasite is transmitted to another mammalian host through an infected mosquito bite [1]. Gametocytes therefore provide a link in the transmission of malaria from the mammalian host to the mosquito, thereby making them prime targets for transmission-blocking intervention strategies. These strategies rely on either vaccines or drugs, which target the gametocyte or the mosquito midgut stages to block malaria transmission from the human to the mosquito, thereby preventing the spread of the disease.

Despite their essential role in maintaining the parasite life cycle, research on gametocytes has been very much left out of the limelight. Several reasons could be accounted for this: first, gametocytes cause no clinical manifestation in their host as opposed to the asexual blood stages that are responsible for the clinical features of malaria. Second, it has been a great challenge to culture gametocytes because of the cost and time-consuming cultivation procedure, and finally, it has been a hurdle to obtain pure gametocytes for molecular and metabolic studies as well as drug screening purposes. However, in the last decade, the rapid emergence of drug-resistant parasites and mosquitoes, together with the absence of a malaria vaccine, has rekindled the interest of researchers on alternative measures aimed at interrupting the parasite life cycle by targeting gametocytes. This interest has led to the improvement of gametocyte cultivation and purification methods, which have enabled a greater understanding of the gametocyte biology.

In this chapter, we focus on key aspects of the gametocyte biology such as gametocyte commitment, maturation (gametocytogenesis), metabolism and gametogenesis. This will deepen our understanding on the biology of gametocytes and thereby open up more avenues for the development of malaria transmission-blocking intervention strategies.

2. Gametocyte commitment

The asexual blood stage parasites produce the clinical form of malaria due to destruction of the erythrocytes, while replicating in the mammalian host. However, these asexual blood stages cannot be transmitted to the mosquito to continue the life cycle of the parasite. For this reason, a subset of the asexual blood stages is able to switch to the sexual pathway, resulting in the formation of the sexual precursor cells, the gametocytes. The process of switching from the asexual blood stage to the gametocyte is referred to as gametocyte commitment.

Commitment to gametocyte development is believed to take place at some point before schizogony, in which each individual schizont produces a progeny of merozoites that develop into either sexual forms or asexual blood stage parasites, which continue the erythrocytic cycle [2, 3] (**Figure 1**). In addition, merozoites released from a single sexually committed schizont can either become male or female gametocytes and the characteristic female-biased sex ratio observed in the malaria parasite is due to the production of a higher percentage of committed female schizonts than their male counterpart [3, 4].

Until recently, gametocyte commitment was mainly assigned to stress factors such as high parasitaemia, anaemia, host immune response or drug treatment, with an overwhelming amount of studies to justify these facts. A study by Chaubey and colleagues suggested that the malaria parasite reacts to endoplasmic reticulum stress by switching to gametocytes [5]. The treatment of mice with phenylhydrazine, which induces hyper-reticulocyte formation, stimulates gametocyte formation when infected with *P. chabaudi* [6]. Lymphocyte and serum from Gambian children have also been shown to induce *P. falciparum* gametocyte production [7]. Another study showed that *P. falciparum* cultures grown in reticulocyte-rich blood from patients with sickle cell anaemia result in enhanced gametocyte formation as compared to normal blood [8]. Haemolysis of infected erythrocytes also triggers the formation of *P. falciparum* gametocytes [9]. The treatment of the malaria parasite with drugs such as steroid hormones [10], fansidar [11] and chloroquine or sulfadoxine-pyrimethamine [12] also enhances gametocyte production.

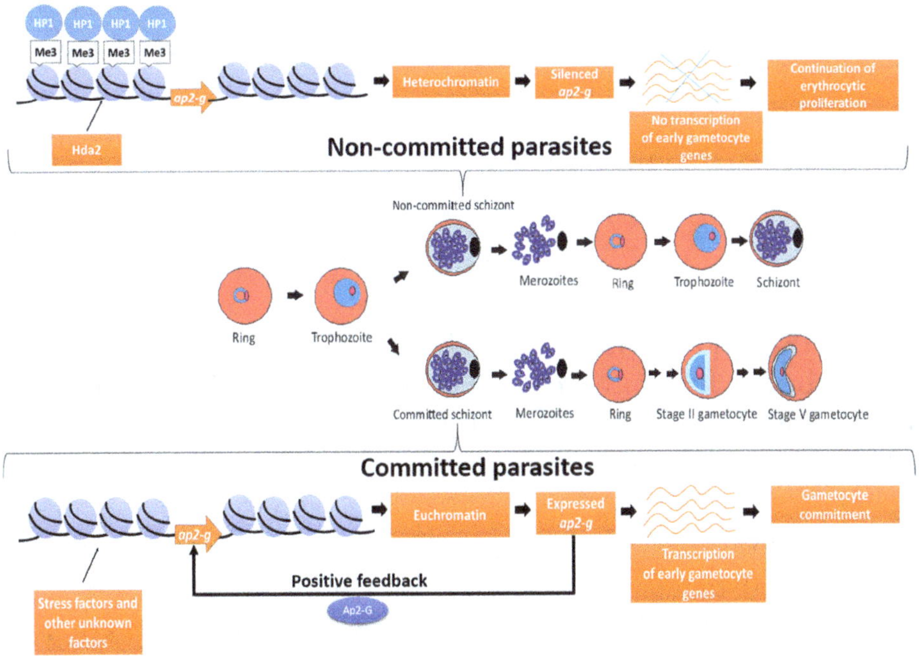

Figure 1. Proposed mechanism of gametocyte commitment. During the erythrocyte cycle, epigenetic and transcriptional regulation work hand in hand to control gametocyte commitment. Two populations of blood stage parasites exist. Non-committed parasites continue the erythrocytic replication of the parasite, and committed parasites are able to differentiate to gametocytes.

However, despite the knowledge that gametocyte commitment can be enhanced by stress factors, the mechanism by which stress induces this process is not well understood. Recent studies have also associated gametocyte commitment to the concerted action of epigenetics and transcriptional regulation.

2.1. Epigenetic mechanism of gametocyte commitment

Epigenetic mechanisms through histone modifications have been shown to regulate gene expression of important proteins in the malaria parasite [13, 14]. In *P. falciparum*, two master players in gene silencing, *P. falciparum* heterochromatin protein 1 (PfHP1) and *P. falciparum* histone deacetylase 2 (PfHda2) were demonstrated to be implicated in the epigenetic regulation of gametocyte commitment [15, 16].

Heterochromatin protein 1 (HP1) was initially described in *Drosophila* as the main suppressor of position-effect variegation and the major component of heterochromatin gene silencing [17]. Brancucci and colleagues [16] reported that in *P. falciparum*, PfHP1 binds to histone H3-trimethylated residues on lysine 9 (H3K9me3) to maintain heterochromatin gene silencing, which results in the suppression of gametocyte commitment and variegated expression of *var* genes. *Var* genes encode for a family of 60 parasite virulent proteins in *P. falciparum* named *P. falciparum* erythrocyte membrane protein 1 (PfEMP1). PfEMP1 is present on surface of the *P. falciparum*-infected erythrocyte of which only one is expressed at a time and this phenomenon is associated with antigenic variation. Conditional depletion of PfHP1 results in the hyper-induction of viable gametocytes, thereby demonstrating a role of PfHP1 in suppressing gametocyte commitment. Depletion of PfHP1 also results in derepression of the *ap2-g* gene, which encodes for the AP2-G transcription factor, the only member of the ApiAP2 family shown to associate with PfHP1 [18]. AP2-G was demonstrated to be important in gametocyte commitment in both *P. falciparum* and the rodent malaria parasite *P. berghei* by acting as a transcriptional switch that controls gametocyte differentiation through activating the transcription of early gametocyte genes [19, 20].

Histone deacetylases are histone-modifying enzymes that promote transcriptional silencing by removing acetyl groups from histones. The removal of the acetyl groups facilitates histone methylation and HP1 binding [18, 21, 22], thereby resulting in reduced accessibility for transcriptional factors and heterochromatin formation. A study by Coleman and colleagues [15], which complements the results of Brancucci et al. [16], showed an essential role of PfHda2 in the global silencing of *var* genes as well as controlling gametocyte commitment in *P. falciparum*. Knockdown of PfHda2 results in up-regulation of gene expression of genes associated with gametocytogenesis leading to an increase in gametocyte production. It also results in derepression of the *ap2-g* gene. The authors further reported that most of the genes dysregulated following PfHda2 knockdown were bound to PfHP1, and both proteins localize together with PfHda2-regulated genes, which were significantly enriched in H3K9me3, indicating an interaction between PfHda2 and PfHP1. The two studies therefore provide a link between PfHda2 and PfHP1 in controlling gametocyte commitment.

2.2. Transcriptional regulation of gametocyte commitment

AP2-G is a member of the apicomplexan AP2 DNA-binding protein family, characterized by the presence of an Apetala2/ethylene response factor (AP2/ERF) DNA-binding domain [23]. In the malaria parasite, other AP2 proteins have been assigned to the stage-specific transition during parasite development, for example, the development of midgut, sporozoite and liver stages [24–27].

Two studies in *P. falciparum* and *P. berghei* have shown that AP2-G triggers a transcription cascade that initiates gametocyte commitment [14, 19, 20]. To determine initially, if AP2-G is essential for gametocyte commitment and production, both studies sequenced and analysed the *ap2-g* gene from specific gametocyte-less producing strains for single nucleotide polymorphisms, insertions or mutations. Their results showed nonsense or missense mutations in the *ap2-g* gene providing an explanation for the inability of the strains to commit and produce gametocytes. Their initial findings were further confirmed by targeted disruption of the *ap2-g* locus in both *P. falciparum* and *P. berghei,* which resulted in the loss of sexual commitment and gametocyte production. The disruption of the *ap2-g* locus also resulted in the down-regulation of many genes highly expressed in early gametocytes such as *Pfs16* and *Pfg25/27*. The DNA motif involved in AP2-G-binding was identified as GTAC and shown to be located upstream of many genes associated with gametocytogenesis [19, 20, 28]. Because the *ap2-g* gene also possesses the GTAC domain on its promoter region, this suggests that it regulates itself through a feedback mechanism. The AP2-G DNA-binding motif was shown to interact with gametocyte-associated gene promoters in a motif-dependent manner. Mutations of the motif in the promoter region result in a blockage of the gene expression of the gametocyte-associated genes, thereby indicating that AP2-G induces the expression of genes containing the AP2-G DNA motif by binding to it at the promoter region [19].

During the malaria life cycle, therefore, two populations of the malaria parasite exist. Non-committed parasites, which continue the erythrocytic cycle, and committed parasites that form gametocytes. In the case of non-committed parasites, PHP1 binds to H3K9me3 residues thereby maintaining the *ap2-g* locus at a heterochromatic state resulting in silencing of the *ap2-g* expression. This silencing leads to the inability to initiate transcription of genes important for gametocyte commitment; therefore, the parasite continues with erythrocytic replication. PHda2 is also involved in the silencing of the *ap2-g* gene expression in non-committed parasites, probably by the removal of acetylated histone residues allowing for their methylation leading to the binding of PHP1. In committed parasites, stress factors and other unknown factors cause the removal of the histone H3 trimethylation mark, thereby preventing PHP1 from binding to the histone and therefore maintaining the *ap2-g* locus at an active state, resulting in AP2-G expression. The expression of AP2-G promotes the transcription of early gametocyte genes, which leads to gametocyte commitment and formation (**Figure 1**).

3. Gametocyte maturation

3.1. Gametocyte morphology

The morphology of gametocytes varies among the *Plasmodium* species. While mature gametocytes from *P. ovale, P. malariae, P. vivax* and *P. knowlesi* possess a round to oval shape, *P. falciparum* adopts a crescent or falciform shape when matured [29–31].

P. falciparum is named from the crescent or falciform shape of its mature stage. During gametocyte development, the parasite undergoes five distinct morphological stages (I–V) (**Figure 2**). The first observations on the morphology of *P. falciparum* gametocytes were made in the 1950s, when the five development stages were defined [30]. Later studies using light and electron microscopic approaches have defined the shape and time of appearance [32, 33]. Studies have shown that stages I–IV are sequestered into the bone marrow, while stage V circulates in the peripheral blood vessels [34–36]. Stage I gametocyte has a rounded shape, which is indistinguishable from the young asexual trophozoite. Stage IIa, on the other hand, can be distinguished from the trophozoite by its large round format and granular distribution of pigment in several food vacuoles. In stage IIb, the parasite starts to elongate and a D-shape can be observed. Stage III gametocytes adopt an oval shape with the red blood cell slightly distorted due to further elongated of the parasite. In stage IV, it is possible to distinguish between male and female gametocytes. Both genders have an elongate thin format with pointed tips. In male gametocytes, the pigment tends to be scattered while in female it is denser. The stage V gametocyte is the most distinguishable among all stages due to the crescent or falciform shape. While the male gametocyte is thicker and the cytoplasm appears pale blue following Giemsa staining, the female is more elongate and curved with a blue-stained cytoplasm. This stage is visible in the periphery circulation after 10–12 days of maturation [29].

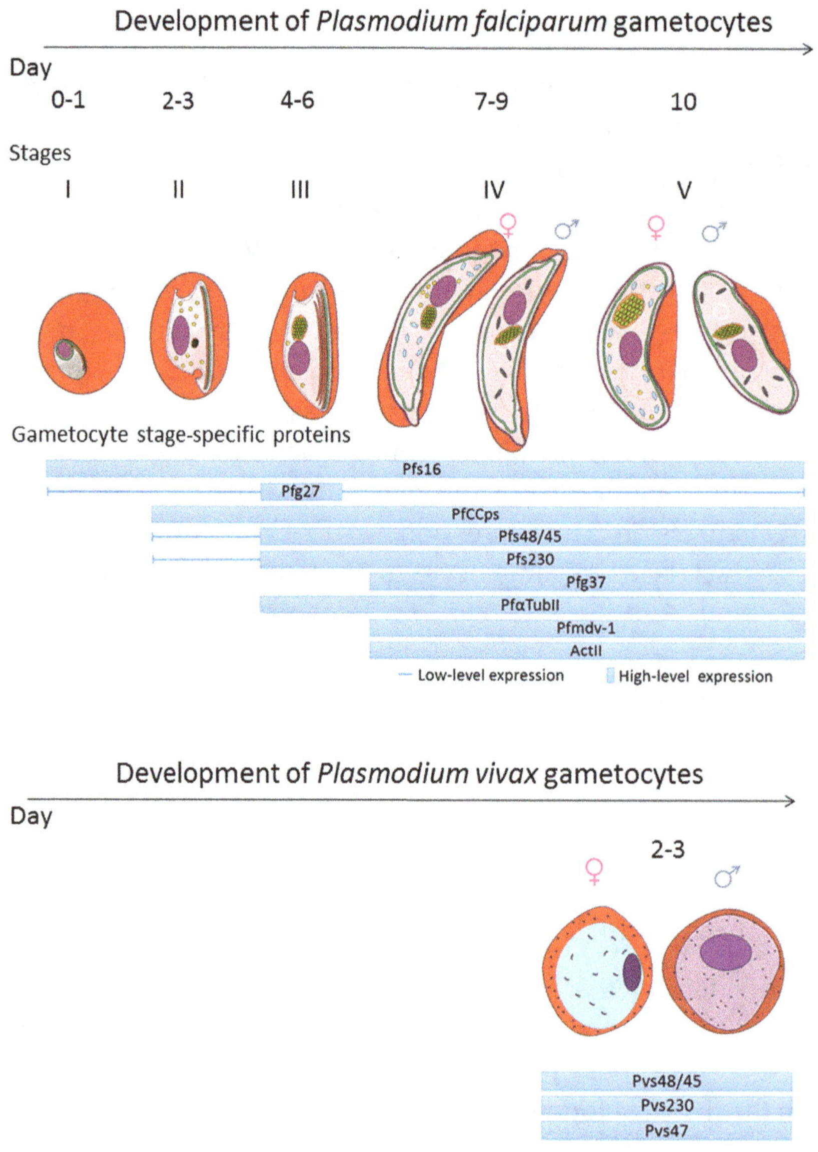

Figure 2. *P. falciparum* and *P. vivax* stage-specific protein expression during gametocyte development. The bar represents high-level expression and full line low-level expression. Only gene products were in included in this figure.

Among the other species of malaria, *P. vivax* is the most important because of its high impact on human health in South and Central America and South Asia [37]. The gametocytes of *P. vivax* are different from *P. falciparum* in their biology, dynamics and their formation, which occur within 2–3 days after asexual blood stage appearance in the circulation [38]. The male and female gametocytes of *P. vivax* possess a round shape as it is observed in *P. malariae, P. ovale* and *P. knowlesi*, but it is only in *P. vivax* that the parasite fills an enlarged red blood cell (**Figure 2**). In Giemsa-stained thin blood smears, female gametocytes have a blue-stained cytoplasm, and the chromatin is a purplish mass with a peripheral distribution, while male gametocytes possess a large and loose chromatin mass.

One remarkable morphological feature of gametocytes is the presence of the inner membrane complex (IMC), which underlies the plasmalemma and consists of flat membranous sacs called alveoli that are coupled to a supporting cytoskeletal network. The IMC was originally assigned to the invasive stages of *Plasmodium* as part of actin-myosin motor complex, and thus, the IMC is important for motility [39]. Recently, it was confirmed that gametocytes also possess an IMC [40–42], which is thought to be required for the stability of the crescent shape. The outer alveolar membrane contains complexes of the gliding-associated proteins GAP40, GAP45 and GAP50, which facilitate binding of myosin to this membrane. The gametocyte alveoli are subtended by a subpellicular network of interwoven alveoli filaments linked to the alveoli via intramembranous particles [39–41, 43]. Underneath the subpellicular network, an array of longitudinally oriented microtubules and F-actin fibrils are found that become reorganized in stage V gametocytes, leading to rounding-up of the gametocyte tips [44].

3.2. Gametocyte-specific proteins

Approximately 20% of all plasmodial genes are specifically expressed in the sexual stages [45, 46]. In *P. falciparum* gametocytes, the proteins are expressed at different levels in the five distinct developmental stages (**Figure 2**). Most of these proteins are associated with gametocyte development, integrity and preparation for fertilization. Furthermore, gender-related proteins are expressed in the later stages in order to support the gametes for fertilization in the mosquito midgut [1, 47–49].

In the early stage I–II gametocytes, important proteins such as Pfs16, Pfg27 and the six LCCL-domain proteins are expressed [50]. Pfs16 is present in all gametocyte stages, but it is initially expressed in stage I. It is localized in the parasitophorous vacuole (PV) where it plays a role in gametocyte development [51–53]. The main function of Pfs16 is unknown, but its disruption leads to a decrease in gametocyte production and an impairment in the ability of microgametocyte to exflagellate [54]. The protein Pfg27 is a phosphoprotein that starts to be expressed from stage II. It is known that Pfg27 forms a homodimer to act as single-stranded RNA-binding proteins *in vitro* and its gene deletion leads to the formation of abnormal gametocytes [55, 56]. The six LCCL-domain proteins (termed CCp in *P. falciparum* and LAP in *P. berghei*) possess adhesive properties and expression begins from stage II. In *P. falciparum* gametocytes, CCp proteins are localized within the PV, but after gamete emergence, the proteins are associated with the surface of gametes [47, 48, 57, 58].

Starting from stage IIb, well-known sexual-stage proteins such as the 6-cys proteins Pfs48/45 and Pfs230 and the osmiophilic body protein Pfg377 and Pfmdv-1 or sexual stage-specific cytoskeletal proteins such as α-tubII (tubulin II) and actin II are synthesized [50]. Similar to the six LCCL-domain proteins, the surface proteins Pfs48/45 and Pfs230 have adhesive properties and gene disruption of both proteins impair male gamete fertility [59, 60]. Pfg377 is known to be associated with osmiophilic bodies in female gametocyte of *P. falciparum*, and gene disruption demonstrates a fundamental role in the formation of osmiophilic bodies [61, 62]. The Pfmdv-1 protein, also known as Pfpeg3, is highly expressed in early gametocyte until stage V afterwards reaching a low level of expression. The function of *Pfmdv-1* is still unknown although disruption of the *Pfmdv-1* encoding gene leads to a 20-fold decrease in the production of male gametocytes [63]. The cytoskeletal proteins α-tubulin II and actin II are sexual stage-specific, and both are shown to be predominantly present in male gametocytes [64–66]. While α-tubulin II has been described to incorporate to axonemes of emerging male gametes, the function of actin II is still unclear, but gene disruption of both proteins leads to an impairment of male gametogenesis [65, 66]. In the mature microgametocyte, the protein PfB0400w, also known as PfMR5, can be observed. Although its function is still unknown, the expression of PfB0400w in male stage V gametocyte indicates that it may play a role in preparing gametocytes for exflagellation [50, 67].

In the gametocytes of *P. vivax*, three sexual stage-specific proteins have hitherto been identified, i.e. the 6-cys proteins Pvs230, Pvs48/45 and Pvs47, all of which are orthologues of those present in *P. falciparum* (**Figure 2**). Pvs230 has been characterized as an antigen on the surface of gametocytes and gametes while Pvs48/45 and Pvs47 have been studied recently as potential candidates for transmission-blocking vaccines. Following direct membrane feeding assays, anti-Pvs48/45 and anti-Pvs47 antibodies significantly reduced oocyst numbers in the mosquito midgut [68–70].

4. The gametocyte metabolism

During gametocytogenesis, *P. falciparum* parasites undergo intense metabolic processes including energy production as well as synthesis and degradation of various molecules such as lipids and proteins. These processes are essentials for the survival of the malaria parasite and ensure gametocyte stage development, drug resistance and transmission to the mosquito vector [30, 71, 72].

As vital molecules, lipids are responsible for many functions such as cell signalling, energy storage and the stability of membranes. Furthermore, during the various stages of the *Plasmodium* life cycle, lipids play a crucial role in the growth and proliferation of the parasite [73]. Among asexual blood stages and gametocytes, there are more than 300 lipids with known and unknown functions [74]. Although not reflected in all classes of lipids, the amount of lipids would more than double during gametocytogenesis [75]. The lipid composition of all developmental stages differs, including during gametocyte maturation. It is known that sphingolipids involved in ceramide metabolism are enriched during gametocyte maturation and the inhibition of the ceramide biosynthetic pathway might kill gametocytes. In addition, phosphatidylserine is also highly expressed during gametocytogenesis and together with ceramides leads to gametocyte induction [74]. Neutral lipids such as cholesteryl ester and diacylglycerol (DAG) have also been shown to be significantly increased during gametocyte maturation; however, more data to better understand the metabolism and function of these lipids during gametocytogenesis are required [75].

In gametocytes, no DNA-replication occurs [76] and the nucleic acid synthesis is exclusive for RNA production. The production of RNA ceases from around day 6 of gametocytogenesis, thus the RNA and protein synthesis are more important in the early than late gametocyte stages [77, 78]. One interesting feature of malaria parasites is the expression of small subunit ribosomal RNA (SSU rRNA) genes [79], seven of them are synthesized in *P. falciparum* and one (S-type, formally known as C-type) is exclusively expressed in gametocytes. Proteomics identified 931 different proteins (72.2% of the proteins identified in *P. falciparum*) in gametocytes and within these proteins include conserved, stage-specific, secreted and membrane-associated proteins [46]. It is also known that protein expression differs between gender, female gametocytes synthetize proteins required for mitochondria and ribosomes, while male gametocytes only need proteins for DNA synthesis, axoneme formation and exflagellation [29, 80].

In eukaryotes, the mitochondria have many vital roles such as ATP synthesis, calcium homeostasis, lipid metabolism and synthesis of ion-sulphate clusters. The malaria parasites only possess a single mitochondrion and during parasite development it is observed that the mitochondria of gametocytes are longer and possess more cristae when compare to the ones of the asexual blood stages. This suggests that ATP synthesis via the electron transport chain is the main mechanism of energy production in gametocytes [29, 33]. Indeed the sexual stages appear to have seven times more cytochrome b than the asexual blood stages [81]. The cytochrome bc1 complex feeds the electron transport chain with more protons, which creates a gradient that drives ATP synthesis [82]. The cytochrome bc1 is a prime target for the antimalarial drug atovaquone that inhibits ubiquinone leading to the inhibition of *Plasmodium* cytochrome bc1 activity and loss of mitochondrial function [83–85]. Other drugs such as primaquine and the primaquine analogue bulaquine have been shown to exhibit gametocytocidal activities and primaquine is suggested to have the site of action in the mitochondria by causing its deformation. Although the mode of action is poorly understood, these drugs reduce gametocytemia in infection by *P. falciparum* and have an effect against the exo-erythrocytic stages of *P. vivax* [86].

Despite the fact that the mitochondria have been well characterized in other organisms, many mitochondrion-associated events in *P. falciparum* are still not well understood. Initially, *P. falciparum* blood stage parasites were thought to be glucose- and glycolysis-dependent for carbon metabolism, ATP production and survival [87]. However, recent reports have also shown the importance of the tricarboxylic acid (TCA) cycle for energy production, especially in gametocytes [88]. The gametocyte utilizes mitochondrial TCA to catabolize host glucose and glutamine. The carbon skeleton derived from these molecules enters in the TCA cycle via acetyl-CoA to generate proton flux and ATP via the ATP synthase. Due to the role of the TCA cycle in parasite development, inhibition of this metabolic pathway leads to defects in gametocytogenesis. In addition, many mitochondrial enzymes involved in metabolic pathways can be targets for drug development [88].

5. Gametocyte activation and gametogenesis

5.1. The signalling cascade of gametocyte activation

The mature stage V gametocytes, which circulate in the blood of the mammalian host, are picked up by the female *Anopheles* mosquito during a bite and enter the midgut together with the blood meal. During the process, the gametocytes receive environmental signals, which indicate the switch from the warm-blooded host to the insect vector. The perception of these signals results in the immediate activation of the gametocytes followed by the onset of gametogenesis. Signals inducing gamete formation include a decrease in temperature by approximately 5°C, which is mandatory for gametocyte activation, and the presence of the mosquito-derived molecule xanthurenic acid (XA), a by-product of eye pigment synthesis [89–91].

While the plasmodial receptor or receptors important for signal perception are still unknown, the signalling pathway resulting in gametogenesis has partially been deciphered (**Figure 3**). It has previously been shown that male gametogenesis, during which the activated male microgametocyte forms eight motile flagellar microgametes (a process termed exflagellation), involves a fast increase in intracellular calcium and the second messenger cGMP [92, 93]. Two membrane-integrated guanylyl cyclases (GCα and GCβ) were identified in *Plasmodium*; however, only GCα appears to be important for cGMP synthesis in activated gametocytes [94–97]. The guanylyl cyclase can be stimulated by addition of XA. It has to be clarified, though, if XA acts directly or indirectly on GCα.

While in eukaryotes, cGMP is synthesized by guanylyl cyclases, phosphodiesterases (PDEs), which hydrolyse cGMP to GMP, are in general required for fast down-regulation of the second messenger. In *Plasmodium*, four PDEs, termed PDEα-δ, were identified, and PDEδ is highly expressed in gametocytes [98]. Zaprinast, a PDE inhibitor, is able to stimulate gametogenesis in the absence of XA due to increased cGMP levels [99]. Disruption of the gene encoding for PDEδ, however, impaired egress of *P. falciparum* gametocytes, indicating that a tight regulation of cGMP levels is important for gametogenesis [97].

The increase in cGMP activates the cGMP-dependent protein kinase PKG and chemical inhibition of PKG impairs rounding-up of the activated gametocytes. Since rounding-up is a calcium-independent step and cannot be inhibited by calcium chelators (see below), PKG acts prior to calcium increase in the activated gametocytes [97]. Gametocyte activation further leads to the generation of the second messenger molecules DAG and inositol-(1,4,5)-trisphosphate (IP_3) from phosphatidylinositol-(4,5)-bisphosphate (PIP_2) via the plasmodial phospholipase PI-PLC activity (**Figure 3**), as shown in *P. berghei*. IP_3 synthesis results in a rapid mobilization of calcium from the endoplasmic reticulum [100, 101]. PI-PLC activity itself appears to be regulated by calcium, since it can be impaired by calcium ionophores, pointing to a calcium-regulated feedback mechanism. The increase in cytoplasmic calcium levels is further dependent on PKG activity and quantitative phosphoproteomics demonstrated that PKG is able to phosphorylate enzymes involved in the inositol phospholipid metabolism such as phosphatidylinositol-4-kinase (PI4K) and phosphoatidlyinositol-4-phosphate-5-kinase (PIP5K), which are involved in the synthesis of PIP_2 from phosphatidyl-1D-*myo*-inositol (PI) via phosphatidylinositol-4-phosphate (PI4P) [102].

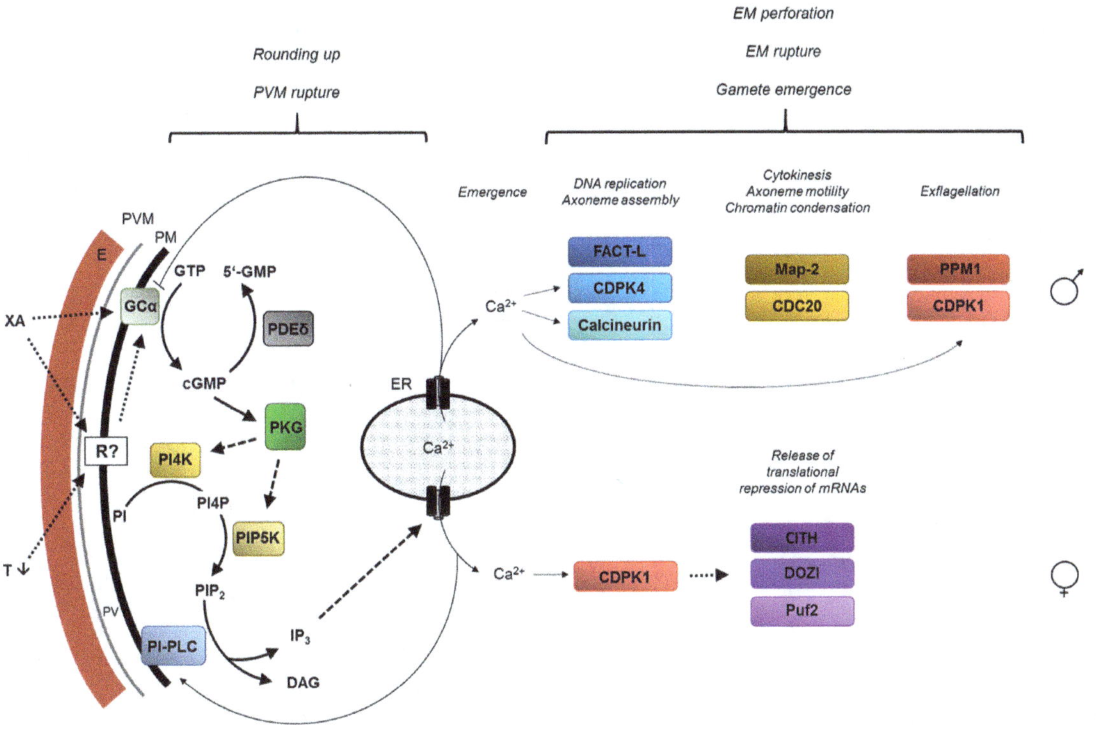

Figure 3. The signalling pathway involved in gametogenesis. Ca^{2+}, calcium ion; CDC20, cell division cycle protein 20; CDPK, calcium-dependent protein kinase; cGMP, cyclic guanosine monophosphate; CITH, homolog of worm CAR-I and fly Trailer Hitch; DAG, diacylglycerol; DNA, deoxyribonucleic acid; DOZI, development of zygote inhibited; E, erythrocyte; EM, erythrocyte membrane; ER endoplasmic reticulum; FACT-L, facilitates chromatin transcription protein L; GC, guanylyl cyclase; 5′-GMP, guanosine monophosphate; GTP, guanosine triphosphate; IP_3, inositol triphosphate; Map-2, mitogen-activated protein kinase 2; mRNA, messenger ribonucleic acid; PDE, phosphodiesterase; PI, phosphatidyl-1D-*myo*-inositol; PI4K, phosphatidylinositol-4-kinase; PI4P, phosphatidylinosito-4-phosphate; PIP_2, phosphatidylinositol-4,5-bisphosphate; PIP5K, phosphatidylinositol-5-kinase; PKG, cGMP-dependent protein kinase; PPM1, metallo-dependent protein phosphatase 1; Puf2, pumilio/FBF (fem-3 binding factor) family protein 2; PV, parasitophorous vacuole; PVM, parasitophorous vacuole membrane; R, receptor; T, temperature; XA, xanthurenic acid.

In activated *P. berghei* microgametocytes, the increase in intracellular calcium was shown to activate the calcium-dependent protein kinases CDPK1 and CDPK4 and parasites lacking CDPK4 are not able to undergo DNA synthesis [103] (**Figure 3**). Further linked to this process is plasmodial FACT-L (facilitates chromatin transcription) [104]. Downstream of DNA replication two more proteins become activated, the mitogen-activated protein kinase MAP2 and the cell division cycle protein CDC20. Loss of MAP2 or CDC20 interferes with chromatin condensation, axoneme motility and cytokinesis [105–107]. Furthermore, depletion of the metallo-dependent protein phosphatase PPM1 or the calcium-dependent phosphatase calcineurin as well as knock-down of CDPK1 result in impaired exflagellation [108–110]. While these combined studies pinpoint some key regulators of gametogenesis, the detailed pathway leading to gametocyte-to-gamete conversion is not known yet.

In female macrogametocytes, activation results in a sudden onset of protein synthesis, which is due to the CDPK1-regulated release of translational repression of messenger RNAs (mRNAs) [108]. In *P. berghei,* a total of 731 mRNAs are associated with two proteins of regulatory ribonucleoprotein complexes, i.e. the RNA helicase DOZI (development of zygote inhibited) and the Sm-like factor CITH (homolog of worm CAR-I and fly Trailer Hitch), which function in translational repression of these transcripts (**Figure 3**). These include the mRNAs encoding for P25, GAP45 and GAP50 [111–113]. For *P. falciparum,* translational repression of mRNAs was shown to involve the Pumilio/FBF (Puf) family RNA-binding protein Puf2 that is required for controlling a number of transcripts in gametocytes including those encoding for P25 and P28 [114]. The repressed mRNAs mostly encode for components of the later ookinete stage.

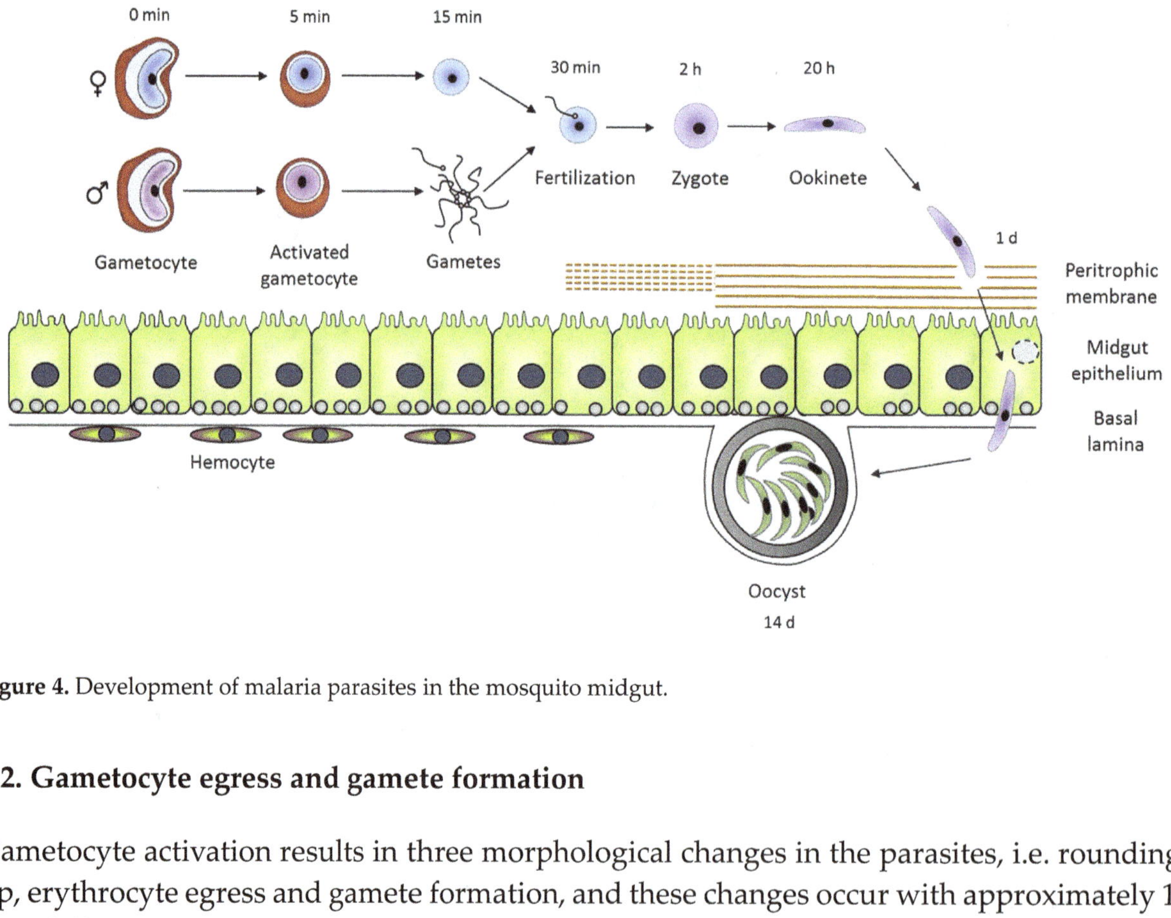

Figure 4. Development of malaria parasites in the mosquito midgut.

5.2. Gametocyte egress and gamete formation

Gametocyte activation results in three morphological changes in the parasites, i.e. rounding-up, erythrocyte egress and gamete formation, and these changes occur with approximately 15 min following perception of the environmental signals (**Figure 4**). Gametocytes exit the erythrocyte via an inside-out mode, during which the parasitophorous vacuolar membrane (PVM) ruptures prior to the opening of the erythrocyte membrane (EM). Rupture of the PVM occurs at multiple sites less than 2 min following signal perception and is accompanied by the rounding-up of the parasite. Both events are calcium-independent [91, 99]. It is suggested that the PVM rupture is linked to the discharge of the osmiophilic body content into the PV, since an accumulation of osmiophilic bodies can be observed underneath the rupture sites [91, 115].

In a second, a calcium-dependent step, another type of vesicle discharges its content into the cytoplasm of the host erythrocyte, which includes the plasmodial pore-forming perforin PPLP2. This perforin is able to permeate the EM, resulting in the release the erythrocyte cytoplasm, eventually leaving the forming gamete enclosed by the EM [115–117]. While EM permeabilization occurs approximately 6 min post-activation, its rupture takes place 9 min later. Here, the EM opens at a single pore and releases the fertile gamete [91, 117].

The IMC disintegrates shortly after onset of gametogenesis, eventually resulting in gametes solely confined by the plasmalemma. It was shown that the transmembrane protein GAP50, which in gametocytes, is located in the outer membrane of the alveoli, relocates to the gamete plasmalemma during gametogenesis. During relocation, the N-terminal part of GAP50 becomes extracellularly exposed and once the gametes have freed from the EM binds complement factor H from the blood meal, a step crucial to protect the newly formed gametes from lysis by human complement factors [42]. Coevally with the IMC degradation long membranous tubules, termed tunneling nanotubes (TNTs), form, which protrude from the gamete surface. TNTs represent long-distance cell-to-cell connections, which were proposed to mediate intercellular contacts between gametes as a pre-requisite for mating [118]. While the question of the origin of the membranous tubules remains unanswered, one might stipulate that after IMC disintegration the alveoli membranes are used for TNT formation.

Upon activation, the male microgametocyte replicates its genome three times and mitotically produces eight flagellar microgametes [119] (**Figure 4**). Flagellum formation requires the axonemal assembly from basal bodies, which involves the centriole/basal body protein SAS-6 [120], while axoneme motility is regulated by the conserved armadillo-repeat protein PF16 [121]. Exflagellating microgametes typically adhere avidly to neighbouring erythrocytes and are hidden within such rosettes. During exflagellation, the microgamete detaches from the residual body and is freely motile in search of a female macrogamete. Once adhering to a macrogamete, fertilization begins by the fusion of the two gamete plasma membranes, and the axoneme and attached male nucleus enter the female cytoplasm. While the exact proteins involved in initial binding of male and female gametes are yet unknown, gamete fusion is mediated by the microgamete-specific protein GCS1 (generative cell specific 1), also termed HAP2 [122, 123]. Over the next 3 hours, meiosis occurs and the zygote becomes tetraploid [119]. The transformation of the zygote into an ookinete is completed at 19–36 hours post-blood meal, and the ookinete then rapidly exits the midgut lumen to settle down at the basal site of the midgut epithelium and to differentiate into an oocyst [124–127]. Parasite tetraploidy persists until sporozoite budding in the oocyst restores the haploid state [119].

6. Conclusion

Although our knowledge of the biology of gametocytes is not as advanced as that of the asexual blood stages, the great interest by researchers in recent years has considerably deepened our understanding of the gametocyte biology. Advances in gametocyte cultivation, isolation and purification techniques as well as the impressive amount of data gained from genome-wide analyses, proteomics and microarray studies have led to the identification of some gametocyte stage-specific antigens as well as sex-specific proteins, which may be exploited as targets for malaria transmission-blocking intervention strategies. In addition, the recent discoveries on the molecular mechanism of gametocyte commitment have greatly improved our knowledge on how sexual differentiation is initiated and regulated in the malaria parasite. However, several questions are still to be answered regarding the biology of gametocytes. The mechanism by which stress factors are perceived to enhance gametocyte commitment is not well understood. Some components of the signalling cascade of gametocyte activation are yet unknown such as the receptor or receptors responsible for signal perception following gametocyte activation by XA. How gametocyte sequestration in the bone marrow takes place as well as the molecular mechanism underlying this phenomenon has to been deciphered. Also, a proper understanding of the mechanism by which the gametocyte rapidly adapts once in the mosquito vector and the basis of fertilization is needed. Furthermore, not much is known about the metabolism of gametocytes. Most of the metabolic pathways have not been described. A proper understanding of these aspects in the biology of gametocytes would greatly improve strategies aimed to target gametocytes.

Author details

Che Julius Ngwa*, Thiago F. de A. Rosa and Gabriele Pradel

*Address all correspondence to: ngwa.che@bio2.rwth-aachen.de

Division of Cellular and Applied Infection Biology, Institute of Zoology, RWTH Aachen University, Aachen, Germany

References

[1] Kuehn A, Pradel G. The coming-out of malaria gametocytes. J Biomed Biotechnol [Internet]. 2010;2010:976827. Available from: http://www.pubmedcentral.nih.gov/articlerender.fcgi?artid=2810480&tool=pmcentrez&rendertype=abstract

[2] Bruce MC, Alano P, Duthie S, Carter R. Commitment of the malaria parasite *Plasmodium falciparum* to sexual and asexual development. Parasitology [Internet]. 1990 Apr [cited 2015 Dec 29];100(Pt 2):191–200. Available from: http://www.ncbi.nlm.nih.gov/pubmed/2189114

[3] Smith TG, Lourenço P, Carter R, Walliker D, Ranford-Cartwright LC. Commitment to sexual differentiation in the human malaria parasite, *Plasmodium falciparum*. Parasitology. 2000;121:127–33.

[4] Silvestrini F, Alano P, Williams JL. Commitment to the production of male and female gametocytes in the human malaria parasite *Plasmodium falciparum*. Parasitology [Internet]. 2000 Nov [cited 2016 Jan 19];121(Pt 5):465–71. Available from: http://www.ncbi.nlm.nih.gov/pubmed/11128797

[5] Chaubey S, Grover M, Tatu U. Endoplasmic reticulum stress triggers gametocytogenesis in the malaria parasite. J Biol Chem. 2014;289(24):16662–74.

[6] Gautret P, Miltgen F, Gantier JC, Chabaud AG, Landau I. Enhanced gametocyte formation by *Plasmodium chabaudi* in immature erythrocytes: pattern of production, sequestration, and infectivity to mosquitoes. J Parasitol [Internet]. 1996 Dec [cited 2016 Apr 5];82(6):900–6. Available from: http://www.ncbi.nlm.nih.gov/pubmed/8973397

[7] Smalley ME, Brown J. *Plasmodium falciparum* gametocytogenesis stimulated by lymphocytes and serum from infected Gambian children. Trans R Soc Trop Med Hyg [Internet]. 1981 Jan [cited 2015 Nov 25];75(2):316–7. Available from: http://www.ncbi.nlm.nih.gov/pubmed/7029805

[8] Trager W, Gill GS. Enhanced gametocyte formation in young erythrocytes by *Plasmodium falciparum* in vitro. J Protozool [Internet]. 1992 Jan [cited 2016 Apr 5];39(3):429–32. Available from: http://www.ncbi.nlm.nih.gov/pubmed/1640389

[9] Schneweis S, Maier WA, Seitz HM. Haemolysis of infected erythrocytes – a trigger for formation of *Plasmodium falciparum* gametocytes? Parasitol Res [Internet]. 1991 Jan [cited 2016 Feb 4];77(5):458–60. Available from: http://www.ncbi.nlm.nih.gov/pubmed/1891456

[10] Lingnau A, Margos G, Maier WA, Seitz HM. The effects of hormones on the gametocytogenesis of *Plasmodium falciparum* in vitro. Appl Parasitol [Internet]. 1993 Sep [cited 2016 Feb 4];34(3):153–60. Available from: http://www.ncbi.nlm.nih.gov/pubmed/8220571

[11] Puta C, Manyando C. Enhanced gametocyte production in Fansidar-treated *Plasmodium falciparum* malaria patients: implications for malaria transmission control programmes. Trop Med Int Health [Internet]. 1997 Mar [cited 2016 Feb 4];2(3):227–9. Available from: http://www.ncbi.nlm.nih.gov/pubmed/9491100

[12] Talman AM, Paul REL, Sokhna CS, Domarle O, Ariey F, Trape J-F, et al. Influence of chemotherapy on the Plasmodium gametocyte sex ratio of mice and humans. Am J Trop Med Hyg [Internet]. 2004 Dec [cited 2016 Feb 4];71(6):739–44. Available from: http://www.ncbi.nlm.nih.gov/pubmed/15642963

[13] Duffy MF, Selvarajah SA, Josling GA, Petter M. Epigenetic regulation of the *Plasmodium falciparum* genome. Brief Funct Genomics. 2014;13(3):203–16.

[14] Josling GA, Llinás M. Sexual development in Plasmodium parasites: knowing when it's time to commit. Nat Rev Microbiol [Internet]. 2015;13(9):573–87. Available from: http://www.ncbi.nlm.nih.gov/pubmed/26272409

[15] Coleman BI, Skillman KM, Jiang RHY, Childs LM, Altenhofen LM, Ganter M, et al. A *Plasmodium falciparum* histone deacetylase regulates antigenic variation and gametocyte conversion. Cell Host Microbe [Internet]. 2014;16(2):177–86. Available from: http://www.sciencedirect.com/science/article/pii/S1931312814002625

[16] Brancucci NMB, Bertschi NL, Zhu L, Niederwieser I, Chin WH, Wampfler R, et al. Heterochromatin protein 1 secures survival and transmission of malaria parasites. Cell Host and Microbe. 2014;16(2):165–76. Available from: http://ac.els-cdn.com/S1931312814002583/1-s2.0-S1931312814002583-main.pdf?_tid=858c21fc-6d44-11e5-9c59-00000aab0f26&acdnat=1444257857_991a4915b9e0c23b300a77dbed1a4edb

[17] Eissenberg JC, James TC, Foster-Hartnett DM, Hartnett T, Ngan V, Elgin SC. Mutation in a heterochromatin-specific chromosomal protein is associated with suppression of position-effect variegation in Drosophila melanogaster. Proc Natl Acad Sci U S A [Internet]. 1990 Dec [cited 2016 Apr 5];87(24):9923–7. Available from: http://www.pubmedcentral.nih.gov/articlerender.fcgi?artid=55286&tool=pmcentrez&rendertype=abstract

[18] Flueck C, Bartfai R, Volz J, Niederwieser I, Salcedo-Amaya AM, Alako BTF, et al. Plasmodium falciparum heterochromatin protein 1 marks genomic loci linked to phenotypic variation of exported virulence factors. PLoS Pathog. 2009;5(9) e1000569.

[19] Kafsack BFC, Rovira-Graells N, Clark TG, Bancells C, Crowley VM, Campino SG, et al. A transcriptional switch underlies commitment to sexual development in malaria parasites. Nature [Internet]. 2014;507(7491):248–52. Available from: http://www.ncbi.nlm.nih.gov/pubmed/24572369

[20] Sinha A, Hughes KR, Modrzynska KK, Otto TD, Pfander C, Dickens NJ, et al. A cascade of DNA-binding proteins for sexual commitment and development in Plasmodium. Nature [Internet]. 2014;507(7491):253–7. Available from: http://www.ncbi.nlm.nih.gov/pubmed/24572359

[21] Lopez-Rubio J-J, Mancio-Silva L, Scherf A. Genome-wide analysis of heterochromatin associates clonally variant gene regulation with perinuclear repressive centers in malaria parasites. Cell Host Microbe [Internet]. 2009 Feb 19 [cited 2016 Apr 5];5(2):179–90. Available from: http://www.ncbi.nlm.nih.gov/pubmed/19218088

[22] Pérez-Toledo K, Rojas-Meza AP, Mancio-Silva L, Hernández-Cuevas NA, Delgadillo DM, Vargas M, et al. Plasmodium falciparum heterochromatin protein 1 binds to tri-methylated histone 3 lysine 9 and is linked to mutually exclusive expression of var genes. Nucleic Acids Res [Internet]. 2009 May [cited 2016 Apr 5];37(8):2596–606. Available from: http://www.pubmedcentral.nih.gov/articlerender.fcgi?artid=2677873&tool=pmcentrez&rendertype=abstract

[23] Balaji S, Babu MM, Iyer LM, Aravind L. Discovery of the principal specific transcription factors of Apicomplexa and their implication for the evolution of the AP2-integrase DNA binding domains. Nucleic Acids Res [Internet]. 2005 Jan [cited 2016 Mar 16];

33(13):3994–4006. Available from: http://www.pubmedcentral.nih.gov/articlerender.fcgi?artid=1178005&tool=pmcentrez&rendertype=abstract

[24] Yuda M, Iwanaga S, Shigenobu S, Mair GR, Janse CJ, Waters AP, et al. Identification of a transcription factor in the mosquito-invasive stage of malaria parasites. Mol Microbiol [Internet]. 2009 Mar [cited 2016 Feb 15];71(6):1402–14. Available from: http://www.ncbi.nlm.nih.gov/pubmed/19220746

[25] Yuda M, Iwanaga S, Shigenobu S, Kato T, Kaneko I. Transcription factor AP2-Sp and its target genes in malarial sporozoites. Mol Microbiol [Internet]. 2010 Feb [cited 2016 Apr 5];75(4):854–63. Available from: http://www.ncbi.nlm.nih.gov/pubmed/20025671

[26] Painter HJ, Campbell TL, Llinás M. The Apicomplexan AP2 family: integral factors regulating Plasmodium development. Mol Biochem Parasitol [Internet]. 2011 Mar [cited 2016 Apr 5];176(1):1–7. Available from: http://www.pubmedcentral.nih.gov/articlerender.fcgi?artid=3026892&tool=pmcentrez&rendertype=abstract

[27] Iwanaga S, Kaneko I, Kato T, Yuda M. Identification of an AP2-family protein that is critical for malaria liver stage development. PLoS One [Internet]. 2012 Jan [cited 2016 Feb 15];7(11):e47557. Available from: http://www.pubmedcentral.nih.gov/articlerender.fcgi?artid=3492389&tool=pmcentrez&rendertype=abstract

[28] Campbell TL, De Silva EK, Olszewski KL, Elemento O, Llinás M. Identification and genome-wide prediction of DNA binding specificities for the ApiAP2 family of regulators from the malaria parasite. PLoS Pathog [Internet]. 2010 Jan [cited 2016 Apr 5];6(10):e1001165. Available from: http://www.pubmedcentral.nih.gov/articlerender.fcgi?artid=2965767&tool=pmcentrez&rendertype=abstract

[29] Sinden RE. Gametocytogenesis of Plasmodium falciparum in vitro: an electron microscopic study. Parasitology [Internet]. 1982 Feb [cited 2016 Apr 6];84(1):1–11. Available from: http://www.ncbi.nlm.nih.gov/pubmed/7038594

[30] Day KP, Hayward RE, Dyer M. The biology of *Plasmodium falciparum* transmission stages. Parasitology [Internet]. 1998;116(Supplement S1):S95–109. Available from: href="http://dx.doi.org/10.1017/S0031182000084985

[31] Dixon MWA, Thompson J, Gardiner DL, Trenholme KR. Sex in Plasmodium: a sign of commitment. Trends Parasitol. 2008;24(4):168–75.

[32] Hawking F, Wilson ME, Gammage K. Evidence for cyclic development and short-lived maturity in the gametocytes of Plasmodium falciparum. Trans R Soc Trop Med Hyg [Internet]. 1971 Jan [cited 2016 Feb 19];65(5):549–59. Available from: http://www.ncbi.nlm.nih.gov/pubmed/5003557

[33] Langreth SG, Jensen JB, Reese RT, Trager W. Fine structure of human malaria in vitro. J Protozool [Internet]. 1978 Nov [cited 2016 Apr 6];25(4):443–52. Available from: http://www.ncbi.nlm.nih.gov/pubmed/105129

[34] Tibúrcio M, Silvestrini F, Bertuccini L, Sander AF, Turner L, Lavstsen T, et al. Early gametocytes of the malaria parasite Plasmodium falciparum specifically remodel the

adhesive properties of infected erythrocyte surface. Cell Microbiol [Internet]. 2013 Apr [cited 2016 Apr 6];15(4):647–59. Available from: http://www.ncbi.nlm.nih.gov/pubmed/23114006

[35] Aguilar R, Magallon-Tejada A, Achtman AH, Moraleda C, Joice R, Cisteró P, et al. Molecular evidence for the localization of Plasmodium falciparum immature gametocytes in bone marrow. Blood [Internet]. 2014 Feb 13 [cited 2016 Apr 6]; 123(7):959–66. Available from: http://www.pubmedcentral.nih.gov/articlerender.fcgi?artid=4067503&tool=pmcentrez&rendertype=abstract

[36] Joice R, Nilsson SK, Montgomery J, Dankwa S, Egan E, Morahan B, et al. Plasmodium falciparum transmission stages accumulate in the human bone marrow. Sci Transl Med [Internet]. 2014 Jul 9 [cited 2016 Feb 19];6(244):244re5. Available from: http://www.pubmedcentral.nih.gov/articlerender.fcgi?artid=4175394&tool=pmcentrez&rendertype=abstract

[37] Guerra CA, Howes RE, Patil AP, Gething PW, Van Boeckel TP, Temperley WH, et al. The international limits and population at risk of Plasmodium vivax transmission in 2009. PLoS Negl Trop Dis [Internet]. 2010 Jan [cited 2016 Feb 26];4(8):e774. Available from: http://www.pubmedcentral.nih.gov/articlerender.fcgi?artid=2914753&tool=pmcentrez&rendertype=abstract

[38] Bousema T, Drakeley C. Epidemiology and infectivity of Plasmodium falciparum and Plasmodium vivax gametocytes in relation to malaria control and elimination. Clin Microbiol Rev [Internet]. 2011;24(2):377–410. Available from: http://cmr.asm.org/cgi/doi/10.1128/CMR.00051-10

[39] Harding CR, Meissner M. The inner membrane complex through development of Toxoplasma gondii and Plasmodium. Cell Microbiol [Internet]. 2014 May [cited 2016 Feb 19];16(5):632–41. Available from: http://www.pubmedcentral.nih.gov/articlerender.fcgi?artid=4286798&tool=pmcentrez&rendertype=abstract

[40] Dearnley MK, Yeoman JA, Hanssen E, Kenny S, Turnbull L, Whitchurch CB, et al. Origin, composition, organization and function of the inner membrane complex of Plasmodium falciparum gametocytes. J Cell Sci [Internet]. 2012 Apr 15 [cited 2016 Apr 7];125(Pt 8):2053–63. Available from: http://www.ncbi.nlm.nih.gov/pubmed/22328505

[41] Kono M, Herrmann S, Loughran NB, Cabrera A, Engelberg K, Lehmann C, et al. Evolution and architecture of the inner membrane complex in asexual and sexual stages of the malaria parasite. Mol Biol Evol [Internet]. 2012;29(9):2113–32. Available from: http://mbe.oxfordjournals.org/cgi/doi/10.1093/molbev/mss081

[42] Simon N, Lasonder E, Scheuermayer M, Kuehn A, Tews S, Fischer R, et al. Malaria parasites co-opt human factor h to prevent complement-mediated lysis in the mosquito midgut. Cell Host Microbe [Internet]. 2013;13(1):29–41. Available from: http://dx.doi.org/10.1016/j.chom.2012.11.013

[43] Boucher LE, Bosch J. The apicomplexan glideosome and adhesins – structures and function. J Struct Biol [Internet]. 2015 May [cited 2015 Jun 25];190(2):93–114. Available from: http://www.ncbi.nlm.nih.gov/pubmed/25764948

[44] Hliscs M, Millet C, Dixon MW, Siden-Kiamos I, McMillan P, Tilley L. Organization and function of an actin cytoskeleton in Plasmodium falciparum gametocytes. Cell Microbiol [Internet]. 2015 Feb [cited 2016 Apr 7];17(2):207–25. Available from: http://www.ncbi.nlm.nih.gov/pubmed/25224798

[45] Florens L, Washburn MP, Raine JD, Anthony RM, Grainger M, Haynes JD, et al. A proteomic view of the Plasmodium falciparum life cycle. Nature [Internet]. 2002;419(6906):520–6. Available from: http://www.ncbi.nlm.nih.gov/pubmed/12368866

[46] Lasonder E, Ishihama Y, Andersen JS, Vermunt AMW, Pain A, Sauerwein RW, et al. Analysis of the Plasmodium falciparum proteome by high-accuracy mass spectrometry. Nature [Internet]. 2002 Oct 3 [cited 2016 Apr 7];419(6906):537–42. Available from: http://www.ncbi.nlm.nih.gov/pubmed/12368870

[47] Scholz SM, Simon N, Lavazec C, Dude MA, Templeton TJ, Pradel G. PfCCp proteins of Plasmodium falciparum: gametocyte-specific expression and role in complement-mediated inhibition of exflagellation. Int J Parasitol. 2008;38(3–4):327–40.

[48] Simon N, Scholz SM, Moreira CK, Templeton TJ, Kuehn A, Dude M-A, et al. Sexual stage adhesion proteins form multi-protein complexes in the malaria parasite Plasmodium falciparum. J Biol Chem [Internet]. 2009;284(21):14537–46. Available from: http://www.pubmedcentral.nih.gov/articlerender.fcgi?artid=2682902&tool=pmcentrez&rendertype=abstract

[49] Kuehn A, Simon N, Pradel G. Family members stick together: multi-protein complexes of malaria parasites. Med Microbiol Immunol. 2010;199(3):209–26.

[50] Pradel G. Proteins of the malaria parasite sexual stages: expression, function and potential for transmission blocking strategies. Parasitology. 2007;134(Pt. 14):1911–29.

[51] Moelans II, Meis JF, Kocken C, Konings RN, Schoenmakers JG. A novel protein antigen of the malaria parasite Plasmodium falciparum, located on the surface of gametes and sporozoites. Mol Biochem Parasitol [Internet]. 1991 Apr [cited 2016 Apr 7];45(2):193–204. Available from: http://www.ncbi.nlm.nih.gov/pubmed/2038355

[52] Bruce MC, Carter RN, Nakamura K, Aikawa M, Carter R. Cellular location and temporal expression of the Plasmodium falciparum sexual stage antigen Pfs16. Mol Biochem Parasitol [Internet]. 1994 May [cited 2016 Apr 7];65(1):11–22. Available from: http://www.ncbi.nlm.nih.gov/pubmed/7935618

[53] Baker DA, Daramola O, McCrossan MV, Harmer J, Targett GA. Subcellular localization of Pfs16, a Plasmodium falciparum gametocyte antigen. Parasitology [Internet]. 1994 Feb [cited 2016 Apr 7];108(Pt 2):129–37. Available from: http://www.ncbi.nlm.nih.gov/pubmed/8159458

[54] Kongkasuriyachai D, Fujioka H, Kumar N. Functional analysis of Plasmodium falciparum parasitophorous vacuole membrane protein (Pfs16) during gametocytogenesis and gametogenesis by targeted gene disruption. Mol Biochem Parasitol [Internet]. 2004 Feb [cited 2016 Apr 7];133(2):275–85. Available from: http://www.ncbi.nlm.nih.gov/pubmed/14698439

[55] Sharma A, Sharma I, Kogkasuriyachai D, Kumar N. Structure of a gametocyte protein essential for sexual development in Plasmodium falciparum. Nat Struct Biol [Internet]. 2003 Mar [cited 2016 Apr 7];10(3):197–203. Available from: http://www.ncbi.nlm.nih.gov/pubmed/12577051

[56] Olivieri A, Camarda G, Bertuccini L, van de Vegte-Bolmer M, Luty AJF, Sauerwein R, et al. The Plasmodium falciparum protein Pfg27 is dispensable for gametocyte and gamete production, but contributes to cell integrity during gametocytogenesis. Mol Microbiol [Internet]. 2009 Jul [cited 2016 Apr 7];73(2):180–93. Available from: http://www.ncbi.nlm.nih.gov/pubmed/19570101

[57] Pradel G. A multidomain adhesion protein family expressed in plasmodium falciparum is essential for transmission to the mosquito. J Exp Med [Internet]. 2004;199(11):1533–44. Available from: http://www.jem.org/cgi/doi/10.1084/jem.20031274

[58] Pradel G, Wagner C, Mejia C, Templeton TJ. Plasmodium falciparum: co-dependent expression and co-localization of the PfCCp multi-adhesion domain proteins. Exp Parasitol [Internet]. 2006;112(4):263–8. Available from: http://www.ncbi.nlm.nih.gov/pubmed/16388802

[59] van Dijk MR, Janse CJ, Thompson J, Waters AP, Braks JA, Dodemont HJ, et al. A central role for P48/45 in malaria parasite male gamete fertility. Cell [Internet]. 2001 Jan 12 [cited 2016 Apr 7];104(1):153–64. Available from: http://www.ncbi.nlm.nih.gov/pubmed/11163248

[60] Eksi S, Czesny B, van Gemert G-J, Sauerwein RW, Eling W, Williamson KC. Malaria transmission-blocking antigen, Pfs230, mediates human red blood cell binding to exflagellating male parasites and oocyst production. Mol Microbiol [Internet]. 2006;61(4):991–8. Available from: http://doi.wiley.com/10.1111/j.1365-2958.2006.05284.x

[61] de Koning-Ward TF, Olivieri A, Bertuccini L, Hood A, Silvestrini F, Charvalias K, et al. The role of osmiophilic bodies and Pfg377 expression in female gametocyte emergence and mosquito infectivity in the human malaria parasite Plasmodium falciparum. Mol Microbiol [Internet]. 2008 Jan [cited 2016 Apr 7];67(2):278–90. Available from: http://www.ncbi.nlm.nih.gov/pubmed/18086189

[62] Suaréz-Cortés P, Silvestrini F, Alano P. A fast, non-invasive, quantitative staining protocol provides insights in Plasmodium falciparum gamete egress and in the role of osmiophilic bodies. Malar J [Internet]. 2014 Jan [cited

2016 Apr 6];13:389. Available from: http://www.pubmedcentral.nih.gov/articlerender.fcgi?artid=4194377&tool=pmcentrez&rendertype=abstract

[63] Furuya T, Mu J, Hayton K, Liu A, Duan J, Nkrumah L, et al. Disruption of a Plasmodium falciparum gene linked to male sexual development causes early arrest in gametocytogenesis. Proc Natl Acad Sci U S A [Internet]. 2005 Nov 15 [cited 2016 Apr 6];102(46): 16813–8. Available from: http://www.pubmedcentral.nih.gov/articlerender.fcgi?artid=1277966&tool=pmcentrez&rendertype=abstract

[64] Rawlings DJ, Fujioka H, Fried M, Keister DB, Aikawa M, Kaslow DC. Alpha-tubulin II is a male-specific protein in Plasmodium falciparum. Mol Biochem Parasitol [Internet]. 1992 Dec [cited 2016 Apr 7];56(2):239–50. Available from: http://www.ncbi.nlm.nih.gov/pubmed/1484548

[65] Guinet F, Dvorak JA, Fujioka H, Keister DB, Muratova O, Kaslow DC, et al. A developmental defect in Plasmodium falciparum male gametogenesis. J Cell Biol [Internet]. 1996 Oct [cited 2016 Apr 7];135(1):269–78. Available from: http://www.pubmedcentral.nih.gov/articlerender.fcgi?artid=2121010&tool=pmcentrez&rendertype=abstract

[66] Deligianni E, Morgan RN, Bertuccini L, Kooij TW, Laforge A, Nahar C, et al. Critical role for a stage-specific actin in male exflagellation of the malaria parasite. Cell Microbiol [Internet]. 2011;13(11):1714–30. Available from: http://www.ncbi.nlm.nih.gov/pubmed/21790945

[67] Eksi S, Williamson KC. Male-specific expression of the paralog of malaria transmission-blocking target antigen Pfs230, PfB0400w. Mol Biochem Parasitol [Internet]. 2002 Jul [cited 2016 Apr 7];122(2):127–30. Available from: http://www.ncbi.nlm.nih.gov/pubmed/12106866

[68] Doi M, Tanabe K, Tachibana S-I, Hamai M, Tachibana M, Mita T, et al. Worldwide sequence conservation of transmission-blocking vaccine candidate Pvs230 in Plasmodium vivax. Vaccine [Internet]. 2011 Jun 10 [cited 2016 Apr 26];29(26):4308–15. Available from: http://www.pubmedcentral.nih.gov/articlerender.fcgi?artid=3130600&tool=pmcentrez&rendertype=abstract

[69] Tachibana M, Sato C, Otsuki H, Sattabongkot J, Kaneko O, Torii M, et al. Plasmodium vivax gametocyte protein Pvs230 is a transmission-blocking vaccine candidate. Vaccine [Internet]. 2012;30(10):1807–12. Available from: http://linkinghub.elsevier.com/retrieve/pii/S0264410X12000047

[70] Tachibana M, Suwanabun N, Kaneko O, Iriko H, Otsuki H, Sattabongkot J, et al. Plasmodium vivax gametocyte proteins, Pvs48/45 and Pvs47, induce transmission-reducing antibodies by DNA immunization. Vaccine [Internet]. 2015 Apr 15 [cited 2016 Apr 26];33(16):1901–8. Available from: http://www.ncbi.nlm.nih.gov/pubmed/25765968

[71] Talman AM, Domarle O, McKenzie FE, Ariey F, Robert V. Gametocytogenesis: the puberty of Plasmodium falciparum. Malar J [Internet]. 2004 Jul 14 [cited 2016 Apr 7];

3:24. Available from: http://www.pubmedcentral.nih.gov/articlerender.fcgi?artid=497046&tool=pmcentrez&rendertype=abstract

[72] Baker DA. Malaria gametocytogenesis. Mol Biochem Parasitol [Internet]. 2010;172(2): 57–65. Available from: http://dx.doi.org/10.1016/j.molbiopara.2010.03.019

[73] Ben Mamoun C, Prigge ST, Vial H. Targeting the lipid metabolic pathways for the treatment of malaria. Drug Dev Res [Internet]. 2010 Feb [cited 2016 Apr 7];71(1):44–55. Available from: http://www.pubmedcentral.nih.gov/articlerender.fcgi?artid=2886290&tool=pmcentrez&rendertype=abstract

[74] Gulati S, Ekland EH, Ruggles KV, Chan RB, Jayabalasingham B, Zhou B, et al. Profiling the essential nature of lipid metabolism in asexual blood and gametocyte stages of Plasmodium falciparum. Cell Host Microbe [Internet]. 2015 Sep 9 [cited 2016 Mar 27];18(3):371–81. Available from: http://www.ncbi.nlm.nih.gov/pubmed/26355219

[75] Tran PN, Brown SHJ, Rug M, Ridgway MC, Mitchell TW, Maier AG. Changes in lipid composition during sexual development of the malaria parasite Plasmodium falciparum. Malar J [Internet]. 2016 Jan [cited 2016 Apr 7];15(1):73. Available from: http://www.pubmedcentral.nih.gov/articlerender.fcgi?artid=4744411&tool=pmcentrez&rendertype=abstract

[76] Raabe AC, Billker O, Vial HJ, Wengelnik K. Quantitative assessment of DNA replication to monitor microgametogenesis in Plasmodium berghei. Mol Biochem Parasitol [Internet]. 2009 Dec [cited 2016 Apr 7];168(2):172–6. Available from: http://www.pubmedcentral.nih.gov/articlerender.fcgi?artid=2789244&tool=pmcentrez&rendertype=abstract

[77] Canning EU, Sinden RE. Nuclear organisation in gametocytes of Plasmodium and Hepatocystis: a cytochemical study. Zeitschrift für Parasitenkd (Berlin, Ger [Internet]. 1975 Jul 16 [cited 2016 Apr 7];46(4):297–9. Available from: http://www.ncbi.nlm.nih.gov/pubmed/812282

[78] Sinden RE, Canning EU, Bray RS, Smalley ME. Gametocyte and gamete development in Plasmodium falciparum. Proc R Soc London Ser B, Biol Sci [Internet]. 1978 Jun 5 [cited 2016 Apr 7];201(1145):375–99. Available from: http://www.ncbi.nlm.nih.gov/pubmed/27809

[79] Waters AP, Syin C, McCutchan TF. Developmental regulation of stage-specific ribosome populations in Plasmodium. Nature [Internet]. 1989 Nov 23 [cited 2016 Apr 7];342(6248):438–40. Available from: http://www.ncbi.nlm.nih.gov/pubmed/2586613

[80] Khan SM, Franke-Fayard B, Mair GR, Lasonder E, Janse CJ, Mann M, et al. Proteome analysis of separated male and female gametocytes reveals novel sex-specific Plasmodium biology. Cell [Internet]. 2005;121(5):675–87. Available from: http://linkinghub.elsevier.com/retrieve/pii/S0092867405002990

[81] Petmitr S, Krungkrai J. Mitochondrial cytochrome b gene in two developmental stages of human malarial parasite Plasmodium falciparum. Southeast Asian J Trop Med Public Health [Internet]. 1995 Dec [cited 2016 Apr 7];26(4):600–5. Available from: http://www.ncbi.nlm.nih.gov/pubmed/9139360

[82] Crofts AR. The cytochrome bc1 complex: function in the context of structure. Annu Rev Physiol [Internet]. 2004 Jan [cited 2016 Apr 7];66:689–733. Available from: http://www.ncbi.nlm.nih.gov/pubmed/14977419

[83] Fry M, Pudney M. Site of action of the antimalarial hydroxynaphthoquinone, 2-[trans-4-(4′-chlorophenyl) cyclohexyl]-3-hydroxy-1,4-naphthoquinone (566C80). Biochem Pharmacol [Internet]. 1992 Apr 1 [cited 2016 Apr 7];43(7):1545–53. Available from: http://www.ncbi.nlm.nih.gov/pubmed/1314606

[84] Fisher N, Abd Majid R, Antoine T, Al-Helal M, Warman AJ, Johnson DJ, et al. Cytochrome b mutation Y268S conferring atovaquone resistance phenotype in malaria parasite results in reduced parasite bc1 catalytic turnover and protein expression. J Biol Chem [Internet]. 2012 Mar 23 [cited 2016 Mar 13];287(13):9731–41. Available from: http://www.pubmedcentral.nih.gov/articlerender.fcgi?artid=3322985&tool=pmcentrez&rendertype=abstract

[85] Siregar JE, Kurisu G, Kobayashi T, Matsuzaki M, Sakamoto K, Mi-ichi F, et al. Direct evidence for the atovaquone action on the Plasmodium cytochrome bc1 complex. Parasitol Int [Internet]. 2015 Jun [cited 2016 Mar 22];64(3):295–300. Available from: http://www.ncbi.nlm.nih.gov/pubmed/25264100

[86] Butterworth AS, Skinner-Adams TS, Gardiner DL, Trenholme KR. Plasmodium falciparum gametocytes: with a view to a kill. Parasitology [Internet]. 2013 Dec [cited 2016 Apr 7];140(14):1718–34. Available from: http://www.ncbi.nlm.nih.gov/pubmed/23953486

[87] Sherman IW. Biochemistry of Plasmodium (malarial parasites). Microbiol Rev [Internet]. 1979 Dec [cited 2016 Apr 7];43(4):453–95. Available from: http://www.pubmedcentral.nih.gov/articlerender.fcgi?artid=281489&tool=pmcentrez&rendertype=abstract

[88] MacRae JI, Dixon MW, Dearnley MK, Chua HH, Chambers JM, Kenny S, et al. Mitochondrial metabolism of sexual and asexual blood stages of the malaria parasite Plasmodium falciparum. BMC Biol [Internet]. 2013 Jan [cited 2016 Apr 7];11:67. Available from: http://www.pubmedcentral.nih.gov/articlerender.fcgi?artid=3704724&tool=pmcentrez&rendertype=abstract

[89] Billker O, Lindo V, Panico M, Etienne AE, Paxton T, Dell A, et al. Identification of xanthurenic acid as the putative inducer of malaria development in the mosquito. Nature [Internet]. 1998 Mar 19 [cited 2016 Apr 5];392(6673):289–92. Available from: http://www.ncbi.nlm.nih.gov/pubmed/9521324

[90] Garcia GE, Wirtz RA, Barr JR, Woolfitt A, Rosenberg R. Xanthurenic acid induces gametogenesis in Plasmodium, the malaria parasite. J Biol Chem [Internet]. 1998 May

15 [cited 2016 Apr 5];273(20):12003–5. Available from: http://www.ncbi.nlm.nih.gov/pubmed/9575140

[91] Sologub L, Kuehn A, Kern S, Przyborski J, Schillig R, Pradel G. Malaria proteases mediate inside-out egress of gametocytes from red blood cells following parasite transmission to the mosquito. Cell Microbiol. 2011;13(6):897–912.

[92] Kawamoto F, Alejo-Blanco R, Fleck SL, Kawamoto Y, Sinden RE. Possible roles of Ca2+ and cGMP as mediators of the exflagellation of Plasmodium berghei and Plasmodium falciparum. Mol Biochem Parasitol [Internet]. 1990 Aug [cited 2016 Apr 5];42(1):101–8. Available from: http://www.ncbi.nlm.nih.gov/pubmed/2172816

[93] Kawamoto F, Fujioka H, Murakami R, Syafruddin, Hagiwara M, Ishikawa T, et al. The roles of Ca2+/calmodulin- and cGMP-dependent pathways in gametogenesis of a rodent malaria parasite, Plasmodium berghei. Eur J Cell Biol [Internet]. 1993 Feb [cited 2016 Apr 5];60(1):101–7. Available from: http://www.ncbi.nlm.nih.gov/pubmed/8385016

[94] Carucci DJ, Witney AA, Muhia DK, Warhurst DC, Schaap P, Meima M, et al. Guanylyl cyclase activity associated with putative bifunctional integral membrane proteins in Plasmodium falciparum. J Biol Chem [Internet]. 2000 Jul 21 [cited 2016 Apr 5];275(29): 22147–56. Available from: http://www.ncbi.nlm.nih.gov/pubmed/10747978

[95] Muhia DK, Swales CA, Deng W, Kelly JM, Baker DA. The gametocyte-activating factor xanthurenic acid stimulates an increase in membrane-associated guanylyl cyclase activity in the human malaria parasite Plasmodium falciparum. Mol Microbiol [Internet]. 2001 Oct [cited 2016 Apr 5];42(2):553–60. Available from: http://www.ncbi.nlm.nih.gov/pubmed/11703675

[96] Hirai M, Arai M, Kawai S, Matsuoka H. PbGCbeta is essential for Plasmodium ookinete motility to invade midgut cell and for successful completion of parasite life cycle in mosquitoes. J Biochem [Internet]. 2006 Nov [cited 2016 Apr 5];140(5):747–57. Available from: http://www.ncbi.nlm.nih.gov/pubmed/17030505

[97] Taylor CJ, McRobert L, Baker DA. Disruption of a Plasmodium falciparum cyclic nucleotide phosphodiesterase gene causes aberrant gametogenesis. Mol Microbiol [Internet]. 2008 Jul [cited 2016 Apr 5];69(1):110–8. Available from: http://www.pubmedcentral.nih.gov/articlerender.fcgi?artid=2615252&tool=pmcentrez&rendertype=abstract

[98] Young JA, Fivelman QL, Blair PL, de la Vega P, Le Roch KG, Zhou Y, et al. The Plasmodium falciparum sexual development transcriptome: a microarray analysis using ontology-based pattern identification. Mol Biochem Parasitol [Internet]. 2005;143(1): 67–79. Available from: http://linkinghub.elsevier.com/retrieve/pii/S0166685105001623

[99] McRobert L, Taylor CJ, Deng W, Fivelman QL, Cummings RM, Polley SD, et al. Gametogenesis in malaria parasites is mediated by the cGMP-dependent protein

kinase. PLoS Biol [Internet]. 2008;6(6):e139. Available from: http://biology.plosjournals.org/perlserv/?request=get-document&doi=10.1371/journal.pbio.0060139

[100] Martin JV, Nagele RG, Lee HY. Temporal changes in intracellular free calcium levels in the developing neuroepithelium during neurulation in the chick. Comp Biochem Physiol Comp Physiol [Internet]. 1994 Apr [cited 2016 Apr 5];107(4):655–9. Available from: http://www.ncbi.nlm.nih.gov/pubmed/7911410

[101] Raabe A, Berry L, Sollelis L, Cerdan R, Tawk L, Vial HJ, et al. Genetic and transcriptional analysis of phosphoinositide-specific phospholipase C in Plasmodium. Exp Parasitol [Internet]. 2011 Sep [cited 2016 Apr 5];129(1):75–80. Available from: http://www.ncbi.nlm.nih.gov/pubmed/21651909

[102] Brochet M, Collins MO, Smith TK, Thompson E, Sebastian S, Volkmann K, et al. Phosphoinositide metabolism links cGMP-dependent protein kinase G to essential Ca^{2+} signals at key decision points in the life cycle of malaria parasites. PLoS Biol [Internet]. 2014 Mar [cited 2016 Mar 24];12(3):e1001806. Available from: http://www.pubmedcentral.nih.gov/articlerender.fcgi?artid=3942320&tool=pmcentrez&rendertype=abstract

[103] Billker O, Dechamps S, Tewari R, Wenig G, Franke-Fayard B, Brinkmann V. Calcium and a calcium-dependent protein kinase regulate gamete formation and mosquito transmission in a malaria parasite. Cell. 2004;117(4):503–14.

[104] Laurentino EC, Taylor S, Mair GR, Lasonder E, Bartfai R, Stunnenberg HG, et al. Experimentally controlled downregulation of the histone chaperone FACT in Plasmodium berghei reveals that it is critical to male gamete fertility. Cell Microbiol [Internet]. 2011 Dec [cited 2016 Apr 5];13(12):1956–74. Available from: http://www.pubmedcentral.nih.gov/articlerender.fcgi?artid=3429858&tool=pmcentrez&rendertype=abstract

[105] Rangarajan R, Bei AK, Jethwaney D, Maldonado P, Dorin D, Sultan AA, et al. A mitogen-activated protein kinase regulates male gametogenesis and transmission of the malaria parasite Plasmodium berghei. EMBO Rep [Internet]. 2005 May [cited 2016 Apr 6];6(5):464–9. Available from: http://www.pubmedcentral.nih.gov/articlerender.fcgi?artid=1299310&tool=pmcentrez&rendertype=abstract

[106] Tewari R, Dorin D, Moon R, Doerig C, Billker O. An atypical mitogen-activated protein kinase controls cytokinesis and flagellar motility during male gamete formation in a malaria parasite. Mol Microbiol. 2005;58(5):1253–63.

[107] Guttery DS, Ferguson DJP, Poulin B, Xu Z, Straschil U, Klop O, et al. A putative homologue of CDC20/CDH1 in the malaria parasite is essential for male gamete development. PLoS Pathog [Internet]. 2012 Feb [cited 2016 Apr 6];8(2):e1002554. Available from: http://www.pubmedcentral.nih.gov/articlerender.fcgi?artid=3285604&tool=pmcentrez&rendertype=abstract

[108] Sebastian S, Brochet M, Collins MO, Schwach F, Jones ML, Goulding D, et al. A Plasmodium calcium-dependent protein kinase controls zygote development and

transmission by translationally activating pepressed mRNAs. Cell Host Microbe. 2012;12(1):9–19.

[109] Guttery DS, Poulin B, Ramaprasad A, Wall RJ, Ferguson DJP, Brady D, et al. Genome-wide functional analysis of Plasmodium protein phosphatases reveals key regulators of parasite development and differentiation. Cell Host Microbe [Internet]. 2014 Jul 9 [cited 2016 Apr 6];16(1):128–40. Available from: http://www.pubmedcentral.nih.gov/articlerender.fcgi?artid=4094981&tool=pmcentrez&rendertype=abstract

[110] Philip N, Waters AP. Conditional degradation of Plasmodium calcineurin reveals functions in parasite colonization of both host and vector. Cell Host Microbe [Internet]. 2015 Jul 8 [cited 2015 Dec 29];18(1):122–31. Available from: http://www.pubmedcentral.nih.gov/articlerender.fcgi?artid=4509507&tool=pmcentrez&rendertype=abstract

[111] Mair GR. Regulation of sexual development of plasmodium by translational repression. Science (80-) [Internet]. 2006;313(5787):667–9. Available from: http://www.sciencemag.org/cgi/doi/10.1126/science.1125129

[112] Mair GR, Lasonder E, Garver LS, Franke-Fayard BMD, Carret CK, Wiegant JCAG, et al. Universal features of post-transcriptional gene regulation are critical for plasmodium zygote development. PLoS Pathog [Internet]. 2010;6(2):e1000767. Available from: http://dx.plos.org/10.1371/journal.ppat.1000767

[113] Guerreiro A, Deligianni E, Santos JM, Silva PAGC, Louis C, Pain A, et al. Genome-wide RIP-Chip analysis of translational repressor-bound mRNAs in the Plasmodium gametocyte. Genome Biol [Internet]. 2014 Jan [cited 2016 Apr 6]; 15(11):493. Available from: http://www.pubmedcentral.nih.gov/articlerender.fcgi?artid=4234863&tool=pmcentrez&rendertype=abstract

[114] Miao J, Fan Q, Parker D, Li X, Li J, Cui L. Puf mediates translation repression of transmission-blocking vaccine candidates in malaria parasites. PLoS Pathog [Internet]. 2013 Jan [cited 2016 Apr 6];9(4):e1003268. Available from: http://www.pubmedcentral.nih.gov/articlerender.fcgi?artid=3630172&tool=pmcentrez&rendertype=abstract

[115] Wirth CC, Pradel G. Molecular mechanisms of host cell egress by malaria parasites. Int J Med Microbiol [Internet]. 2012;302(4–5):172–8. Available from: http://linkinghub.elsevier.com/retrieve/pii/S1438422112000318

[116] Deligianni E, Morgan RN, Bertuccini L, Wirth CC, Silmon de Monerri NC, Spanos L, et al. A perforin-like protein mediates disruption of the erythrocyte membrane during egress of Plasmodium berghei male gametocytes. Cell Microbiol [Internet]. 2013 Aug [cited 2016 Apr 6];15(8):1438–55. Available from: http://www.ncbi.nlm.nih.gov/pubmed/23461714

[117] Wirth CC, Glushakova S, Scheuermayer M, Repnik U, Garg S, Schaack D, et al. Perforin-like protein PPLP2 permeabilizes the red blood cell membrane during egress of Plasmodium falciparum gametocytes. Cell Microbiol. 2014;16(5):709–33.

[118] Rupp I, Sologub L, Williamson KC, Scheuermayer M, Reininger L, Doerig C, et al. Malaria parasites form filamentous cell-to-cell connections during reproduction in the mosquito midgut. Cell Res [Internet]. 2011;21(4):683–96. Available from: http://www.pubmedcentral.nih.gov/articlerender.fcgi?artid=3072464&tool=pmcentrez&rendertype=abstract\nhttp://dx.doi.org/10.1038/cr.2010.176

[119] Janse CJ, Van der Klooster PF, Van der Kaay HJ, Van der Ploeg M, Overdulve JP. Rapid repeated DNA replication during microgametogenesis and DNA synthesis in young zygotes of Plasmodium berghei. Trans R Soc Trop Med Hyg [Internet]. 1986 Jan [cited 2016 Apr 6];80(1):154–7. Available from: http://www.ncbi.nlm.nih.gov/pubmed/3088783

[120] Marques SR, Ramakrishnan C, Carzaniga R, Blagborough AM, Delves MJ, Talman AM, et al. An essential role of the basal body protein SAS-6 in Plasmodium male gamete development and malaria transmission. Cell Microbiol [Internet]. 2015 Feb [cited 2016 Apr 6];17(2):191–206. Available from: http://www.pubmedcentral.nih.gov/articlerender.fcgi?artid=4441282&tool=pmcentrez&rendertype=abstract

[121] Straschil U, Talman AM, Ferguson DJP, Bunting KA, Xu Z, Bailes E, et al. The Armadillo repeat protein PF16 is essential for flagellar structure and function in Plasmodium male gametes. PLoS One [Internet]. 2010 Jan [cited 2016 Apr 6];5(9):e12901. Available from: http://www.pubmedcentral.nih.gov/articlerender.fcgi?artid=2944832&tool=pmcentrez&rendertype=abstract

[122] Hirai M, Arai M, Mori T, Miyagishima S-Y, Kawai S, Kita K, et al. Male fertility of malaria parasites is determined by GCS1, a plant-type reproduction factor. Curr Biol [Internet]. 2008 Apr 22 [cited 2016 Apr 6];18(8):607–13. Available from: http://www.ncbi.nlm.nih.gov/pubmed/18403203

[123] Liu Y, Tewari R, Ning J, Blagborough AM, Garbom S, Pei J, et al. The conserved plant sterility gene HAP2 functions after attachment of fusogenic membranes in Chlamydomonas and Plasmodium gametes. Genes Dev [Internet]. 2008 Apr 15 [cited 2016 Apr 6];22(8):1051–68. Available from: http://www.pubmedcentral.nih.gov/articlerender.fcgi?artid=2335326&tool=pmcentrez&rendertype=abstract

[124] Aikawa M, Schwartz A, Uni S, Nussenzweig R, Hollingdale M. Ultrastructure of in vitro cultured exoerythrocytic stage of Plasmodium berghei in a hepatoma cell line. Am J Trop Med Hyg [Internet]. 1984 Sep [cited 2016 Apr 6];33(5):792–9. Available from: http://www.ncbi.nlm.nih.gov/pubmed/6091467

[125] Sinden RE. Molecular interactions between Plasmodium and its insect vectors. Cell Microbiol [Internet]. 2002 Nov [cited 2016 Apr 6];4(11):713–24. Available from: http://www.ncbi.nlm.nih.gov/pubmed/12427094

[126] Sinden RE, Hartley RH, Winger L. The development of Plasmodium ookinetes in vitro: an ultrastructural study including a description of meiotic division. Parasitology

[Internet]. 1985 Oct [cited 2016 Feb 22];91(Pt 2):227–44. Available from: http://www.ncbi.nlm.nih.gov/pubmed/3906519

[127] Vlachou D, Zimmermann T, Cantera R, Janse CJ, Waters AP, Kafatos FC. Real-time, in vivo analysis of malaria ookinete locomotion and mosquito midgut invasion. Cell Microbiol [Internet]. 2004 Jul [cited 2016 Feb 11];6(7):671–85. Available from: http://www.ncbi.nlm.nih.gov/pubmed/15186403

9

Resting Behaviour of Deltamethrin-Resistant Malaria Vectors, *Anopheles arabiensis* and *Anopheles coluzzii*, from North Cameroon: Upshots from a Two-Level Ordinary Logit Model

Josiane Etang, Betrand Fesuh Nono,
Parfait Awono-Ambene, Jude Bigoga,
Wolfgang Ekoko Eyisap, Michael Piameu,
Jean-Claude Toto, Eugène Patrice Ndong Nguema,
Henri Gwet, Etienne Fondjo and
Abraham Peter Mnzava

Abstract

The current study was conducted in Garoua, Pitoa, and Mayo-Oulo health districts of north Cameroon, in order to investigate the resting behaviour of deltamethrin-resistant *Anopheles* (*An.*) *gambiae s.l.* populations and build a model of their response to the use of Permanet 2.0 long-lasting insecticidal nets (LLINs). Adult mosquitoes were collected in October and November 2011, using spray catches and window exit traps in 29 clusters with LLINs in use. Sampled *An. gambiae s.l.* were identified down to species and analysed for blood-meal origin, physiological and circumsporozoite protein status. Deltamethrin resistance was assessed using World Health Organization's (WHO's) standard protocol. A two-level ordinary logit model was used to relate the resting behaviour and deltamethrin resistance. Identified species of the *An. gambiae* complex included *An. arabiensis* (90.6%), *An. coluzzii* (7.1%) and *An. gambiae s.s.* (2.3%). They displayed 1.1–4.8% infection rates, 80% indoor-resting density and 56–80% human blood index. Eleven *An. gambiae s.l.* populations over the 15 tested were resistant to deltamethrin (51–89.5% mortality rates). Model results showed a significant dependence of indoor vector density on increasing deltamethrin resistance (p-value of <0.01). These behavioural and resistance patterns may lead to increasing malaria transmission in study health districts.

Keywords: north cameroon, long-lasting insecticidal nets, malaria vectors behaviour, insecticide resistance, two-level analysis

1. Introduction

Malaria still remains a priority problem in the world today. According to the latest estimates, there were about 214 million cases of malaria in 2015 (with an uncertainty range of 205–316 million) and an estimated 438,000 deaths (with an uncertainty range of 236,000–635,000) [1]. People living in the poorest countries are the most exposed to malaria, with 90% of deaths occurring in the African region, mostly among children [1]. The emergence of vector resistance to insecticides is a serious threat in the fight against malaria, since the general use of insecticides in indoor residual spraying (IRS) or in long-lasting insecticidal nets (LLINs) constitutes the only means of mass prevention [2]. In many sub-Saharan African countries, vector resistance to all classes of insecticides has been reported [3–5]. Some studies conducted in south western Chad (close to the North Region of Cameroon), where insecticide-treated nets (ITNs) and LLINs are used in large scale, have revealed deltamethrin resistance in the *Anopheles (An.). gambiae s.l.* populations [3, 6]. Given that the successes in the reduction of malaria burden acquired in the long run may strongly be compromised by vector resistance to insecticides, it is necessary to elaborate strategies for the management of this phenomenon.

In Cameroon, malaria is responsible for 30% of morbidity cases, 36% of outpatient consultation, 67% of childhood mortality and 48% of hospital admissions [7]. Malaria infection is essentially due to *Plasmodium falciparum*, followed by *P. ovale and P. malariae* [8]. Seven anopheline species play major roles in *Plasmodium* parasite transmission, among which are *An arabiensis, An. gambiae* and *An. coluzzii*, three sibling species of the *An. gambiae* complex [9]. However, several studies have reported insecticide resistance in these three mosquito species, threatening the progress towards malaria elimination in the country [10–12]. Field observations have shown that the emergence of insecticide resistance is favoured by the abusive and anarchic use of pesticides in public health and/or in agriculture [11, 13]. The regions that are mostly concerned with resistance are the North, Centre, Littoral, West and North West. Two resistance mechanisms have been noticed, *metabolic*- and *kdr*-based insecticide resistance. *Metabolic*-based resistance is due to altered levels of detoxifying enzymes such as P450s, esterases and glutathione S-transferases, whose expression levels may well be modulated by variation in many genes, making it a quantitative genetic trait [14, 15]. The *kdr*-based insecticide resistance results from a single leucine to phenylalanine or serine amino acid mutation at the voltage gate sodium channel which is the target side of dichlorodiphenyltricholoroethane (DDT) and pyrethroid insecticides [5]. *Metabolic*-based resistance is the major mechanism in the northern tropical regions of Cameroon, whereas multiple insecticide resistance, including *metabolic*- and *kdr*-based resistance mechanisms, is widespread in the southern equatorial regions [16–18].

However, while the major mechanisms of insecticide resistance in malaria vectors are more and more documented, an important research gap remains on detailed understanding of the likely genetic basis of specific behavioural traits, and how surveillance programs should be implemented to best monitor changes in these traits. In other words, how insecticide resistance might interact with vector behavioural response to interventions is very poorly known.

The current study was carried out in three health districts in the North of Cameroon, namely Pitoa, Garoua and Mayo-Oulo, where *metabolic*-based resistance to deltamethrin was reported in *An. gambiae* s.s. and the twin species *An. arabiensis*. These species are the major malaria vectors in the North Region, malaria incidence in these districts (46–62%) is among the highest of the 12 health districts of northern Cameroon region [19, 20]. Deltamethrin LLINs (Permanet 2.0) were distributed there at universal coverage in 2010, for malaria mass prevention. The aim of the study was to assess the resting behaviour of local *An. gambiae s.l.* populations when control interventions are put in place, with respect to their insecticide resistance status.

2. Main body

2.1. Experiments

2.1.1. Study area

The field survey was carried out in the North Region of Cameroon from October 2011 to November 2011 in 27 villages in three health districts: Garoua, the regional capital city (9° 30N; 13°40E), Pitoa (9°21N; 13°31E), situated 15 km from Garoua, and Mayo-Oulo (9°46N; 13° 44E), 140 km from Garoua. This is a cotton-cultivated area where there is an extensive use of LLINs for human protection with approximately 87% of households having at least one net and 69% of households having at least one net per two people [21]. The North Region of Cameroon makes up 66,090 km^2 of the Northern half of the Republic of Cameroon with a population density of 13 people/km^2. Neighbouring territories include the Far North Region to the north, the Adamawa Region to the south, Nigeria to the west, Chad to the east and Central African Republic to the south-east. The districts and their study clusters are given in **Figure 1**.

2.1.2. Mosquito collection

Mosquitoes were collected during a cross-sectional survey in 29 clusters including 12 clusters in the Garoua health district, 10 clusters in the Pitoa health district and seven clusters in the Mayo-Oulo health district (**Table 1**). Two separate data sets were collected: one on mosquito's resting behaviour while another was collected on insecticide resistance. For the resting behaviour data, two techniques of adult mosquito collection were used: window exit traps (WETs) and indoor spray catches (ISCs).

WET were placed over the windows of bedrooms to collect mosquitoes that attempt to escape during the night [22]. Ten rooms per cluster were used to collect mosquitoes during two consecutive nights. WETs were placed at 6.00 pm over the windows of each bedroom till 6.00

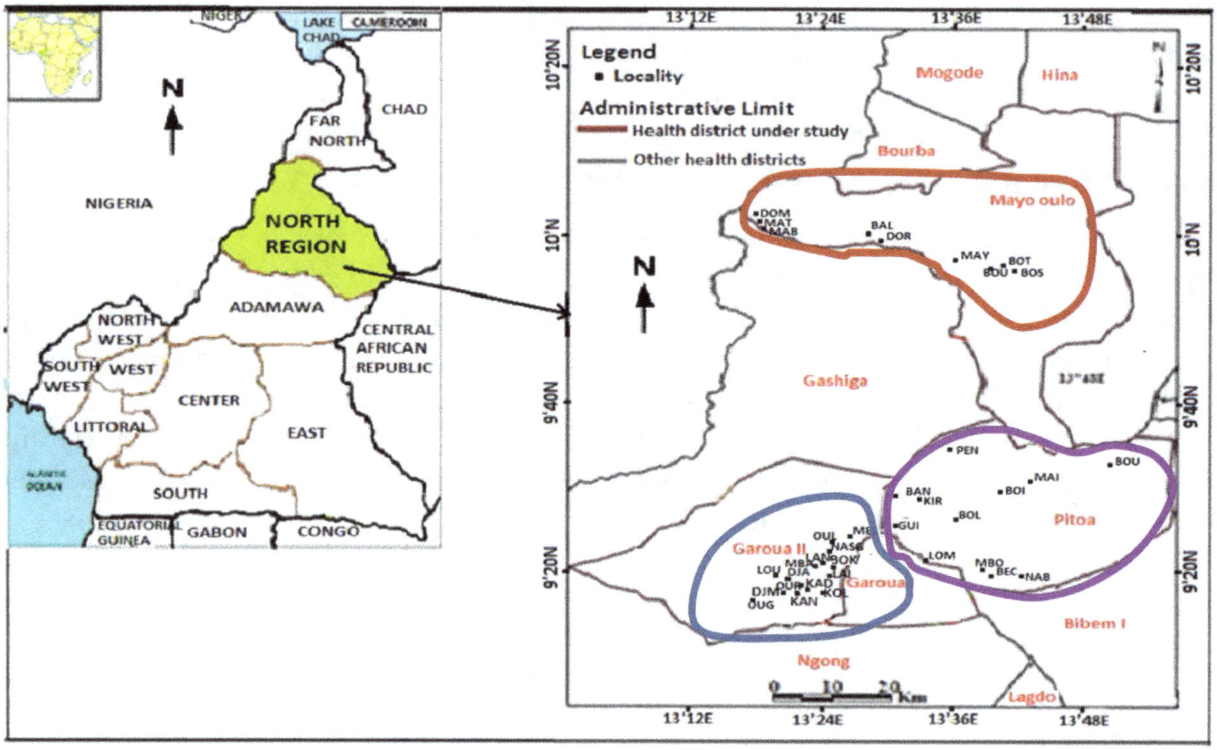

Figure 1. Map of Cameroon showing the study region, health districts and study clusters. The red chart encloses cluster of the Mayo-Oulo Health District (MAY: Mayo-Oulo; BOU: Bouyoum; BOT: Batoum; BOS: Bossoum; DOR: Dourbaye; MAB: Maboni; BAL: Balla). The purple chart encloses cluster of the Pitoa Health District (MAL: Mayo Lebri; BEC: Be Centre; BOI: Boula-Ibbi; BOL: Boulgou; BOUS: Boussa GUI: Guizigaré; NASP: Nassarao; MBO: Mbolom; PEN: Pena KIR; Kirombo). The blue chart encloses cluster of the Garoua Health Districts (DJA: Djamboutou I; DJM: Djamboutou II; KAD: Kanadi II; KAN: Kanadi I; LAN: Laïndé II; LOU: Loundérou; MBA: Mboum-aviation; MBI: Mbilga; BOK: Bocki; NASG: Nassarao; OUL: Oulo Lawane; OUG: Ouro-Garga).

am. Mosquitoes were then collected inside the trap in the morning, between 6 and 8 am using a mouth aspirator.

ISCs were done in the morning, from 6 to 8 pm, to sample mosquitoes resting inside rooms used for WETs. After spreading white sheets to cover the entire floor space and objects, rooms were sprayed with commercial aerosols containing pyrethroids. Mosquitoes fall on to the white sheets 10 min after spraying and were carefully picked up.

Female anophelines collected from WET and ISCs were morphologically identified using identification keys [23, 24]; they were separated according to their physiological status (unfed, freshly fed, half gravid and gravid) and individually preserved in tubes with desiccant for subsequent laboratory analyses.

For insecticide resistance testing, samples of anopheline larvae and pupae were collected from the maximum number of breeding sites. In each cluster, all open water bodies were inspected. Samples of immature anophelines were collected from active breeding sites by the dipping method [22]; they were pooled per cluster and brought to a local insectary, then reared in spring water. Larvae were fed on Tetramin Fish Food (Tetra Werke Company, Inc., Blacksburg, VA, USA) and pupae were kept in a cage to emerge into adults. Emerging adults were

Health district	Population of district	Selected health areas	Distance to headquarters (km)	Human population	Clusters
		Pitoa	0	32,327	GUI, BOL
		Banaye	13	6296	PEN, KIR
Pitoa	108,611	Be Centre	22	4341	BEC, MBO, NASP
		Bouba Ibib	40	15,262	BOI, MAL, BOUS
Total				**58,226**	
		Kolleré	0	27,692	KAD, KAN
		Nassarao	12	7224	NASG, BOK, MBI
Garoua	316,957	Laïndé	10	56,569	LAN, OUL, MBA
		Djamboutou	7	40,122	DJA, DJM, OUG, LOU
Total				**165,212**	
		Mayo-Oulo	0	28,203	MAY, BOT, BOU
Mayo-Oulo	91,501	Dourbaye	10	16,106	DOR, BAL, MAB
		Doumo	42	8502	BOS
Total				**52,811**	

BAL: Balla; BEC: Be Centre; BOI: Boula-Ibbi; BOK: Bocki; BOL: Boulgou; BOS: Bossoum; BOUS: Boussa; BOU: Bouyoum; BOT: Batoum; DOR: Dourbaye; GUI: Guizigaré; DJA: Djamboutou I; DJM: Djamboutou II; KAD: Kanadi II; KAN: Kanadi I; KIR: Kirombo; LAN: Laïndé II; LOU: Loundérou; MAB: Maboni; MAY: Mayo-Oulo; MBA: Mboum-aviation; MBO: Mbolom; MAL: Mayo Lebri; MBI: Mbilga; NASG: Nassarao; OUL: Oulo Lawane; NASP: Nassarao; OUG: Ouro-Garga; PEN: Pena.

Table 1. Health districts and study clusters in the north Cameroon region.

maintained on 10% sugar solution. Adult anophelines were then morphologically identified as belonging to the *An. gambiae* complex by means of reference keys [23, 24] and used for susceptibility tests.

2.1.3. Insecticide susceptibility test

Insecticide susceptibility tests were performed on mosquitoes aged 2–4 days, emerged from field-collected larvae and pupae. *An. gambiae s.l.* females were exposed for 1 h to 0.05% deltamethrin-impregnated papers using WHO susceptibility test kits and standard protocol for adult mosquitoes [25] under ambient room temperature (25–28°C) and 70–80% relative humidity. Test kits including deltamethrin-impregnated papers, test tubes and accessories were supplied by the Vector Control and Research Unit, University Sains Malaysia (Penang, Malaysia). Filter paper sheets (12 × 15 cm, Whatman N°1) were impregnated with the discriminating dosage of deltamethrin (0.05%) (pyrethroid insecticide), mixed with acetone and silicon oil. Other batches of filter paper sheets were impregnated with acetone + silicon solution for use as control. Acetone acted as the solvent and silicon oil as a carrier. The purchased impregnated papers were stored at 4°C until the date of the test.

Each full set of bioassays was performed with five batches of 20–25 non-blood fed, 2–4-day-old females: four batches were exposed to insecticide-impregnated filter papers and one batch was exposed to untreated filter paper and served as a control. The number of mosquitoes knocked down was recorded at 5-min interval during the 1-h long exposure to deltamethrin-impregnated papers. After exposure to insecticide-impregnated papers or control papers, mosquitoes were transferred to holding tubes and provided with cotton pads soaked with 10% sugar solution. The mortality rates were determined 24 h post exposure.

The resistance status in the mosquito populations was determined according to WHO's criteria [25]:

- A mortality rate in the range of 98–100% indicates susceptibility;
- A mortality rate between 90 and 97% suggests possible resistance to be confirmed;
- A mortality rate less than 90% indicates resistance.

The above criteria are recommended on the grounds that a greater than 2% survival at the diagnostic concentration is considered unlikely to be due to chance alone, and provided that all the test conditions are met.

Tests with mortality of the controls greater than 20% were taken all over again.

2.1.4. *Laboratory analysis*

The head and thorax of field-collected female *An. gambiae s.l.* were examined for *P. falciparum* circumsporozoite protein (CSP) by enzyme-linked immunosorbent assay (ELISA) [26, 27]. Sporozoite rates were determined as the number of anophelines positive for circumsporozoite protein ÷ the total number of specimens tested by ELISA CSP.

Blood-meal sources were identified by ELISA [28]. The technique identifies human, bovine, ovine (sheep and goat), equine (horse and donkey), pig or chicken hosts. Human blood index (HBI) was determined for each species, that is, the proportion of female anophelines that were found with human blood in their stomachs thereby giving an indication of anthropophilic rate. The HBI was determined as the number of human feeds ÷ (number of human feeds + number of animal feeds).

Genomic DNA was extracted from each selected *An. gambiae s.l.* specimen as described by Collins et al. [29] and each individual was identified to the species level using polymerase chain reaction-restriction fragment length polymorphism (PCR-RFLP) [30]. This method allows simultaneous identification of species of the *An. gambiae* complex.

2.2. Statistical analysis

2.2.1. *Descriptive analysis*

Pareto charts were used for univariate analysis of the qualitative variables *species, district, locality, phy. status* (physiological status), *csp* (circumsporozoite protein status) and *behaviour* (resting behaviour). Box plots were used to see the distribution of the susceptibility variable (*loc. suscep*) vis-à-vis the modalities of the qualitative variables and results obtained were tested using the Kruskal-Wallis rank sum test.

2.2.2. Missing data

The k-nearest neighbour method of classification with random assignment was used to impute missing observations in the data set, so the missing value in a variable on an individual was imputed by one of its k-nearest neighbours picked at random. As a result of this randomness in imputations, constructed models were implemented each on 10 imputed data sets and parameter estimates were obtained for each model by taking the average over the respective 10 imputed data sets estimates [31].

2.2.3. Model specification

A two-level ordinary logit model was used to establish a relationship between *An. gambiae* species caught indoors and at exit traps and the status of deltamethrin resistance in *An. gambiae s.l.* from the same clusters [31]. This model was used because mosquitoes, which were considered as level-1 units, were clustered within localities, considered as level-2 units and measurements were taken at level 1 and 2 units. The model was interested in the effect of resistance on the odds of the probability that a given species k in locality j will be found indoors against the probability that it will be found at the level of the exit trap. The model therefore has the form: where

$$\log\left[\frac{\Pr(\text{behavior}_{jk}=1|x_{jk},z_j,\mu_j)}{1\text{–Prbehavior}_{jk}=1|x_{jk},z_j,\mu_j)}\right]=\gamma+\beta_{\text{res}}\text{loc.suscep}_j+\beta_{A.gamM}1_{\text{species}_{jk}=A.gamM}+ \\ \beta_{A.gamS}1_{\text{species}_{jk}=A.gamS}+\beta_P 1_{csp_{jk}=P}+\beta_{\text{Gravid}}1_{phy.status_{jk}=\text{Gravid}}+\beta_{H.grav}1_{phy.status_{jk}=H.grav} \\ +\beta_{\text{Unfed}}1_{phy.status_{jk}=\text{Unfed}}+\text{loc.ran.effect}_j, \tag{1}$$

- x_{jk} is a realization of the vector of level-1 covariates (*species, csp* and *physiological status*) for a mosquito k in locality j,
- z_j is a realization of the level-2 covariate (*locality susceptibility*). It is the percentage of deltamethrin susceptibility of locality j,
- μ_j = loc.ran.effect$_j$ is the locality j's random effect in the model assumed to follow a normal distribution with mean 0 and variance σ^2,
- γ, β_{res}, $\beta_{A.gam\ M}$, $\beta_{A.gam\ S}$ β_p, β_{Gravid}, $\beta_{H.grav}$ β_{Unfed} *and* σ^2 are the model parameters to be estimated and
- $1_{X_{jk}=x}=\begin{cases}1 & \text{if} X_{jk}=x\\ 0 & \text{otherwise}\end{cases}$

2.2.4. Estimation of parameters

The maximum marginal likelihood method was used to estimate the parameters of the model. Solutions to the likelihood equations were approximated using Fisher's method of scoring with numerical approximations of integrals obtained using the Gauss- Hermite quadrature (GHQ) method [31]. Analyses were done in EXCEL and in *R*, using the *R*-function *sabre* in the *R*-package *sabreR* [31–33].

2.3. Results

2.3.1. Vector densities, infection rates and blood-meal origins

A total of 1135 *Anopheline* mosquitoes were collected from October 2011 to November 2011 in 29 clusters across the three study health districts (Garoua, Pitoa and Mayo-Oulo). On the bases of morphological identification, 10 anopheline species were identified in collected mosquito samples, including:

- -three species of the *An. gambiae s.l.* complex representing more than half of the total population of *anopheles* vectors (609/1135= 53.7%),
- -*An. funestus* group (408/1135 = 35.9%),
- -*An. rufipes* (82/1135 = 7.2%),
- -*An. pharoensis, An. nili, An. coustani, An. maculipalpis* and *An. paludis* representing each less than 5% of the total analysed samples.

Among the samples belonging to the *An. gambiae* complex, 299/374 (80%) specimens were successfully identified down to species using PCR-RFLP. *An. arabiensis* was the predominant species (271/299 = 90.6%), followed by *An. coluzzii* (21/299 = 7.1%) and *An. gambiae* s.s. (7/299 = 2.3%) (**Table 2**).

A total of 6/696 anopheline mosquitoes tested by ELISA CSP showed the presence of the circumsporozoite protein, corresponding to 0.86% global infection rate. These specimens belonged to three species: *An. coluzzii, An. arabiensis* and *An. funestus*. The infection rates per

		Physiological status (or gonotrophic state) (%)				
Species	**Point of collection**	**Unfed**	**Freshly fed**	**Half gravid**	**Gravid**	**Total (%)**
An. arabiensis	Indoors	55 (70.5)	99 (84.6)	18 (62.1)	45 (95.7)	217 (80.2)
	Exit traps	23 (29.5)	18 (15.4)	11 (37.9)	2 (4.3)	54 (19.8)
An. coluzzii	Indoors	3 (75.0)	15 (88.2)	0	0	18 (85.7)
	Exit traps	1 (25.0)	2 (11.8)	0	0	3 (14.3)
An. gambiae	Indoors	1 (50.0)	3 (60.0)	0	0	4 (57.1)
	Exit traps	1 (50.0)	2 (40.0)	0	0	3 (42.9)
Total	Indoors	59 (92.2)	117 (84.2)	18 (62.8)	45 (95.7)	239 (79.9)
	Exit traps	25 (7.8)	22 (15.8)	11 (37.9)	2 (4.3)	60 (20.2)

Table 2. Residual and exit trap faunas in relation to species of the *Anopheles gambiae* complex and physiological status. %: proportion of mosquitoes collected indoors versus exit traps.

species were 4.8% (1/21), 1.1% (3/271) and 0.5% (2/408) for *An. coluzzii, An. arabiensis* and *An. funestus*, respectively.

Four hundred and ninety-seven (497) anophelines were tested for blood-meal origins, among which 229 meals were successfully determined. They included 55.5% (127/229) meals from human, 31.4% (72/229) from cattle and 4.8% (7/229) from sheep and pig (**Table 2**). There were 8.3% (21/229) mixed blood meals from human + pig, human + cattle, human + cattle + sheep, cattle + sheep, cattle + pig and cattle + sheep + pig. The three species of the *An. gambiae* complex (*An. arabiensis, An. coluzzii* and *An. gambiae s.s.*) displayed high human blood indexes (HBI), ranging from 0.56 to 0.8, suggesting high anthropophagic tendencies compared with *An. funestus* (HBI = 0.42, $p < 0.005$) (**Table 3**).

Species	H	C	S	P	H/C	H/P	H/C/S	C/S	C/P	C/S/P	Total	HBI
An. arabiensis	94	39	2	2	1	5	1	2	0	0	146	0.69
An. coluzzii	7	3	1	3	2	0	0	0	0	0	16	0.56
An. gambiae	4	1	0	0	0	0	0	0	0	0	5	0.80
An. funestus	22	29	1	2	0	3	1	1	1	2	62	0.42
Total	127	72	4	7	3	8	2	3	1	2	229	0.62
(%)	55.5	31.4	1.7	3.1	1.3	3.5	0.9	1.3	0.4	0.9	100	

H: human; C: cattle; S: sheep; P: pig; H/P: human + pig; H/C: human + cattle; H/C/S: human + cattle + sheep, C/S: cattle + sheep, C/P: cattle + pig; C/S/P: cattle + sheep + pig.

Table 3. Origin of blood meals of the four major malaria vectors in the study health districts.

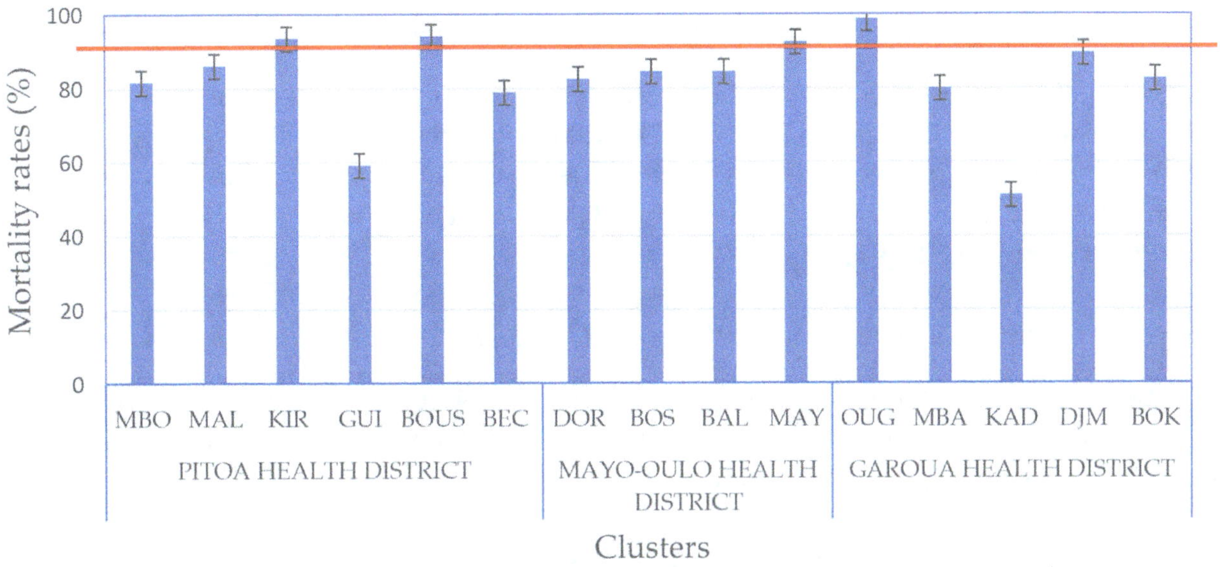

Figure 2. Mortality rates of *Anopheles gambiae s.l.* populations 24 h post exposure to 0.05% deltamethrin-impregnated papers. The red line at 90% mortality rate indicates the threshold below which a mosquito population is classified as resistant to the insecticide used for susceptibility test [25]. BAL: Balla; BEC: Be Centre; BOK: Bocki; BOS: Bossoum; BOUS: Boussa; DOR: Dourbaye; GUI: Guizigaré; DJM: Djamboutou II; KIR: Kirombo; MAY: Mayo-Oulo; MBA: Mboum-aviation; MBO: Mbolom; MAL: Mayo Lebri; OUG: Ouro-Garga.

2.3.2. *Status of deltamethrin resistance in An. gambiae s.l. populations*

One thousand two hundred and thirteen (1213) females of the *An. gambiae s.l.* were tested for their susceptibility to deltamethrin. They were from 15 field populations, including six from the Pitoa health district, four from the Mayo-Oulo health district and five from the Garoua health district. Recorded mortality rates are presented in **Figure 2**. According to WHO's criteria, 11 populations among the 15 tested were found resistant to deltamethrin with mortality rates ranging from 51 to 89.5%. Resistance was suspected in three populations, that is, those from Kirambo and Boussa in the Pitoa health district and Mayo-Oulo in the Mayo-Oulo health district, with 92–94% mortality rate. Only the Ouro-Garga population was found susceptible to deltamethrin. These data showed that deltamethrin resistance was widespread in the three study health districts.

2.3.3. *Resting behaviour and physiological statuses of the species of the An. gambiae complex*

Among the three identified sibling species of the *An. gambiae* complex, high proportions of *An. arabiensis* (217/271 = 80%) and *An. coluzzii* (18/21 = 86%) samples were caught indoors compared with exit traps collection (20 and 14%, respectively), showing their high endophilic behaviour in the study areas (**Table 2**). These proportions were not significantly different between the two species (p-value = 0.25). However, similar rates of *An. gambiae* s.s. specimens were caught indoors versus in exit traps, although the sample size was very small.

Considering the physiological status of collected mosquitoes, all the four gonotrophic states (unfed, freshly fed, half gravid and gravid) were found in *An. arabiensis* samples collected indoors or in exit traps, with freshly fed and unfed mosquitoes being predominant. Meanwhile, only unfed and freshly fed gonotrophic states were found in analysed *An. coluzzii* and *An. gambiae s.s.* samples, raising the question about the behavioural patterns (endophilic/exiting) of half gravid and gravid mosquitoes of these two species.

The overall indoor-resting rate for the three species of the *An. gambiae* complex was 80% (239/299), increasing from half gravid (18/29 = 62%), to freshly fed (117/239 = 84.2%), unfed (59/84 = 92%) and gravid mosquitoes (45/47 = 96%) (**Table 2**). Conversely, the highest rate of exiting mosquitoes was recorded among the half gravid samples (11/29 = 40%) and the lowest among the gravid samples (2/47 = 4%).

2.3.4. *Effect of deltamethrin resistance on the resting behaviour*

The two level logit regression analysis given in **Table 4** showed a statistically significant dependence of resting behaviour on deltamethrin resistance. Fitting the mean parameter estimates in the model, we obtained the following:

$$log\left[\frac{\Pr(\text{behavior}_{jk}=1|x_{jk},z_j,\mu_j)}{1-\Pr(\text{behavior}_{jk}=1|x_{jk},z_j,\mu_j)}\right] = -14.4626 + 0.1398\text{loc.suscep}_j - 2.36991_{\text{species}_{jk}=A.gamM} - 2.0974\_1_{phy.status_{jk}=\text{Gravid}} + 1.29431_{phy.status_{jk}=\text{Unfed}} + \text{loc.ran.effect}_j \quad (2)$$

This model showed that the estimated coefficient of the locality resistance variable (*loc.suscep*)

Variable	Mean estimate of parameter	Variance of imputation method	Standard error estimate	Signal-to-noise ratio	95% C.I. Approximation	Approximated *P*-value
Threshold intercept	−14.463	4.662	2.265	6.385	(−18.902, −0.0232)	0.000
Resistance *loc. suscept*	0.140	0.000701	0.0271	5.158	(0.0866, 0.193)	0.000
Species cies *(An. Arabiensis* = ref) *A. coluzzii* *A. gambiae s.s.*	−2.370 −0.301	0.199 0.711	0.470 0.885	5.0471 0.340	(−3.290, −1.450) (−2.0357, 1.434)	0.000 0.734
csp (Abs = ref) Presence	−16.865	0.265	355.814	0.0474	(−14.259, 680.531)	0.962
Phy.Status (Freshly fed = ref) Gravid Half Gravid Unfed	−2.0974 −0.678 1.294	0.0615 0.185 0.0855	0.264 0.451 0.307	7.936 1.502 4.210	(−2.615, −1.580) (−1.563, 0.207) (0.691, 1.897)	0.000 0.133 0.000
Variance of locality random effect (σ^2)	3.673	0.0864	0.311	11.803	(3.0627, 4.283)	0.000

Table 4. Mean of estimates of parameters in the two-level logit regression model and their corresponding precisions.

	***p*-Value**					
	Behaviour	*Locality*	*District*	*Species*	*Physiological status*	*csp*
Susceptibility to deltamethrin	0.0041	2.2e–16	2.2e–16	0.18	4.1e–06	Observations in same group

Table 5. Kruskal-Wallis rank sum tests of independence between the deltamethrin susceptibility variable and the qualitative variables.

has a positive sign, indicating that the species were more likely to be endophilic (stay indoors) with decreasing values of mortality rates to deltamethrin susceptibility test (increasing deltamethrin resistance). The result was significant at the 5% level (*p*-value = 2.502e–07). This result was confirmed by the Kruskal-Wallis rank sum test (*p*-value = 0.0041) (**Table 5**).

Furthermore, there was varying effect of physiological status on the resting behaviour. **Figure 3** shows the relationships between resting behaviour and deltamethrin resistance for the *An. arabiensis* (A) and *An. coluzzii* species (B) with different physiological statuses.

With specimens of the *An. arabiensis* species, the probability that an unfed specimen was endophilic decreased from 1.00 to 0.31, as the mortality to susceptibility test increased from 50 to 100% **(Figure 3A)**. The total difference in probability was 1.00–0.31 = 0.69. Thus, when the mortality rate was less than 80%, the probability that the unfed *An. arabiensis* was endophilic was greater than 0.88 and when mortality was greater than 98%, the probability was less than 0.38. The effect gradually decreased on freshly fed (total difference in probability was 1.00 –

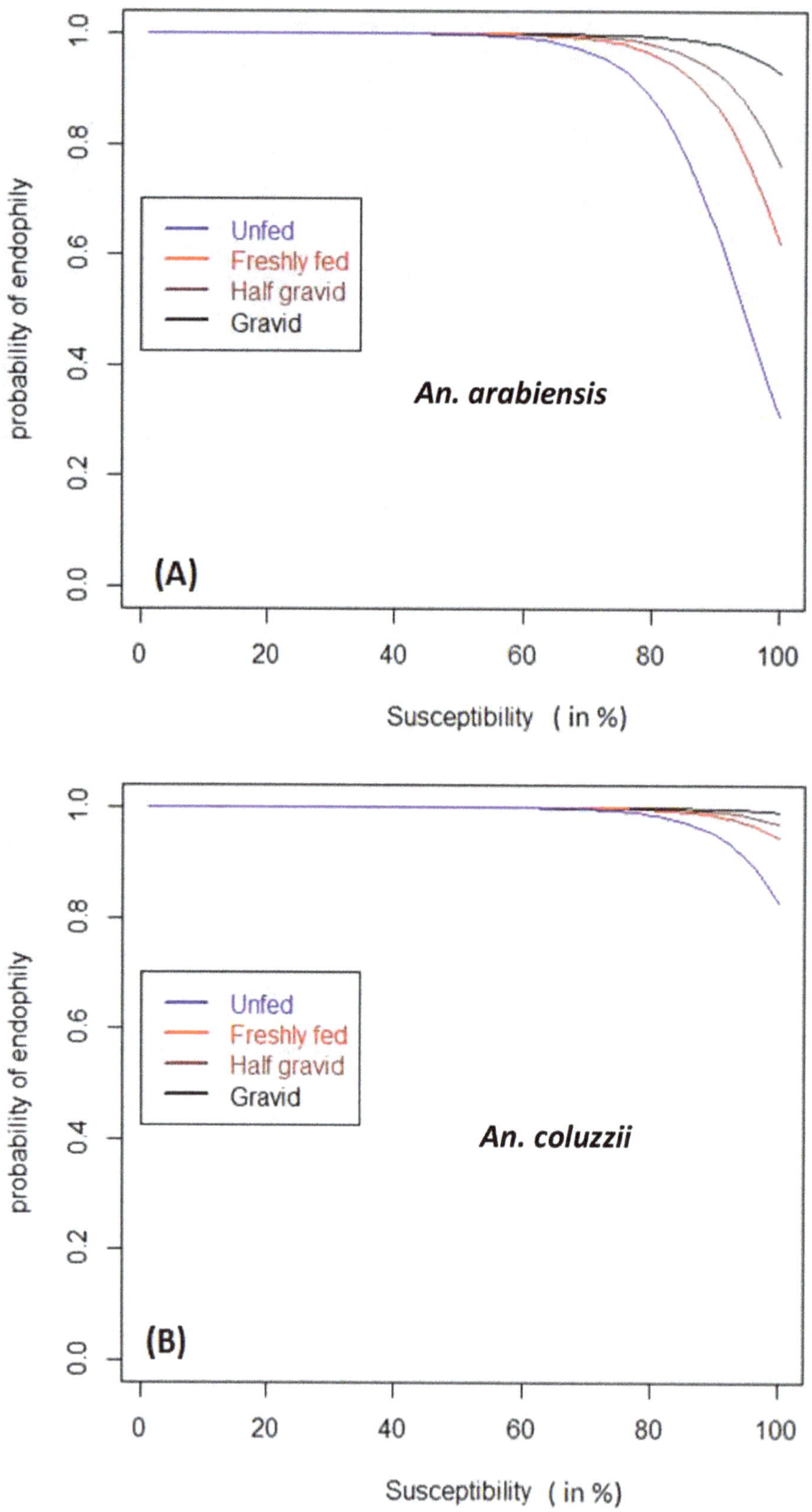

Figure 3. Endophily curves for *An. arabiensis* (A) and *An. coluzzii* (B) in relation to physiological statuses and mortality rates to susceptibility tests.

0.62 = 0.38) and half gravid specimens (total difference in probability was 1.00 − 0.76 = 0.24). The effect of deltamethrin resistance on the resting behaviour of gravid *An. arabiensis* was not significant.

With specimens of the *An. coluzzii* species, the effect of deltamethrin resistance on the resting behaviour was not significant ($p > 0.8$) in general as shown in **Figure 3(B)**. Nevertheless, the probability of endophily in unfed *An. coluzzii* was slightly decreased between 80 and 100% mortality rates.

2.4. Discussion

The current study revealed high indoor densities and an obvious infectivity of deltamethrin-resistant *An. arabiensis* and *An. coluzzii* populations, leading to contact with humans and ongoing malaria transmission in the study districts no matter high coverage of LLINs.

Most important malaria vectors such as *An. gambiae, An. arabiensis* and *An. funestus* [34] prefer to feed in the middle of the night when most humans are typically asleep, immobile and vulnerable to attack. Feeding indoors at night is, therefore, the behaviour that is targeted by the use of LLINs to protect sleeping humans. Indoor feeding is then often followed by resting within the same sheltered domestic structure for one or two nights while the blood meal is digested and eggs are developed. Applications of insecticides to houses by IRS, to kill mosquitoes resting on inner surfaces of the walls and roof after they have fed upon the human occupants, are therefore a highly effective strategy for controlling populations of vectors that rest indoors as a matter of preference. Overall, the community-wide mass effect of LLINs and IRS can have a dramatic impact on the population size of stereotypical vectors that depend heavily upon feeding on humans and resting inside houses [35]. However, there are a number of possible impacts that insecticide use indoors could have on mosquito behaviour including changes in biting phenology, the rate of endophagy and endophily. Therefore, understanding that the limits of IRS, LLINs or any other vector-control strategy are primarily defined by the behavioural traits of mosquitoes [36–38] is fundamental. Patterns of malaria vector behaviours have been examined in quite a good number of studies where vectors undergo modifications on their behaviour to facilitate avoidance or circumvention of insecticides [39]. However, better understanding the interactions between insecticide resistance phenotypes in field malaria vector populations, the resistance mechanisms and subsequent behavioural patterns in the presence of LLINs at household level is essential.

The phenotype of deltamethrin resistance in *An. arabiensis* and *An. coluzzii* recorded in this study was consistent with previous studies conducted in the north Cameroon Region [11, 19, 40]. Furthermore, these data provided evidence of widespread deltamethrin resistance in species of the *An. gambiae* complex from this region. In *An. arabiensis* field populations from Pitoa, a set of constitutively overexpressed antioxidant genes (superoxide dismutases *SOD2* and *SOD3*, the glutathione S-transferase *GSTS1* and the thioredoxin-dependent peroxidase *TPX4*) and a single P450 (*CYP4G16*) were previously associated with increased tolerance to deltamethrin [15]. Indeed, metabolic-based resistance was likely the main DDT and pyrethroid resistance mechanisms in *An. gambiae s.l.* in this area, since the *kdr L1014F* allele, which is recessive, was found at low frequency and heterozygous state in August 2011 just before the current survey [40].

The most abundant species of the *An. gambiae* complex encountered in the three study health districts was the *An. arabiensis*, while *An. coluzzii* and *An. gambiae s.s.* occurred in small ranges. The predominance of *An. arabiensis* in the analysed samples was consistent with the distribution of species of the *An. gambiae* complex in north Cameroon [11, 15, 19]. Since data collection for the current study was done between October and November 2011, the observed distribution of sibling species of *An. gambiae* complex may vary periodically [41]. Significant variations in the relative frequencies of *An. arabiensis* and *An. gambiae* were previously recorded over time and between localities in the north Cameroon. More interestingly, both species were resistant to DDT and deltamethrin, and the resistance steadily increased throughout the rainy season [11]. In other studies, *An. arabiensis* populations have shown some variations in biting or resting behaviour at different locations, with some of these variations being explained by seasons or historical use of insecticides [42].

Substantial variations have also been recorded in the current study. Most of the indoor-collected samples were freshly fed or unfed, suggesting that the vectors might tend to increase the chance of feeding on humans by remaining indoors, regardless of the presence of the LLINs. This behavioural pattern could therefore lead to increasing malaria risk in north Cameroon, since the sporozoite rates in mosquito samples were 4.8 and 1.1% for *An. coluzzii* and *An. arabiensis*, respectively, suggesting regular malaria transmission in households with LLINs. Furthermore, the human blood index was high (56–80%) for the three sibling species, demonstrating their anthropophilic tendencies. Further variations were linked to mosquito physiological status. While all the four gonotrophic states were found in analysed *An. arabiensis* samples (indoors or exiting), only unfed and freshly fed gonotrophic states were found in *An. coluzzii* and *An. gambiae s.s.* samples, suggesting outdoor-resting habit (exophily) for half gravid and gravid mosquitoes of these two species, although the small size of the collected and analysed samples (N = 21 for *An. coluzzii* and N = 7 for *An. gambiae*) precludes any strong conclusion in these cases. Around 40% of half gravid *An. arabiensis* samples were found in exit traps and almost the same proportion of specimens of this species displayed animal blood meals (cattle, pigs and sheep), sometimes mixed with human blood. This variability of resting behaviour of *An. arabiensis* and to a lesser extent *An. coluzzii* was confirmed by the two-level logit regression analysis in relation with deltamethrin resistance. The decrease of insecticide resistance tended to induce exophily in unfed specimens, while the probability for gravid *An. arabiensis* to remain indoors no matter their susceptibility status was high. Although endophily of gravid mosquitoes was consistent with blood digestion and egg development processes, it could also be enhanced in the specimens displaying resistance to deltamethrin.

Data reported in this study put forward a high plasticity of feeding and resting behaviour in the three species of the *An. gambiae* complex from the study areas. Accordingly, resistant malaria vectors, which have developed the capacity of blood feeding or resting in houses in the presence of LLINs, render LLINs useless if they are not in good state (torn, holed or not large enough). The physical integrity of LLINs in the specific context of vector resistance to pyrethroid insecticides is essential for the sustainability of malaria mass prevention. These findings concord with those reported in Benin, where households in the areas with resistant mosquitoes showed high rates of blood feeding, while freshly insecticide-treated nets provided no protection once holed. By contrast, sleeping under a holed LLIN in the location where susceptible mosquitoes were common decreased the odds of being bitten by 66% and the majority of mosquitoes were killed by the treatment [43].

When the LLIN is intact, a side effect of physiological resistance would be the reduction in vector behavioural responsiveness to the insecticide [44–46]. Pyrethroid-resistant mosquitoes showed reduced irritability to insecticides, which allow them to rest on the surface for longer periods than susceptible mosquitoes, thus increasing the dose of insecticide received and likely the subsequent mortality rates [46]. In most cases, the effect of physiological resistance is unquantified and dependent on the mechanism of resistance [45]. The *Kdr* mutation is considered a relatively weak form of resistance compared to metabolic-based resistance, and it is usually only when the *kdr* occurs along with metabolic-based resistance that control fails [47, 48]. Furthermore, the current study has demonstrated that control failure may also result from a cumulative effect of insecticide resistance mechanisms and the profile of physiological status of targeted vector population.

With untreated nets, such effects of insecticide resistance and behavioural traits may not occur, and personal protection may be afforded provided the nets are tucked in, maintained in good condition and sufficiently large so that the sleepers do not make contact with the net [49]. Subsequently, this protection may result in a reduction of malaria morbidity compared with areas without nets at all. However, the obtained level of protection remains lower than that conferred by the LLINs which remain one of the most cost-effective tools for malaria mass prevention, even in some areas where vectors have developed pyrethroid resistance [46, 50, 51].

According to WHO, when insecticide resistance is confirmed, pre-emptive actions must be taken to manage this resistance and to ensure that the effectiveness of insecticides used for malaria vector control is preserved [25]. Trials of the combination of LLINs and IRS with different classes of insecticides (carbamates or organophosphates) as a resistance management strategy are necessary in north Cameroon, in order to guide malaria vector-control strategies in this region.

3. Conclusions

The data generated in the current study provide further evidence for cumulative effects of deltamethrin resistance and physiological status of *An. arabiensis* and to lesser extent *An. coluzzii* populations on the patterns of their behavioural responses to LLINs in north Cameroon. It is unique in drawing a model based on analysis of insecticide resistance, indoors/exiting mosquito densities and physiological statuses data. The high densities of vectors inside houses and regular contact with human may lead to increasing malaria transmission in study health districts regardless of the coverage of LLNs. These findings are valuable for the development of resistance management strategies, and effective tools for malaria control and elimination in the study areas.

Acknowledgements

This study was funded by the Bill and Melinda Gates Foundation (Grant Number 4849901) and the World Health Organization. We wish to thank the communities of the three study health districts in north Cameroon for their active participation in the survey and collaboration with the research team.

Author details

Josiane Etang[1,2]*, Betrand Fesuh Nono[3], Parfait Awono-Ambene[1], Jude Bigoga[4], Wolfgang Ekoko Eyisap[1,5], Michael Piameu[6], Jean-Claude Toto[1], Eugène Patrice Ndong Nguema[3], Henri Gwet[3], Etienne Fondjo[7] and Abraham Peter Mnzava[8]

*Address all correspondence to: josyet2@gmail.com

1 Yaoundé Research Institute, Organisation for the Coordination of Endemic Disease Control in Central Africa, Yaoundé, Cameroon

2 Faculty of Medicine and Pharmaceutical Sciences, University of Douala, Douala, Cameroon

3 National Advanced School of Engineering, University of Yaoundé I, Yaoundé, Cameroon

4 Biotechnology Centre, University of Yaoundé I, Cameroon

5 Laboratory of Animal Biology and Physiology, University of Douala, Cameroon

6 School of Health Sciences, Catholic University of Central Africa, Yaoundé, Cameroon

7 National Malaria Control Programme, Ministry of Public Health, Yaoundé, Cameroon

8 Global Malaria Programme, World Health Organization, Geneva, Switzerland

References

[1] World Health Organization: World Malaria Report 2015. Geneva: World Health Organization; 2016:243.

[2] World Health Organization: Global Plan for Insecticide Resistance Management in Malaria Vectors (GPIRM). In: *WHO/HTM/GMP/20125*. Edited by Organization WH. Geneva, Switzerland: World Health Organization; 2012:130.

[3] Ranson H, Abdallah H, Badolo A, Guelbeogo WM, Kerah-Hinzoumbé C, Yangalbé-Kalnoné E, Sagnon N, Simard F, Coetzee M: Insecticide resistance in *Anopheles gambiae*:

data from the first year of a multi-country study highlight the extent of the problem. *Malar J* 2009, 8:299.

[4] Boussari IDO, Sidick A, Martin T, Ranson H, Chandre F, Akogbéto M, Corbel V: Dynamics of insecticide resistance in malaria vectors in Benin: first evidence of the presence of L1014S kdr mutation in *Anopheles gambiae* from West Africa. *Malar J* 2011, 10:261.

[5] Corbel V, N'Guessan R: Distribution, mechanisms, impact and management of insecticide resistance in malaria vectors: a pragmatic review. In: Manguin S (ed) Anopheles mosquitoes—New insights into malaria vectors. *In Tech* 2013; 579–633, doi: 10.5772/56117.

[6] Kerah-Hinzoumbé C, Péka M, Nwane P, Donan-Gouni I, Etang J, Samè-Ekobo A, Simard F: Insecticide resistance in *Anopheles gambiae* from south-western Chad, Central Africa. *Malar J* 2008, 7:192.

[7] Same-Ekobo A: Aspects épidémiologiques du paludisme au Cameroun. *J Cam Acad Sci* 2005, 5(S1):3–16.

[8] Mouchet J, Carnevale P, Coosemans M, Julvez J, Manguin S, Lenoble RD, Sircoulon J: Biodivesité du paludisme dans le monde. Editions John Libbey Eurotext Paris; 2004: 428.

[9] Antonio-Nkondjio C, Kerah CH, Simard F, Awono-Ambene P, Choua?bou M, Tchuinkam T, Fontenille D: Complexity of the malaria vectorial system in Cameroon: contribution of secondary vectors to malaria transmission. *J Med Entomol* 2006, 43:1215–1221.

[10] Etang J, Manga L, Chandre F, Guillet P, Fondjo E, Mimpfoundi R, Toto JC, Fontenille D: Insecticide susceptibility status of *Anopheles gambiae s.l.* (Diptera: Culicidae) in the Republic of Cameroon. *J Med Entomol* 2003, 40: 491–497.

[11] Chouaïbou M, Etang J, Brevault T, Nwane P, Hinzoumbé CK, Mimpfoundi R, Simard F: Dynamics of insecticide resistance in the malaria vector *Anopheles gambiae s.l.* from an area of extensive cotton cultivation in Northern Cameroon. *Trop Med Int Hlth* 2008, 13:1–11.

[12] Antonio-Nkondjio C, TeneFossog B, Ndo C, MenzeDjantio B, ZebazeTogouet S, Awono-Ambene P, Costantini C, Wondji C, Ranson H: *An. gambiae* distribution and insecticide resistance in the cities of Douala and Yaoundé (Cameroon): influence of urban agriculture and pollution. *Malar J* 2011, 10:154.

[13] Müller P, Chouaibou M, Pignatelli P, Etang J, Walker ED, Donnelly MJ, Simard F, Ranson H: Pyrethroid tolerance associated with elevated expression of antioxidants and agricultural practice in *Anopheles arabiensis* sampled from an area of cotton fields in Northern Cameroon. *Mol Ecol* 2008, 17(4):1145–1155.

[14] Ranson H, Paton MG, Jensen B, McCarroll L, Vaughan A, Hogan JR, Hemingway J, Collins FH: Genetic mapping of genes conferring permethrin resistance in the malaria vector, *Anopheles gambiae*. *Insect Mol Biol* 2004, 13:379–386.

[15] Wondji CS, Irving H, Morgan J, Lobo NF, Collins FH, Hunt RH, Coetzee M, Hemingway J, Ranson H: Two duplicated P450 genes are associated with pyrethroid resistance in *Anopheles funestus*, a major malaria vector. *Genome Res* 2009, 19:452–459.

[16] Etang J, Manga L, Toto JC, Guillet P, Fondjo E, Chandre F: Spectrum of metabolic based resistance to insecticides in *Anopheles gambiae s.l.* populations from Cameroon. *J Vect Ecol* 2007, 32(1):123–133.

[17] Nwane P, Etang J, Chouaïbou M, Toto JC, Mimpfoundi R, Simard F: Kdr-based insecticide resistance in *Anopheles gambiae* s.s populations in Cameroon: spread of the L1014F and L1014S mutations. *BMC Res notes* 2011, 4:463.

[18] Nwane P, Etang J, Chouaïbou M, Toto JC, Koffi A, Mimpfoundi R, Simard F: Multiple insecticide resistance mechanisms in *Anopheles gambiae s.l.* populations from Cameroon, Central Africa. *Paras Vect* 2013, 6:41.

[19] Etang J, Chouaibou M, Toto JC, Faye O, Manga L, Samè-Ekobo A, Awono-Ambene P, Simard F: A preliminary test of the protective efficacy of Permethrin-treated bed nets in an area of *Anopheles gambiae* metabolic resistance to pyrethroids in North Cameroon. *Trans Roy Soc Trop Med Hyg* 2007, 101:881–884.

[20] Antonio-Nkondjio C, Kerah CH, Simard F, Awono-Ambene P, Chouaïbou M, Tchuinkam T, Fontenille D: Complexity of the malaria vectorial system in Cameroon: contribution of secondary vectors to malaria transmission. *J Med Entomol* 2006, 43:1215–1221.

[21] MINSANTE, NMCP, WHO, RBM, UNICEF, ACMS, CHAI, IRESCO, PLAN and CCAM: Cameroon malaria knowledge, attitudes, and practices. Progress from 2011 to 2012. Malaria NO MORE Final Report, August; 2012:17.

[22] Service MW: Mosquito Ecology: Field Sampling Methods. 2nd ed. London: Elsevier; 1993:988.

[23] Gillies MT, De Meillon B: The Anophelinae of Africa South of the Sahara (Ethiopian Zoogeographical Region). 2nd ed. Publications of the South African Institute for Medical Research, Johannesburg; 1968:343.

[24] Gillies MT, Coetzee MA: Supplement to the Anophelinae of Africa South of Sahara. Publication of the South African Institute for Medical Research; 1987:143.

[25] World Health Organization: Test Procedures for Insecticide Resistance Monitoring in Malaria Vectors. Geneva, Switzerland: World Health Organization; 2013:30.

[26] Burkot TR, William JL, Schneider I: Identification of *Plasmodium falciparum* infected mosquitoes by a double antibody enzyme-linked immunosorbent assay. *Am J Trop Med Hyg* 1984, 33:783–788.

[27] Wirtz RA, Zavala F, Charoenvit Y, Campbell GH, Burkot TR, Schneider I, Esser KM, Beaudoin RL, Andre RG: Comparative testing of monoclonal antibodies against *Plasmodium falciparum* sporozoites for ELISA development. *Bull WHO* 1987, 65:39–45.

[28] Beier JC, Perkins PV, Wirtz RA, Koros J, Diggs D, Gargam TPII, Koech DK: Blood meal identification by direct enzyme-linked immunosorbent assay (ELISA) tested on *Anopheles* (Diptera : Culicidae) in Kenya. *J Med Entomol* 1988, 25:9–16.

[29] Collins FH, Mendez MA, Razmussen MO, Mehaffey PC, Besansky NJ, Finnerty VA. Ribosomal RNA gene probe differentiates member species of *Anopheles gambiae* complex. *Am J Trop Med Hyg* 1987, 37:37–41.

[30] Fanello C, Santolamazza F, Della Tore A: A simultaneous identification of species and molecular forms of the *Anopheles gambiae* complex by PCR-RFLP. *Med Vet Entomol* 2002, 16:461–465.

[31] Fesuh NB: Modelling the effects of physiological status and insecticide resistance on the resting behaviour of malaria vectors in North Cameroon [MSc thesis]. Ecole Polytechnique: University of Yaounde I Cameroon; 2012:95.

[32] Crouchley R: R Package sabreR for Multivariate Generalized Linear Mixed Models. Centre for e-Science Lancaster University; 2012.

[33] R version 2.15.0: The R Foundation for Statistical Computing. ISBN 3-900051-07-0, Copyright (C) 2012, Platform: i386-pc-mingw32/i386 (32-bit).

[34] Huho BJ, Briët O, Seyoum A, Sikaala CH, Bayoh N, Gimnig JE, Okumu FO, Diallo D, Abdulla S, Smith TA, Killeen GF: Consistently high estimates for the proportion of human exposure to malaria vector populations occurring indoors in rural Africa. *Int J Epidemiol* 2013, 42:235–247.

[35] Killeen GF, Seyoum A, Sikaala CH, Zomboko AS, Gimnig JE, Govella NJ, White MT: Eliminating malaria vectors. *Paras Vect* 2013, 6:172.

[36] Durnez L, Coosemans M: Residual transmission of malaria: an old issue for new approaches. In *Anopheles* Mosquitoes—New Insights into Malaria Vectors (Manguin. Sth edition). Rijeka: *Intech* 2013:671–704.

[37] Ferguson HM, Dornhaus A, Beeche A, Borgemeister C, Gottlieb M, Mulla MS, Gimnig JE, Fish D, Killeen GF: Ecology: a prerequisite for malaria elimination and eradication. *PLoS Med* 2010, 7:e1000303.

[38] Govella NJ, Chaki PP, Killeen GF: Entomological surveillance of behavioural resilience and resistance in residual malaria vector populations. *Malar J* 2013, 12:124.

[39] Killeen GF: Characterizing, controlling and eliminating residual malaria transmission. *Malar J* 2014, 13:330.

[40] Etang J, Pennetier C, Piameu M, Bouraima A, Chandre F, Awono-Ambene P, Coosemans M, Corbel V: When intensity of deltamethrin resistance in *Anopheles gambiae s.l.* leads to loss of long lasting insecticidal nets efficacy: a case study in North Cameroon. *Paras Vect* 2016, 9:132.

[41] Hunt RH, Fuseini G, Knowles S, Stiles-Ocran J, Verster R, Kaiser ML, Kwang SC, Koekemoer LL, Coetzee M: Insecticide resistance in malaria vector mosquitoes at four localities in Ghana, West Africa. *Paras Vect* 2011, 4:107.

[42] Gatton ML, Chitnis N, Churcher T, Donnelly MJ, Ghani AC, Godfray H, Charles J, Gould F, Hastings I, Marshall J, Ranson H, Rowland M, Shaman J, Lindsay SW: The importance

of mosquito behavioural adaptation to malaria control in Africa. *Outlook Evol Soc* 2013, doi:10.1111/evo.12063.

[43] Asidi A, N'Guessan R, Akogbeto M, Curtis C, Rowland M: Loss of household protection from use of insecticide-treated nets against pyrethroid-resistant mosquitoes, Benin. ISBN. *Emerg Infect Dis* 2012, 18:1101–1106.

[44] Rowland M: Flight activity of insecticide resistant and susceptible *Anopheles stephensi* mosquitoes in actograph chambers lined with malathion, γHCH or dieldrin. *Med Vet Entomol* 1990, 4:397–404.

[45] Hodjati MH, Curtis CF: Dosage differential effects of Permethrin impregnated into bednets on pyrethroid resistant and susceptible genotypes of the mosquito *Anopheles stephensi*. *Med Vet Entomol* 1997,11:368–372.

[46] Henry MC, Assi SB, Rogier C, Dossou-Yovo J, Chandre F, Guillet P, et al.: Protective efficacy of lambda-cyhalothrin treated nets in *Anopheles gambiae* pyrethroid resistance areas of Cote d'Ivoire. *Am J Trop Med Hyg* 2005, 73(5):859–864.

[47] Hargreaves K, Koekemoer LL, Brooke BD, Hunt RH, Mthembu J, Coetzee M: *Anopheles funestus* resistant to pyrethroid insecticides in South Africa. *Med Vet Entomol* 2000, 14:181–189.

[48] Rivero A, Vezilier J, Weill M, Read AF, Gandon S: Insecticide control of vector-borne diseases: when is insecticide resistance a problem? *PLoS Pathog* 2010, 6: e1001000.

[49] Lindsay SW, Shenton FC, Snow RW, Greenwood BM: Responses of *Anopheles gambiae* complex mosquitoes to the use of untreated bed nets in the Gambia. *Med Vet Entomol* 1989, 3:253–262.

[50] Magesa SM, Wilkes TJ, Mnzava AEP et al.: Trial of pyrethroid impregnated bed nets in an area of Tanzania holoendemic for malaria vector population. Part 2. Effects on the malaria vector population. *Acta Trop* 1991, 49:97–108.

[51] Maxwell CA, Myamba J, Njunwa KJ, Greenwood BM, Curtis CF: Comparison of bed nets impregnated with different pyrethroids for their impact on mosquitoes and on re-infection with malaria after clearance of pre-existing infections with chlorproguanil-dapsone. *Trans Roy Soc Trop Med Hyg* 1999, 93, 4–11.

10

Tertian Fevers in Catalonia in the Late Eighteenth Centuries: The Case of Barcelona (1783–1786)

A Methodological Proposal to Develop Studies over Endemic and Epidemic Malaria in Past Societies

Kevin Pometti

Abstract

In this chapter, we propose a broad perspective of the sources available for the development of studies of endemic and epidemic malaria in past societies. The complexity of malaria as a disease is related to a variety of elements (environment, climatic oscillations, and human production and cultivation patterns). Historically, the study of malaria was integrated into the study of fevers in general. Indeed, malaria is a protean disease that interacts in positive, negative, and synergetic ways with other eukaryotic, viral, and bacterial diseases. Because of that, the word "fevers" conflates a wide range of diseases and symptoms that can also help us to detect the prevalence of malaria and relationships between the disease and environmental factors. Terms such as fevers, intermittent fevers, agues, and marshland fevers can be easily found in historical sources, print sources, and a large amount of documentation produced by state-municipal authorities, by physicians, and found in burial records. In sum, these represent the diversity of points of view involved in our research. Using as an example the case of Barcelona in the late eighteenth century, we show some results based on a methodology with a strong interdisciplinary basis.

Keywords: malaria, environment, Spain, Barcelona, disease

1. Introduction

In the late eighteenth century, we find a general context in Catalonia in which institutions, sanitation, and society adapted to political changes marked by the application of the "Real

Decreto de Nueva Planta" [1], one of the most important consequences of the Spanish Succession War. This law was elaborated and applied in 1717 by Bourbon authorities to control traditional Catalan institutions, modify the pre-existing legislation, and also reshuffle the pre-existing structures to create a new assembly according to the interests of the new monarchy. At the same time, the "Principado" political model was introduced in Catalonia. This model was similar to that prevalent in the majority of European countries, in which the sovereign could formulate laws separately from the political community [2]. In this sense, throughout the eighteenth century, the Audience regent in conjunction with the Intendent and the General Captain were the authorities that presided over political decisions throughout the Catalan territories [3].

The city of Barcelona was not an exception concerning the application of the new laws. From December 1718 [4], the consequences were felt in urban structures, the city council, the society, and all sanitation institutions and sanitation professionals. The city fall on 11 September 1714 implied the suppression of the traditional city council (known as "Consell de Cent"), and the construction in 1715 of Ciudadela fortress. This fortification was built to keep the city population under military control (**Figure 1**).

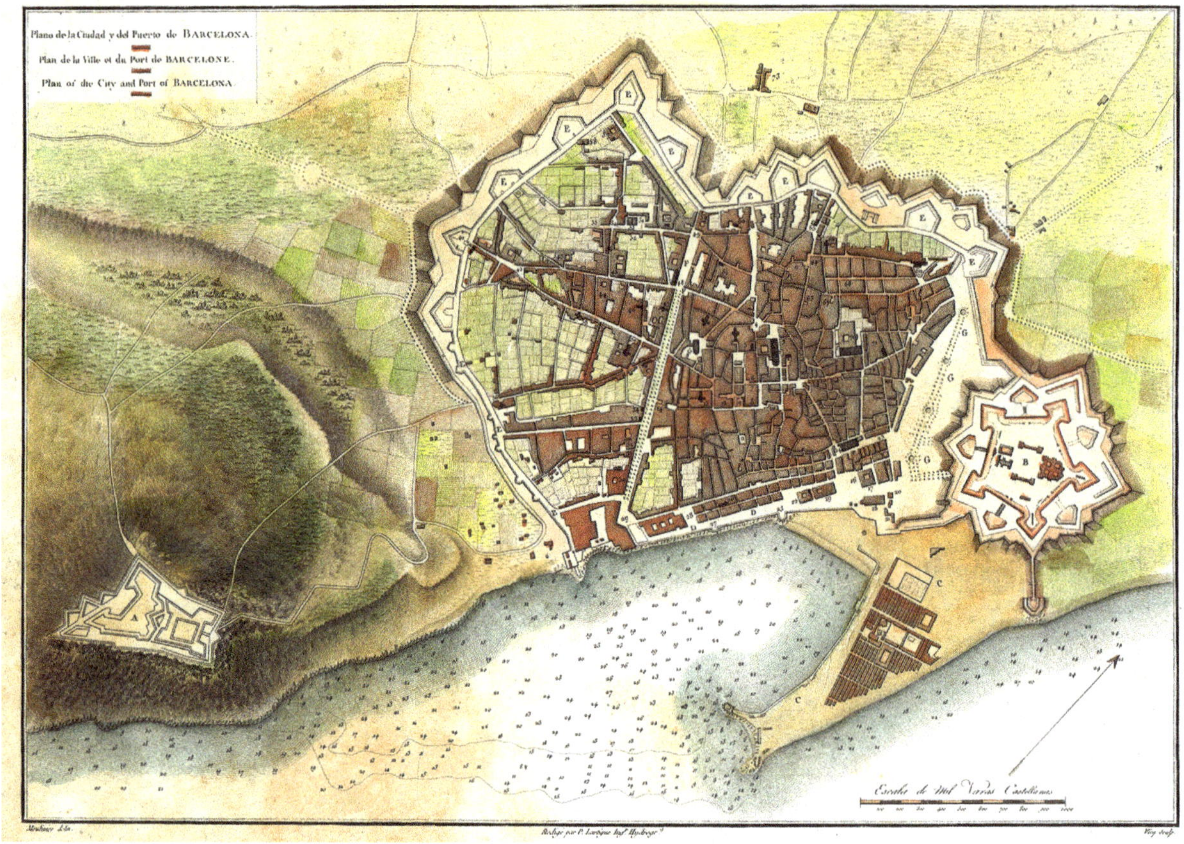

Figure 1. MOULINIER. Plano de la ciudad y Puerto de Barcelona. 1806. ICGC, RM. 19425.

The construction of the Ciudadela fortress also changed the traditional morphological distribution of the city. In fact, 17% of the total urban area [5] was occupied by the fortress, causing 6380 people to be displaced to the most crowded city area, the quarter of Sant Pere i Santa Caterina, and changing the traditional morphology of the "artisan house." The ancient structures were adapted to the necessities of accommodating the displaced population, "There are not so many houses in the city constructed in the present century that don't have three or four rooms, or flats, more of them four, and some even five flats. The referred houses are actually taller than they were in the past. Their interior structures owe more to economics than to health. It is common to form a flat with the essential rooms, including a kitchen, saloon and bed, and a little room. This is seen in places that were commonly used as one room, which now present too many subdivisions. The majority of these rooms have a water well very close to the latrines" [6].

In 1753, a new quarter, designed by the military engineer Jorge Próspero de Verboom, was constructed to take in the population surplus of a crowded city center in which people's quotidian life was quite marked by coexistence with textile industries, stagnant water channels (Rec Comtal), and the unhealthy sanitary conditions of commercial activities. Just 4.2% of the citizens moved to the new Barceloneta. This fact stunned travelers and visitors such as Arthur Young in 1787. "A quarter, called Barceloneta, it is entirely new and regular; their streets cross at right angles. Now: because of the absence of sailors, small businesses and artisans, the houses are low and small. One of the sides faces the docks. The streets are brightened up, but due to the high amount of dust, by a special attention to the wider streets, I cannot say that all of them are provided with flagstone pavement" [7].

The stagnant agriculture patterns of Catalonia in 1750–1760 pushed people to transfer to cities: cities that offered the possibility of importing wheat and export the surplus wine production to maintain the prices [8]. Between 1717 and 1787, the city population increased from 35,928 to 100,160 inhabitants, a 180% enlargement that translated into a population of 114,100 by the end of the century [9]. In consequence, cities like Barcelona saw a considerable increase in and a conflict with infrastructure not adapted to the process of intensive agriculture based on irrigation. Agricultural intensification and specialization had their negative effects in directly favoring the proliferation of unhealthy areas "*We face, as Young noticed, in one of the most advanced agriculture of Europe a dark side: the growth of unhealthy areas with delta fevers as a consequence of irrigation patterns*" [10].

At the end of the century, we find a city adapted to the Bourbon reforms and urbanized with new spaces concerning the construction of Ciudadela and the Ramblas development. The city council from 1784 managed the regulation of the new spaces in which textile industries could be placed—outside the city walls—as we see in the message contained in the Royal Chord of 22 May 1784 "*in attention to the multiplicity of cotton and wool factories that have been built inside this city in recent years, which is currently excessive, and is starting to affect the everyday lives of the citizens and residents of this city*" [11].

The urban reshuffle such as the construction of a new sewage system and the extension of hydraulic infrastructure was considerably restricted due to the reduction of the annual city council budget to a quarter of its previous value [12]. One of the worst consequences was felt in the quality of water, which for the most part was contaminated due to bad insulation conditions of latrines and cesspits. This issue was a common preoccupation for the physicians of the city due to the constant obstruction of an outdated sewer system "*But we have to be very sorry that those sewers have not been continued with the spirit of the first builders. Because of the limited capacity that those sewers currently present, in most streets they cause the presence of stagnant areas in which we often see accumulated a high variety of material and water. In consequence the pollution builds up and all along the vents and particularly the sewers emerge occasionally the putrid vapours that fill the houses and streets with stinking air; and other times the same material overflows, causing an insupportable stench*" [13].

The progressive intensification of the manufacturing activity meant that by 1806 Barcelona took in more than 104 industries with a total of 12,000 workers [14]. These industries crowded Barcelona in the late eighteenth century, particularly in the "prados de indianas" [15] that were placed around the most important rivers. Especially near the Besós [16] River, where in 1784 alone, those industries employed an additional 8638 people [17].

1.1. The pursuit of a medical academy in Barcelona

Sanitation institutions are one of the most important aspects on which we will focus our attention because of the importance of physicians as the principal observers of weather, environment, and diseases of past societies, more importantly in the late eighteenth century. Indeed, sanitation professionals had a strong social position, high importance, and an ancient tradition concerning the application of epidemic prevention policies in Barcelona during the sixteenth and seventeenth centuries [18]. Since the latter half of the sixteenth century, the prestige acquired by the Estudi General—the medical school of Barcelona—signified the inclusion in the citizen oligarchy of the physicians attached to the Col·legi de Doctor en Medicina de Barcelona, the professors of Estudi General, and the ancient Hospital of Santa Creu.

In a more general perspective, the Real Tribunal del Protomedicato [19], founded on 30 March 1477, prevailed as the central state institution to control public health, to regulate medical practice, and to verify the quality of drugs and remedies dispensed by the apothecaries. One of their institutional competences was to collect taxes from exam fees and fines to administer them and the investment of the funds thus obtained. In fact, since the sixteenth century, in the Crown of Aragon, those exposed competences were administered by the traditional institutional structures. Furthermore, an important objective of physicians from Barcelona was to obtain the title of Royal Protomedico.

This institutional position allowed physicians to profit from an important social protection and to maintain the public presence of a medicinal profession open to the arrival of new methods and ideas for the renewal of medicine. The arrival of the new scientific medicine, based on the resurgence of Hippocratism, was the starting point of a change in the way in which epidemics in the latter third of the seventeenth century were confronted and understood [20]. Physicians started to displace the theoretical teaching of medicine to incorporate Hippocrates' aphorisms. From then on, the medicine became an effort to understand nature, naturae conamen, and to expel from patients' bodies all infective material. Physicians had to note carefully all the symptomatology, symptomatum concatenatio, to increase the knowledge of the diversity and variety of illnesses that medicine must face [21]. Physicians Herman Boherhaave or Thomas

Sydenham emphasized the construction of a medical knowledge based on an historical perspective of illnesses. The context of scientific exchanges led to a progressive evolution of medicine to hygienists' policies of the late eighteenth century. These, however, had to face new problems derived from the confluence of supporters and detractors of the new medical improvements, especially at the beginning of the eighteenth century [22].

The consequences of the application of Royal Decrees to sanitation professionals and medical institutions caused the regression of Catalan medicine. The most important effects of these Decrees were the suppression of institutions like the "Estudi General" and the creation of a new university in Cervera [23] (1714–1717). This university did not gain the support of those physicians associated with the former "Estudi General," due to its failure to provide any kind of improvement in medical studies. Debauchery and the loss of institutional control over medical practice drew to Barcelona a considerable number of unlicensed practitioners. This together with the loss of productivity in medical literature, the lack of proper control over medical studies, the decline of medical presence in municipal institutions, and the decline of the social importance of physicians were the principal impulses for physicians to try to recover control of medical practice. Their goal was to instate a medical practice in which professional schools of surgeons and apothecaries prevailed, with the consequent continuous conflicts due to the overlap of institutional competences.

The Junta de Morbo of Barcelona—an institution dedicated to the prevention of epidemics —was also brought under the new institutional laws. In fact, the arrival of the Plague in Marseille in 1720 prompted a reshuffle of the epidemic prevention institutions in the central Superior Council of Sanitation of the Kingdom [24]. This institution, since its foundation on 28 August 1720 by the administration of Felipe V [25], had assumed the local functions of the pre-existing epidemic prevention bodies. In this sense, the diversity of the range of functions of those bodies was, in the case of Barcelona, extremely diversified. The jurisdiction of the Superior Council was considerable, covering Barcelona and the rest of Catalonia at the same time.

This broad purview is explained by the need to build an elaborate network based on the communication of the provincial territorial subdivisions that formed the Superior Council of Sanitation. In the case of Barcelona, the same Royal Audience that proposed city hall members acted as a communication medium between the Superior Council of Sanitation and the municipal city council [26].

In fact, as we can see in the documentation, the communication between physicians, surgeons, and municipal authorities was the principal point that helped to keep an effective prevention system in the city and to apply epidemic prevention laws and observe their effects throughout the territory. At a more local level, the drastic municipal budget reduction of the Bourbon City Council caused serious difficulties and limitations in relation to the executive capabilities of the institution.

The impact of the institutional changes discussed above revealed the importance of the historical trust in physicians and in university medicine as a legitimation of the collective of medical professionals who took part in the public health system. This was one of the objectives of a new generation of physicians, primarily trained at Montpellier University, who arrived in Catalonia in 1740. In the program of the Academia Médico-Práctica de Barcelona, these physicians sought State support and the recognition of the utility of medicine [20].

Philip V's death in 1749 signified a more opportune time to request the reestablishment of University of Barcelona with the consequent opposite interests of the recently founded University of Cervera and the interest of Real Protomedicato. Barcelona in 1760 and 1770 was subject to an institutional impulse that crystallized in the origins of two scientific academies, the Academia Médico Práctica and the Academia de Ciencias y Artes [27]. The origins of both academies were immersed in a context in which European academies were under Royal or manorial protection to develop studies linked to the political interests. The constant failures concerning the reestablishment of the Medical College in 1754, 1769, and 1770 together with the necessity of a medical corporation with teaching responsibilities forced the authorities to suppress those aspects that could present friction or an overlap of competences with the Real Protomedicato [20]. However, the existence of a medical hospital in Barcelona to observe diseases and to collect medical reports brought about the study of the anatomical effects of illnesses by means of dissections. This inclination was one of the pillars of the program of the Academia Médico-Práctica de Barcelona that we can see reflected in the inaugural speech of Dr. Jaume Bonells: "It is not enough to know the causes of illnesses without healing them; only the Government can remedy the origins of those diseases, and it is necessary that the magistrates and physicians work together" [28]. Moreover, Bonells refocused the interest in medical studies over the general interest of a society immersed in a constant development. Those interests included agriculture, cattle raising, and those "useful sciences" from which the economy could profit.

The program elaborated by Bonells is of principal interest for our research in that it concerns the need to observe the relationship between illnesses and the environment and climate [29]. This is in line with the studies proposed by Sydenham and Baglivi, in which a necessary point of observation was the precise moment at which epidemics originated and spread through the territory: "*With the collection of meteorological records of each town, we could have already the medical history of every time and region, and through this medium, Medicine would be in a degree of perfection in which today remains considerably remote*" [28].

This program of the Academia Médico-Práctica was formally proposed by Joan Esteve, lieutenant of the Protomedicato, and Pere Güell, first examiner of Protomedicato, in Catalonia on 29 April 1770. Their proposal obtained the approval of the Royal Audience on 2 July 1770 and was ratified in the first assembly of the Academia Médico-Práctica of Barcelona [30]. The most important recognition is seen in the Royal Decree of 21 September 1786, delivered by Charles III, in which the statutes of the Academia were approved and placed under Royal protection. This recognition gave the Academia the right to use the Royal printer to publish their statutes. Finally, in February 1797, the monarchy granted the chair in Medicine [31] to the Real Academia Médico-Practica de Barcelona; as a consequence, instruction in medicine was officially re-established in Barcelona.

2. Malaria and environment

Malaria and its strong relation to environment becomes one of the most interesting points in relation to develop studies centered on epidemics and their impact over past societies. Paludism is a disease which kept a strong link with landscapes of the past, human productive facilities and agricultural patterns, climatic oscillations, temperature, rainfall, and wind direction [32]. In consequence, we find necessary to offer a general approach to his ethology and symptomatology but, especially, in the particular ways in which the illness interacts with another diseases.

In 2015, *World malaria report*, shows us a regressive impact of the illness in comparison with the estimated values given for the year 2000 (262 million cases of malaria globally—214 million in 2015—and 839,000 deaths—438,000 deaths in 2015) [33]. However, malaria is still present as a resistant illness to vector control measures (insecticides) and to antimalarial treatments (particularly *Plasmodium falciparum*). In fact, malaria is one of the most ancient illnesses known by the humanity with references in China on 2700 BC, Mesopotamia 2000 BC, and Egypt 1570 BC, and in Hindu texts from sixth century BC [34]. An illness whose symptomatology was well known and his relation with environment well specified, as an example, like shows us Hippocrates in 410 BC "*Passed the dog days the fevers became sweat, but behind him did not disappeared; the fevers came back again, with a moderated duration, difficult to attach and without giving to much thirst. In too much patients the fevers stopped in seven and nine days but in others after eleven days, fourteen, seventeen and twenty-two days*" [35].

The link between stagnant waters and malaria is a traditional causal relation present in medical records of the eighteenth century, which worried physicians and authorities by the same way. As an example, Francisco Cerdán said in their *Discursos physico-medicos, politico-morales que tratan ser toda calentura hectica contagiosa, essencia del universal contagio, y medios para precaverlo* (published in 1752) that "*Juan Maria Lancisi, Physician of Clemente XI, testified, that being Aquileya one of the most important cities of Italy... could not to tolerate too much epidemics, caused by the putrid exhalations that came from the stagnant waters*" [36]. In words of Mary Jane Dobson, "*These were the 'silent' fevers creeping from house to house, along the channels of contamination, but eventually revealing their impact on the seasonal, annual and secular graphs of mortality peaks*" [37].

In the case of Barcelona, before and after the epidemic of 1783–1786, we found many proclamations given by the authorities focused in the prevention of flood impact and in the control of marshlands and lagoons, especially, in the two principal rivers that surrounded Barcelona—Besós and Llobregat rivers. In this sense, we have selected three examples in which the first is the proclamation published by order of Jacinto Pazuengos y Zurbarán, Governor of Barcelona, on 8 April 1780 [38]. The principal message transmitted by the Governor was focused on the establishment of preventive hygienist policies to promote the systematic clean of fields, paths, river banks, and stream flows. Due to the constant floods, the necessity to keep river bank boats in good conditions was also mentioned, and building irrigation ditches, building new houses on Besós-Llobregat river banks, and building up embankments on marshlands were specifically prohibited.

On 16 May 1784, Manuel de Terán, General of the Royal Army in Catalonia, [39] published a new proclaim that reminded the authorities about the observations published in the past proclaim of 1780 because *"It is quite common, that the extraordinary rains, and other irregular and violent accidents cause notable injuries to the road paths (…) this happens due to the failure to follow some useful orders to prevent those situations"* [39]. The new and most important measure improved in the municipal proclaim concerns the prohibition to build new cane cultivation rafts. In spite of the efforts of the authorities, it will be problematic to follow the proposed hygienic policies.

On 31 March 1787, Manuel de Terán [40] again published another proclaim. An advice that this time will consist to improve a systematic planting of trees to keep water stream controlled on Besós and Llobregat rivers. However, as we can see through the testimony of Francisco de Zamora the planting of trees was not completely applied in 1789, *"The River banks of the referred rivers and torrents, creeks, streams that run over the center of Barcelona's area, generally, are not planted with trees. There are only few trees planted by the land proprietors of some parts of Besós and Llobregat river bank areas"* [41].

In fact, the relation with malaria and some agricultural patterns based in irrigation has been a common problem all along the sixteenth to eighteenth centuries as we can find in many bibliographical references or through the sources. Especially in the eighteenth and nineteenth centuries, malaria was associated with the rice cultivation [42–44]. This was due to the proliferation of artificial flooded areas that ensured the production of an alimentary resource that could offer a high quantity of food with reduced cost: *"In Europe, rice cultivation areas have been, since their implantation, responsible of the endemics of malaria and also their epidemic forms; although the authorities had tried to limit and avoid this kind of agricultural practice. However the restrictions have been frequently broken, in some cases totally disobeyed because of rice culture was a source of high incomes"* [42]. Unhealthy flooded areas all along peninsular Mediterranean basin that became famous over ages and countries as exemplifies the testimony of Pierre Pauly in his work published in 1874: *"The Mediterranean area of Spain it's all along his basin an important source of epidemics: Intermittent fever, the bilious remittent fever they are common from one side to another, more or less, naturally, by the pass of years; and where a unfortunate meteorological constitution (overcast, cloudy, frequently calm) conjuncts with the active local causes, and epidemic took place, finding a terrain prepared for its development"* [45].

Concerning the etiological aspects of the illness, there are more than 200 types of malaria [46], only four affects to humans: *Plasmodium Falciparum, P. Vivax, P. Ovale,* and *P. Malariae*. Malaria is a eukaryotic disease transmitted through the bite of an *Anopheles* mosquito that starts the infectious process in the human host. However, there are secondary infection forms especially in endemic areas which consist, for example, in mother-to-child transmission [47] causing new-born's weight loss, injuring his immunological system and being children the principal victims of a high range of diseases [46]. Malaria's infectious life cycle starts with an initial stage in which sporozoites flow through the blood circuit until they are installed in liver cells and complete the initial infectious cycle. In the liver cells, sporozoites reproduce themselves through asexual reproduction and through the *lysis*, process in which liberate new merozoites —more than 30,000 merozoites [48]. This is the fact that causes the progressive destruction of blood cells each 24 hours (*P. Falciparum*), 48 hours (*P. Vivax*), and 72 hours (*P. Malariae*) [46]. This process causes malaria's paroxysm in which the most severe fever episodes [49] causing the traditional symptomatology of a malaria infection (chill, fever, and sweat) are concentrated. Malarial fevers can be continuous (if there are no fluctuations higher than 0.5°C in 24 hours), remittent fevers (if the temperature keeps over 1°C or more in 24 hours) or intermittent (if the temperature comes back to normality one or two times in 24 hours) [50].

After that, sexual gametocytes circle along human host blood vessels until another mosquito bites. Inside mosquito's stomach, gametocytes will start the sexual reproduction generating Oocysts if the minimal ambient temperatures are higher than 17°C for *P. vivax* or up to 20°C to *P. falciparum*. This process closes the infectious life cycle when new sporozoites are released into the salivary glands of the mosquito ready to start another asexual reproduction cycle in the human host.

One of the most important consequences of malaria is that it causes the progressive destruction of human blood cells, generating a state of anemia. However, the most common symptomatology of the disease can be similar to less aggressive virus diseases causing abdominal pain, diarrhea, discomfort, fatigue, fever, headache and respiratory disorders in patients. There are also some physical and most appreciable symptoms such as jaundice and splenomegaly. In which the last one appears in adults after a series of malarial relapses but it is faster and easier to detect in kids.

However, the most interesting aspect is the immune system suppression that signifies a high risk of coinfection. A question that should be studied in detail in past societies paying attention to the pathocenosis concept introduced by Mirko G. Grmek. Pathocenosis means that the frequency and distribution of every disease depends, on another endogenous and ecological factors, on the frequency and distribution of all other diseases [51]. In consequence, further studies were developed in ancient societies to better know how malaria interact with other diseases causing a considerable decrease in the health status and interact with the constant flow of history. In words of Eric Faure "*Historically, malaria was probably one the diseases with the greatest opportunity to interact with other diseases because of the extent of the malarious areas, of the level of endemicity and of the fact that humans could be infected during all the duration of their lives*" [52].

Malaria can produce positive or negative effects over the diseases in which the illness interacts in direct or indirect forms. As an example, malaria has been applied as a treatment for syphilitic patients. Moreover, Malaria also interacts with tuberculosis (*Mycobacterium tuberculosis*). In this last example, malaria exacerbates the infection and the last one modulates the host response to malaria. It is also important for this research to focus on positive and synergistic interactions of malaria along other diseases that could have deleterious effects in endemic areas. And positive relations with malaria along illnesses that could have a considerable impact on malarial epidemics along diseases such as virus: flaviviruses as dengue or yellow fever; winter respiratory diseases: influenza or smallpox virus. In addition, malaria can interact in positive forms with bacterial diseases such as cholera (*Vibrio cholerae*), plague (*Yersinia pestis*), shigella, and typhus [46] (*Salmonella enterica* serotype *Typhi*) [52]. In words of Eric Fauré, "*Data from the pre-antibiotic era suggest that malaria increases the host's susceptibility to invasive bacterial infections"* [52].

Finally, in relation to malaria transmission the most complex environmental aspect is found in two principal areas: in *Anopheles* mosquitoes and in sporogonial development inside mosquitoes' stomach. In fact, the link between temperature and oocysts development [53] is essential to know malaria seasonal behavior. As Gustavo Pittaluga said, *"It is not the annual average ambient temperature which determines the degree of endemic (along other conditions), it is more concretely the summer average ambient temperature, the thermal average values of summer, what allows the presence of endemic focus of malaria in temperate climate regions areas"* [54]. In this sense, as mentioned below, through the methodology applied to analyze instrumental meteorological records it varies from minimal temperatures of 17°C for *P. vivax* to 20°C for *P. falciparum* [55, 56]. Our objective is to detect in which years or months malaria epidemics could have a more favorable ambient factor to develop in epidemic forms.

The current problematic for historians' remains in the exactitude to define the variety of Anopheles mosquitoes present in Catalan territories along eighteenth and nineteenth centuries. As a reference, we considered works developed in the first half of the twentieth century such as the Comisión para el Saneamiento de Comarcas Palúdicas (1920–1924) and Comisión Central Antipalúdica (1924–1934) [57]. These works gave us knowledge about the varieties of *Anopheles* that were more common in the Peninsular level until the application of the Proyecto Oficial de Erradicación del Paludismo en España (1959–1962). The works of the zoologist and entomologist Juan Gil Collado inside the campaign led by Gustavo Pittaluga and Sadí de Buen show that from the five varieties that form the complex *Anopheles maculipennis* the variety *labranchiae* was present in Alicante and Murcia. While *Anopheles atroparvus* was the most distributed over Europe [58]. In consequence, we found that our exploratory study focused on examining the relation with environment and *Anopheles* sp. based on the general conditions for "*maculipennis* complex" [59]. Moreover, we analyzed the "superinfection phase" through instrumental meteorological data treatment [60]. The superinfection phase consists of a phase of maximum density of *Anopheles* sp. from April to June. The objective of the study was to focus on those months which present more days with average temperatures less than 25°C [61] and a humidity higher than 40% (fact that was common in all Barcelona area).

One of the possible applications of this historical analysis of malaria over selected Mediterranean areas, regions and cities was to elaborate more precise mathematic models that could help historians to better understand the behavior of the illness in the past. Also, and more important, this analysis could help to develop preventive epidemical models in relation to the current climatic change in which *"Vector-borne diseases are highly sensitive to global warming and associated changes in precipitation"* [62].

3. Sources and methodology

The first question that come to us when we plan to develop studies that involve a high variety and diversity of sources is in relation to which is the most suitable methodology that we must apply. The second question concerns what kind of sources we can manage to achieve our objectives. In fact, due to the variety of names that surrounds endemic and epidemic fevers on past societies (terms such as fevers, intermittent fevers, agues, and marshland fevers), we proposed a methodology to study epidemics, from a historical point of view, that would be open to interdisciplinary approaches from history, biology, geography, demography, and climatology. A proposal that reminds us the work of the team lead by Jean-Paul Desaive [63] or the study developed by Vicente Pérez Moreda [64] with a more demographical perspective. Moreover, we can refer to some works published by authors such as Pablo Giménez-Font [65] from the University de Alicante and Mary Jane Dobson [37] from the Oxford Wellcome Unit for the History of Medicine. In addition, the most recent study conducted by an interdisciplinary team from the Aix-Marseille University [55].

Concerning sources, we parted from a general and specified bibliography (papers, monographs, and theses) that allowed us to focus on compiling the highest and possible amount of information.

The amount of sources and their varieties were relatively large: private sources (diaries and memories), public sources (medical reports, contemporary mortality, and morbidity records), municipal sources (books of acts, municipal proclaims, public health reports, and works on hydraulic or sanitarian issues), ecclesiastical sources (burial and baptisms series, and community books of acts), public and private sanitarian institutional sources (medical reports), print sources (newspapers, Royal Decrees, and contemporary medical reports), cartographical sources, instrumental meteorological data (temperature and rainfall records, and wind direction), and flood-drought monthly proxy data indexes generated from Rogation ceremonies (1780–1800) [66].

In consequence, we will emphasize on the principal sources that can be useful to develop similar research over different times and countries, and a methodology suitable to reconstruct other epidemical cases.

3.1. Municipal sources

All the documentation produced by municipal authorities in past societies has arrived to our current times in many diverse forms and ways. This means that we can find more or less complete archives. However, the most common and complete sources that we can find in municipal archives are, e.g., municipal chords, municipal proclamations, and sanitation expedients.

First, the answer to this source selection rests in the serial and continuous data that we can extract from municipal chords as a first source in which all the information relative to the city and quotidian life is reflected. That is, a conjunct of information compiled from notes taken for the secretary at every municipal session, which contains a variety of typologies: proclamations, design of infrastructures, and accounting documents. The utility in relation to epidemiology remains in the keyword research through the contemporary indexes of municipal chords. The objective is to detect every political measure applied to contain epidemics: burial of clothes, latrine cleaning policies, wheat importations, prices regulation of products affected by commercial blocks or as a consequence of climate instability (carbon, bread, and meat), and police measures applied to guarantee the control of population.

Second, municipal proclamations show the researcher what kind of measures and information were published for the common knowledge, in which data such as urban regulations, advices, prices of essential products, and sanitary policies have a direct impact as measures derived from epidemic situations. After comparing the information extracted from municipal proclamations with the data extracted from municipal chords, the researcher will be able to prove if the municipality had concealed evidences at the time of epidemics.

Finally, sanitarian expedients concentrate all the documents generated or received by the municipal Sanitarian Council. As an example, Barcelona is one of the most complete sanitarian series preserved at the peninsular level with 12 series and 271 independent units providing sanitarian information to the researcher from Barcelona, Catalonia, Spain, and the rest of the world. Although some series are fragmentary, we can obtain data from surveys conducted by physicians, medical records, sanitarian patents, and sanitary chords that can be compared with the information obtained from municipal chords and municipal proclamations.

3.2. Public sources

All the documents from medical institutions such as the Reial Acadèmia de Medicina de Catalunya are another point of interests. The high amount of documentation that we can obtain provides interesting data concerning the symptomatology of the diseases observed at the time of epidemics. In other words, medical topographies conducted by physicians in order to be accepted as partners of the Medical Academy of Barcelona provide interesting data about the common habitudes, landscapes of the past, environmental conditions, and hygienic conditions of the cities analyzed in those works.

On the one hand, medical records were works ordered by municipal authorities in which physicians did an environmental analysis of all the illnesses observed during a concrete chronology. The most interesting aspect we find it in that physicians, following the principles of medical topographies, did a complete study of weather, illnesses, and environmental conditions in every case searching the focus of the illness and the exact time in which epidemics appeared in the cities and villages. A complete work over the urban infrastructures and common people's habits had been corrected through sanitation policy applications.

On the other hand, demographic records collected by physicians in collaboration with ecclesiastic and municipal authorities at the time of epidemics can provide demographic movement of parishes to our research data whose archives are actually inexistent due to the course of history. Another analysis possibility that provides us those demographic tables is to contrast the results with ecclesiastic demographic sources.

Print sources include a high typological diversity and currently the most part is easily accessible through digital repositories. In this sense, the most interesting sources used to complete the information extracted from municipal archives are the medical prescriptions at the time of epidemics and published medical records. In their conjunct, these kinds of print sources (considered as primary sources that were coetaneous published to the period of study) can contribute to better understand the social repercussions of an epidemic and the institutional measures applied to spread the information between common people, authorities and physicians. The historical compilations of epidemics as, e.g., Doctor Joaquin de Villalba's work —military physician of Aragon—are more important concerns, where his message goes directly vinculated to the medical pursuit of the historical reconstruction of endemics, epidemics, and epizootic illnesses *"to show taking as an example past situations to better affront future cases"* [67].

3.3. Ecclesiastical sources

The study on the abundant and variety that present ecclesiastical archives makes to focus research interests on the sources that can have a more sense of utility. Parish books are one of the most important sources to develop historical epidemiology due to the high level of detail and trustworthy information that we can extract from parish baptisms, and death and burial records. In fact, since the Council of Trento (1545–1562) all parishes were obligated to establish parish books to register baptisms (births), deaths, and marriages. Those records, currently, are the well-known kinds of sources which worked in the research fields of demography, historical demography and genetics [68].

As discussed above, the amount of information that can be extracted is significant. Although parish registers can present variations from one parish to another, they usually follow a contained structure. The solid structure of parish registers allow us to extract, taking as example baptism records, information relative to baptism date, name and surname of the newborn, parents' names, and parental professional data and born place. While concerning death and burial records, we can extract homogeneous information concerning death date, name and surname of the deceased, parental information, parental professional data, born place and burial place. Since the beginning of the nineteenth century, it has incorporated another interesting data that concern directly to the principles promoted by the hygienist medicine; this is the cause of death.

Obituary tables elaborated by physician Francisco Salvà, from the Royal Academia of Medicina de Barcelona, are good examples of the interest of physicians to improve the cause of death in parish registers to better study the seasonality of illnesses and detect those epidemics that caused elevated mortality levels. In fact, the latter is a good example in which physicians presented the obituary tables. The problematic work in tables was to exactly delimitate the age group through parish registers, *"Must be necessary that from now on in burial records will be expressed the age of deceased, because otherwise it would follow what currently happens with the name of infants must be understood all those that die until the age of 12, 14 or more years, whatever executed with all the other observations from your H.E. of this illustrious city council obituary tables may again be formed same as those currently made in London, Paris or in other places"* [69].

In fact, the problematic work was the precision of the age group qualified in parish sources as infants continue promoting an intense discussion between historical demographers. It is necessary to refer to the studies developed by Vicente Pérez Moreda, especially, mentioning infants as a collective population comprised of a group of ages from 0 to 7 years old. Moreover, the age group of infants is susceptible, biologically and physically, to succumb to an illness (**Figure 2**) [64].

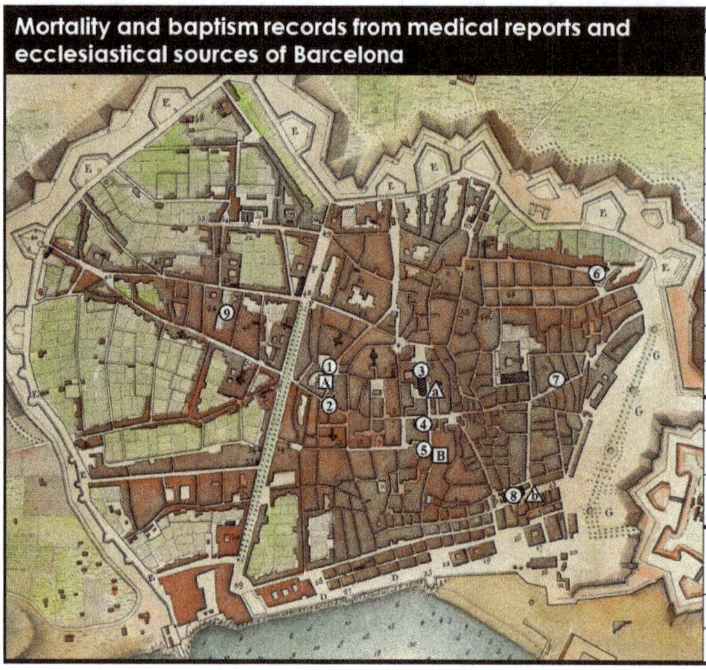

LEGEND				
	Dr. Salvà. Mortality records	**Anual resolution**	**Monthly resolution**	**Daily resolution**
(1)	Sta. Ma. del Pi	1780-86/1797-1803		
(2)	St. Jaume	1780-86/1797-1803		
(3)	Catedral	1780-86/1797-1803	1780-86 1797-1803	
(4)	St. Miquel	1780-86/1797-1803		
(5)	St. Just i Pastor	1780-86/1797-1803		
(6)	St. Pere de les Puel·les	1780-86/1797-1803		
(7)	St. Cugat del Rec	1780-86/1797-1803		
(8)	Sta. Ma. del Mar	1780-86/1797-1803	1780-86 1797-1803	
(9)	Hospital Sta. Creu i Sant Pau		1780-1803	
Dr. Salvà. Baptism records				
(a)	Catedral		1780-86 1797-1803	
(b)	Sta. Ma. del Mar		1780-86 1797-1803	
Mortality parish records: Parish of Santa Maria del Pi (APSMP). Parish of Sant Just I Pastor (APSJP).				
(A)	Sta. Ma. del Pi			1770-1800
(B)	Sant Just i Pastor			1770-1800

Figure 2. Chronologic extreme dates of demographic sources extracted from parish of Santa Maria del Pi, parish of Sant Just i Pastor, and from the Medical Obituary tables created by physician Dr. Francisco Salvà.

As mentioned above, our interest was to focus on obtaining continuous and detailed data series digitized in excel to realize further analysis that will provide us some interesting information about the seasonality of deaths and the age group that was most affected. As an example, we propose to digitize the information extracted from parish records differentiating sex and age in daily resolution to obtain standardized series in monthly or annual resolution through typification statistical process [70]—among other analytic procedures. Other analytic processes such as seasonal mortality patterns can be of great utility to exactly precise in which season's mortality fall in children or adult population. On the other hand, seasonal movements of mortality can be put in relation to the medical records to have a more complete perspective of the diseases present along with detected mortality peaks.

Finally, parish records in spite of their possible discontinuous or fragmentary preservation can be complemented through obituary tables compiled by physicians. Another possibility to sort the disappeared information from some parish archives lies in coetaneous census conducted by state authorities. As an example, the census conducted by Count of Floridablanca in 1787 shows us in the preface that the scrutiny of Catalonia's population was done "*after three years of an epidemic almost general of tertian fevers and putrid fevers, especially in the two Castillas, Aragon Kingdom, and principality of Catalonia, that has resulted in a considerable diminution of their habitants*" [71].

3.4. Instrumental meteorological records

Maldà Oscillation [72] becomes the climatologic context that will have a direct impact on the environmental context generating unhealthy area. A process of climatic instability appeared since 1760 until the end of the eighteenth century. A process of climatic oscillation was marked by the simultaneous emergence of droughts, floods, temperature oscillations, and storms. This phase of climatic change, that reminds us of the current climate problematic, as discussed above, has had repercussions over biological and ecological aspects: proliferation of flooded areas and consequences over the hydraulic resources. This phase also had repercussions over the economy: bad harvests, increase of basic product costs because of bad harvests, and effects on the economic resources.

The relation between climate oscillations and the spread of epidemics was one of the principal interests of physicians because of following the principles of hygienist medicine. Even more, as we observed, the pursuit to elaborate a historical relation of epidemics, to observe and measure the weather, to analyze the environment, and the elaboration of accurate compilations of symptomatological descriptions (clinical histories) fructified into a scientific approach of medicine to another sciences were among other interests. This approach encouraged physicians to develop systematic meteorological observations.

Meteorological tables elaborated by physician Dr. Francisco Salvà i Campillo [73] have denoted a great interest to climate reconstruction [74]. In fact, Dr. Mariano Barriendos together with "Team of Climate Change" from the Climatological Area of the Meteorological Service of Catalonia has digitized those tables in a project of three years of duration. The information contained in those meteorological tables, e.g., atmospheric pressure, temperature (measured each day at 7–14 and 22 hours), and precipitation, has a high potential to develop more accurate predictive models due to the current climate change dynamics through initiatives such as MEDARE (MEditerranean DAta REscue) or ACRE (Atmospheric Circulation Reconstruction over the Earth) [75].

What is even more interesting is the inclusion of medical observances that are focused on the epidemical constitution of every month. In those observations, Dr. Francisco Salvà included an accurate description of the symptomatology observed in their patients. Moreover, the physician searched all the references, at the time of epidemics, to find equal epidemic cases in different countries. This completed some information from contemporary sources in relation to reconstruct the specter of endemic and epidemic fevers at European level.

The utility of instrumental meteorological records opens a high range of possible analysis concerning malaria's relation with climate and environment. In fact, the analysis of temperature records will help us to detect which years presented prolonged warm summers or in which months temperature guaranteed a more considerable presence of *Anopheles* mosquitoes. Furthermore, the conjunction of analyzed annual historical indexes of floods and droughts can detect those years in which cities and village's environment was being affected by an irregular succession of floods and droughts that could have reflected a more propitious terrain for the development of a malaria epidemic. These Concern annual-monthly historical indexes those were generated from rogation ceremonies by Barriendos [66].

Although this methodology requires of further detailed analysis methods, we would like to show some analysis to demonstrate the applicability of this sources to help detect the most favorable conditions for malaria development in past societies. Because malaria is a background disease complex to be identified over the sources, we propose to develop analysis from instrumental meteorological records. The objective is to put together all the direct and indirect conjunct of environmental-climatic elements that can be associated with an epidemic of malaria: warm summers, days that present a highest superinfection phase of *Anopheles* mosquitoes (if temperature is less than 25°C between April and June and humidity is higher than 40%, those years present a large number of *Anopheles* sp.), favorable days for sporogony of *P. vivax* and *P. falciparum* based on the minimal daily temperatures of June-October for all the available and monthly minimum temperatures of June-October for all the period observed (1780–1800).

4. The epidemic context in Catalonia (1783–1786)

The report from Real Tribunal del Protomedicato published in 1785 detailed the constant presence of malaria at Peninsular level "*Tertian fevers have been ever in Spain the dominant illness, and for this reason our authors are the most respectable between the strangers, giving us a clear idea to differentiate over all the forms over tertian fevers those that currently are affecting us*" [76]. This epidemic of malaria, since 1783, is identified in epidemic forms outside its hyperendemic areas (Valencia and Catalonia rice fields and marshlands) along other diseases as typhoid fevers. Tertian fevers and putrid fevers were in fact well known through the Mediterranean littoral areas. Even more, contemporary physicians such as Andrés Piquer noted the strong relation between tertian fevers and rice cultivation or irrigation patterns insisting to the authorities to implement the prohibition of rice cultivation to one league of distance from urban areas. However, the high interests of land proprietors to avoid prohibition or reconcile the legislation to make possible the continuation of rice cultivation was a constant problem (**Figure 3**) [25].

However, tertian fevers epidemic of 1783–1786 could not be compared to precedent equal episodes. In fact, authors such as Vicente Pérez Moreda elevate the impact of the epidemic to a one million affected people and a hundred thousand deaths just in 1786. Moreover, epidemic fevers will spread accompanied by a favorable climatic oscillation and scarcity periods. In words of Pablo Giménez-Font, "*it's possible that a conjunct of favorable conditions, mainly climatic conditions, increased tertian fevers range of impact from hyperendemic areas, such as Valencian ricefields or marshlands close to Cartagena*" [65]. In fact, the relation between the climatic oscillation and the genesis of epidemic fevers was well perceived by contemporary physicians linked to the Real Academia de Medicina de Barcelona as can be seen through the testimony of doctor Juan Tovares "*Too much rain, fogs and snows what they had to give us but rafts, puddles and lagoons, floods, water spills and stagnant waters in embanked landscapes? All this humidity altered vegetation so that fruits, although they were abundant, their quality decreased becoming rot much easier than before (…) propagation of bugs, mosquitoes, and other insects was amazing (…) to this abundance of water in the autumns, winters and springs succeeded the heath of summers, that dissipating the stagnant waters from puddles, lagoons and rafts formed marshes and quagmires filled the atmosphere of vapor and putrid miasmas elevated from the high amount of rotten vegetables and putrefied vermin, and those were the remote causes of the referred epidemic"* [77].

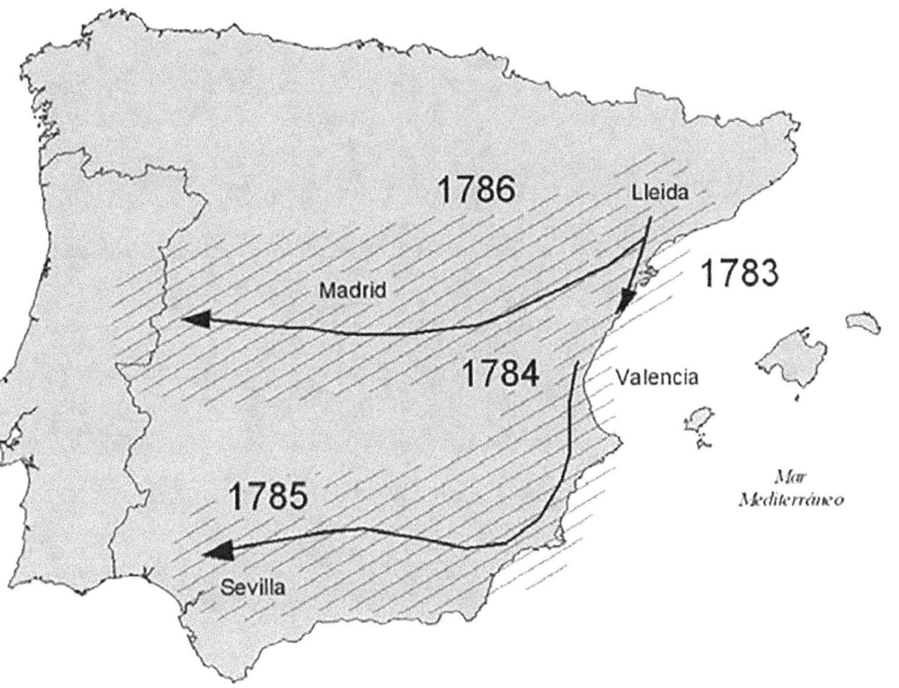

Figure 3. [Extension of tertian fevers epidemic at peninsular level (1783–1786)]. Giménez-Font [65].

Tertian fevers from 1783 onward spread over West, South, and South East of Spain at a peninsular level after being initially declared in Lleida (Catalonia, NE Spain). More importantly, since 1783 until 1785 the principal affected areas were Catalonia, Valencia (SE Spain) and Murcia (SE Spain). While in 1786 the regions that suffered the most damaging effects were Andalusia (South Spain), Castilla la Mancha (South West Spain), and North Sub-Plateau (North center Spain). Once more, physician Juan Tovares pointed that *"by the years 84 and 85 it was especially cruel* [fevers epidemic] *in 86, devastating the major part of our peninsula; but moreover provinces of la Mancha and Alcarria, leaving some villages reduced to a few habitants"* [77]. Fevers with symptomatology, as can be appreciated through the testimony of doctor Christobal Cubillas from Cafez, were commonly detected as a *"fever more or less high with a day of duration. In some cases fevers were extended to two days, just a very few arrived to the third day (...) the fever regularly finished by sweat, and if afterwards sweating continued, this was the greatest success and the lesser evil"* (**Figure 4**) [67].

On 18 May 1783, the message in the letter sent to the physician Josep Masdevall by Floridablanca's Count was explicit. The work entrusted to Masdevall elaborated a memory that contained all the news taken by the physician in relation to the epidemic that spread in Catalan territories since 1783, an epidemic that *"since early past year was discovered in the city of Lérida, spreading through all Urgel plain, Conca de Barberá, fields of Tarragona, Segarra, Manresa, Llusanés, Solsona, until Seu de Urgel and their surroundings, spreading strongly through Igualada, Piera, Vilafranca del Penedès, Martorell and another nearby towns"* [78].

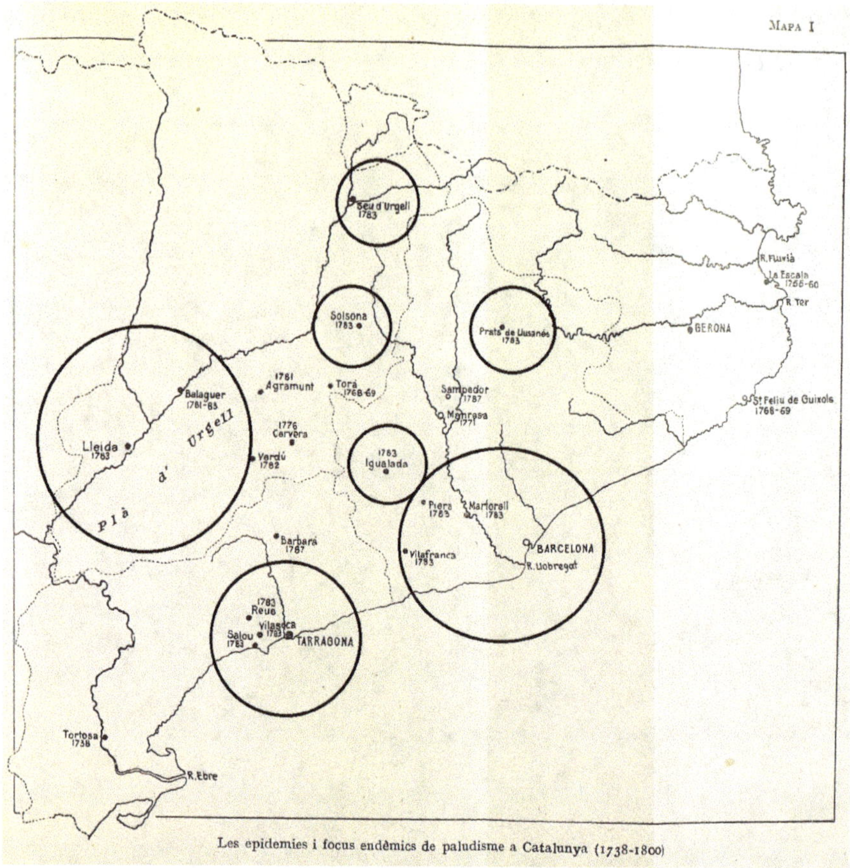

Figure 4. Geographic map elaborated from ancient sources in which is represented the most important epidemical focus of tertian fevers detected in the last years of 18th centuries. Institut de Ciències. Treballs del Servei Tècnic del Paludisme: 1915–1916. Barcelona: Publicacions del Institut de Ciències. 1918, pp. 38–41, 156 p.

In spite of the efforts put by Royal Sanitarian Joint of Barcelona and Royal Sanitarian Joint of Madrid, the efficacy of the lack of practices and remedies stipulated by them did not control the epidemic. Those remedies did not reduce the virulence of the epidemic affected by the illness "*sturdiest people from twenty to fifty years old*" [78]. These epidemic fevers had their origin, following Dr. Masdevall opinion, in the French retry from Portugal in 1764, in the context of the end of the Seven Years' War "*we must confess, that since the retry of French troops we suffer of more malignant fevers and agues than before*" [78] probably favored by the initial climatic oscillations of 1760. Moreover, the retry of French troops supported the opinion of Masdevall that the increased virulence of a preexistent problematic spread silently from one village to another, "*The communication, commerce, friendship and relationship of people's from transit of French troops with the remaining in which they didn't passed, communicated also to them the referred injuries*" [78].

Epidemic fevers that "*started with a sensitive cold, followed by an intense heat, which disappeared through an excessive sweat… Headache was really intense… others presented a bulky abdomen… hand shaking, or convulsions*" [78]. In fact, the epidemic cases detected threatened through the application of the "Antimonial mixture" that caused vomit and increased transpiration, followed by the use of "Opiata" (a chemical remedy in which quine is the principal ingredient).

The relative success of the remedy applied by Masdevall and their efforts were compensated on 30 October 1783 when King Charles III communicated through Count of Floridablanca his promotion as royal physician and Inspector of Epidemics of Spanish kingdom with a salary of 20,000 reals [79].

5. The medical reports of 1783–1786

Through this point, we focus our attention on the interest of physicians to find the origin of epidemic over the most common infectious and proactive areas of Barcelona. Moreover, in both medical reports we find a transition in relation to the search of the environmental cause effect of epidemics and over human productive activities, urban resources… The objective of physicians is to promote a systematic application of hygienic policies to prevent future epidemic situations.

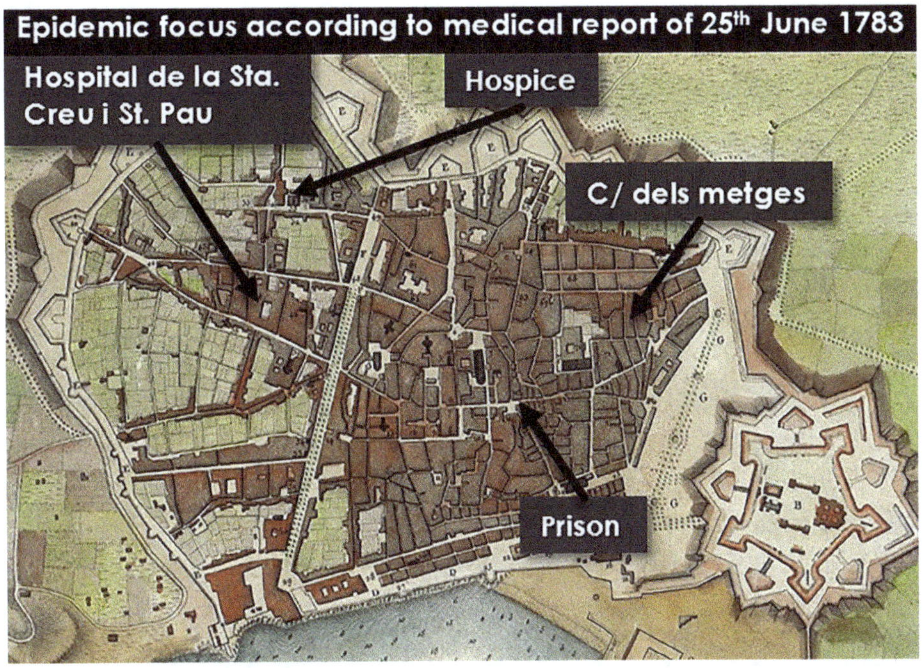

Figure 5. Self-elaborated map from the information provided in the medical report of 25 June 1783. MOULINIER. Plano de la ciudad y Puerto de Barcelona. 1806. ICGC, RM. 19425.

On 19 May 1783, the City Council of Barcelona alerted the presence of tertian fevers in his more immediate areas to the Local Joint of Sanity *"With date of the current 19 may* [1783]*, the City Council of this city assembled in Joint of Sanity show: That some of the surroundings of this Capital reign some diseases that we suspect they are similar or maybe the same illnesses that reign in the part of Lérida"* [80]. In consequence, physicians Buenaventura Milans, Gaspar Balaguer, Pere Güell (Protomedicate tenant), Rafael Steva (Doctor in Public Health), Pablo Balmes, Luis Prats and Benito Pujol elaborated a medical report following the orders of the Supreme Joint of Sanity and the Local Joint of Sanity of Barcelona. A medical report focused on the continuous fevers that spread in Barcelona. More importantly, these fevers were specifically detected on "Metg-es" street, the prison, the hospice, and the Hospital of Santa Creu. In spite of the research effectuated in the most proactive places and areas to be the focus of the epidemic, physicians rejected both houses because before the epidemic was present in the surrounding villages. This illness affected the income of a large number of people of Barcelona's City Hospital (**Figure 5**).

Continuous fevers that "*are currently abundant between poor people of Barcelona, many soldiers, and they become to be present between a few well of people*" [81] with an initial symptomatology quite similar to flu or cold. But the major part of fevers became putrid fevers and, moreover, some of them became malign fevers leaving the major part of the patients prostrated in their beds. Succeeding to the first clinical symptoms of the disease sweat and delirium, "*they become to be delirious, when we least expect it the major part of patients die*" [82]. The relation between tertian fevers and climate-environmental conditions focused on the medical report making reference in the form of benign illnesses that were common in spring and autumn that used to disappear with the summer months. Nonetheless, in 1783, physicians confirmed that these were fevers outside of their seasonal behavior with a considerable preoccupation of doctors who speculated about the possibility of a more increased virulence of fevers during the summer, "*in Lerida fevers have been common as well as in cold or hot seasons. We suspect that with the hot of the terrain will grow up illnesses, which had started to be popular at the arrival of hot weather*" [83].

The pursuit to detect the epidemic origin was the principal objective for the physicians as was mentioned in the records of the first patient who died in the Hospital of Santa Creu. Felip Pujan, who was a soldier of the Royal Walloon Guards, deceased on 21 July 1783 because of typhoid fevers that suspects the possibly of the coexistence of malaria along with typhoid fevers that is denoted as the virulence of the epidemic in the observed period.

One of the interests of physicians was the will of redirecting the hygienic habitudes of inhabitants especially of poor people "*The poor that are abundant in the streets because of the high misery of the Principality. The poverty that can't be repaired because of the consecutive bad harvests. The poor people have been in the major part the victims of the disease (…) this poor day laborers and artisans, in which is the epidemic is abundant, live in wretch rooms. An only room contains a high quantity of dirty beds, a kitchen, a dining room, and everything. Latrines are a conduct in the same room that is never totally clean of excrement and that throw out an unpleasant smell*" [84].

About tertian fever epidemic, physicians proposed the application of a curative methodology essentially based on the systematic application of bleedings, diuretics, emetics, and purges to expel from patients' body all infective material. The most probable effect of this kind of medical treatment in patients affected by malaria could have a silent impact on the public health of the inhabitants of Barcelona. Although had the knowledge of febrifuge attribute of quine, this remedy was only applied in those cases in which fever was really outstanding or if the previously exposed remedies were not completely effective. Otherwise, the use of bad quality quine could not have the expected effect on the related fever epidemics. Moreover, the discussion between traditionalist physicians and chemical remedies will be a constant problem.

Finally in this first medical report, physicians provided a conjunct of hygienic policies that should be applied to preserve the health status in the city and to face on future epidemic cases. These initiatives were specifically made to increase the healthiness level of the city, e.g., stagnant waters of Montjuic and Besós River should be systematically drained on critic epidemic episodes. On the other hand, doctors will focus their interests in helping the authorities to guarantee a better quality of bread increasing alimentation quality of the city inhabitants.

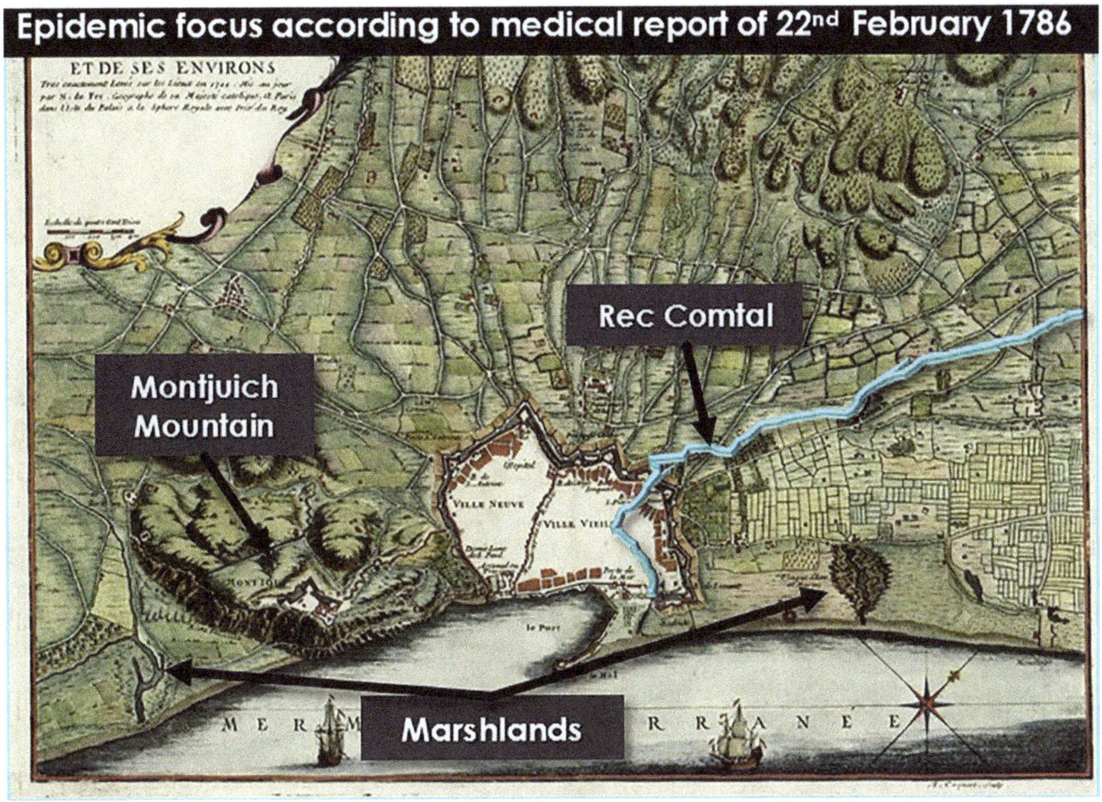

Figure 6. Self-elaborated map from the information provided in the medical report of 22 February 1786. FER, N. Plan de Barcelone et de ses environs, très exactement levés sur les lieux en 1711. Paris: dans l'ile du Palais, à la Sphère Royale. 1711. BNF, GED-1695.

The second medical report presented on 22 February 1786 was another point of interest in which we focused our attention on tertian fever epidemics in Barcelona. This time physicians Rafael Steva, Pablo Balmes, and Lluis Prats answered the order given by Count Campomanes who instigated municipal authorities to spread information that could explain the progression of tertian fevers epidemics in 1785. In the first assessment done by the physicians they admitted that tertian fevers were unusual but more common than in previous years *"but being general in this year tertian fevers over all Kingdom, the fevers have been very rare in the city, but more frequent than in other years"* [85]. But the most preoccupant point was tertian fevers that evolved progressively from benign fevers to putrid fevers *"Have been also particular that inside Barcelona have become malign fevers some that were originally simple, and they keep as such, and benign in some cases. The major parte have been putrid, some of them mixt"* [86].

In this medical report physicians explained the origin of the epidemical cases with an emphasized focus on the irregular climatic behavior of seasons. More importantly, physicians denoted the climatic alteration over the usual behavior of months from June to August. As expressed in physicians' words, "*This year has been particular in the irregularity of the seasons, and being the month of June very heat July and August have been very temperate, rather said fresh, being particular the heat diminution that is noted over our meteorological tables, what maybe is the cause of the major frequency of tertian fevers this year*" [87]. But this time, the origin of the epidemic directly searched upon the environment. That is to say, over the immediate unhealthy areas that surrounded Barcelona in the late eighteenth century.

In consequence, physicians declared Ciudadela, Montjuich Mountain, and Rec Comtal (principal water supply of the most crowded and industrial quarter of Barcelona) and the cotton factories in "Prados de Indianas" and marshlands which is consisted of Barcelona's periphery as unhealthy areas (**Figure 6**).

From the areas exposed above, physicians emphasized to focus authorities' attention on the dangers emanated from stagnant waters. As an example, physicians mentioned the case of the suburban area known as "raval." Because this area fall into the urbanized area of the city it was "*actually very healthy, after having given course to waters that used to be stagnant in the pit that goes from the Puerta de San Antonio to Puerta de Santa Madrona*" [88]. Another interesting case was related to the Ciudadela fortress due to the stagnant waters that were present over all their pits "*and will not be hard to understand why Ciudadela is not healthy, being enough maybe that their pits are double sized, and they are extremely flat that the water remains stagnant* (…) *furthermore we know that inside the fortress there are too much garbage heap which poison the air*" [89].

Moreover, as discussed above, the attention of physicians was focused on the unhealthiest spaces that surrounded the urban area. Insalubrious spaces conditioned the normal development of the city. In fact, Barcelona was a city marked by an infectious suburb in which tertian fevers wreaked upon the civil population generating a constant flow of ill people to the Hospital of Santa Creu. Although there were more the healed than the dead because of the disease, this could have an impact on the presence of indoor malaria between the city walls.

What is a good example are the words that are mentioned in the medical report. Words that denote a high preoccupation of physicians were in fact an illness presented on inhabitants' quotidian life "*Could we look with indifference what means to be surrounded by a source of epidemics in both marines, to be unable to leave to our country estates, to not be able to continue our factories without seeing a constant loose over their offices, their meadows, a high amount of workers. Family men of families that remain orphans. Factories owners that have to rest in the city being not able to go to the offices of their factories when is sometimes interesting to request their presence?*" [90]. In fact, the epidemic focus in this last medical report will be clearly specified on both marines "*It's not difficult to find the origins of insalubrity because both marshlands are insane* (…) *in those marshlands stagnant waters become corrupt when arrives the dry weather* (…) *cane cultivation rafts are really numerous as a consequence of not being followed the hygienic measures that we had exposed to H.E.*" [91]. Those unhealthy areas were not only a consequence of their environmental particularities, but also reported the anthropic impact, the productive activities such as cane cultivation rafts that confer to these areas the meaning of being insalubrious and dangerous for human health.

Because of the problems discussed above, the preventive hygienic measures stipulated on the study directly focused on the periphery of the city, especially concerning hydric resource management. Thus, doctors emphasized the necessity of building more ditches to reroute the stagnant waters present in the coastal region to make them flow in the sea. More importantly, physicians proposed to completely drain both marshlands that surrounded Barcelona *"But above all should be drained both marshlands Remolà and Port, with what is more probable would be very healthy Montjuich"* [92].

Finally, physicians agreed on to follow the medical prescriptions given by the Real Tribunal del Protomedicato. From now on, bleedings were totally avoided in favor of a treatment related to fevers based on the administration of consistent doses of quine and laxatives.

6. The obituary tables from Medical Academy of Barcelona (1783–1786)

Because this is an ongoing research, we would like to show some results of the analyzed mortality series of Barcelona. Due to the fragmentary mortality series obtained through obituary registers from the two of the three currently preserved parish archives of Barcelona (Parish of Santa Maria del Pi and Parish of Sant Just i Sant Pastor), we use as an introduction the mortality records extracted from necrological tables created by physicians of the Real Academia Médico-Práctica de Barcelona. Through this analysis we would like to show some detailed annual results especially focused on detecting parishes that concentrate on the most outstanding children mortality peaks (**Figure** 7).

Through the displayed graph from 1783–1786, we can clearly appreciate the years that presented an anomaly concerning mortality peaks, specifically 1781, 1783, 1785, and 1786. In 1781, in general, burials increased with respect to the previous year. In fact, child mortality exceeded adult mortality in eight Barcelona parishes. In this sense, Barcelona's Cathedral reflects 893 children in contrast to 159 adult people deceased. Moreover, it will be the traditional commercial-artisanal area that will remain the second most elevated value of childish mortality. More importantly, it is the parish of Santa Maria del Mar with 500 children versus the 208 adult bodies registered.

On the other hand, in 1782, mortality over all eight parishes of Barcelona was still being elevated (2724 deceased). In fact, the mortality increment in all parishes of Barcelona is clearly noticed, including the Cathedral, with respect to the previous year. In fact, in the Cathedral child mortality peaks were clearly high with 853 child faced to 168 adult. The conjunction of catastrophic flood events along elevated minimum temperatures and a large number of favorable days for plasmodium development maybe the possible explanation to this continuous over mortality. The constant increase in adult mortality culminates in 1783 with a value of 1.26 standard deviation with respect to the rest of corpses deceased for this series of mortality recovered data. However, although the general lines of mortality are less than in 1781 and 1782, this is because of child population which led the deceleration of the general mortality in 1783. In fact, in 1783 adult corpses surpassed child mortality in all Barcelona's parishes. The exceptions were the parish of Sant Pere (103 adults and 137 children), the Cathedral (192 adults and 700 children), and the parish of Santa María del Mar (299 adults and 308 children). The adult mortality and children mortality that could be in a strong relation to the impact of typhoid fevers together with the presence of endemic and epidemic malaria could have been entered to the city by the affluence of ill people from the suburban areas.

A new minimal mortality peak reappeared in 1784 (2340 total deceased) with almost one standard deviation less than the rest of the mortality values—typical deviation of minus 0.95. The values that proceed after a diminution of childish mortality—typical deviation of minus 0.97—in conjunction with adult mortality—a typical deviation of minus 0.01.

The year 1785 concentrates the maximum conjunct of the absolute mortality values (3276 deaths) with adult and children manifesting the same upward trend in mortality. In this sense, the intensity in which children mortality exceeds adult corpses due to the negative maximum typical deviation of 1784 in 1785—typical deviation of 1.75—is especially noticeable.

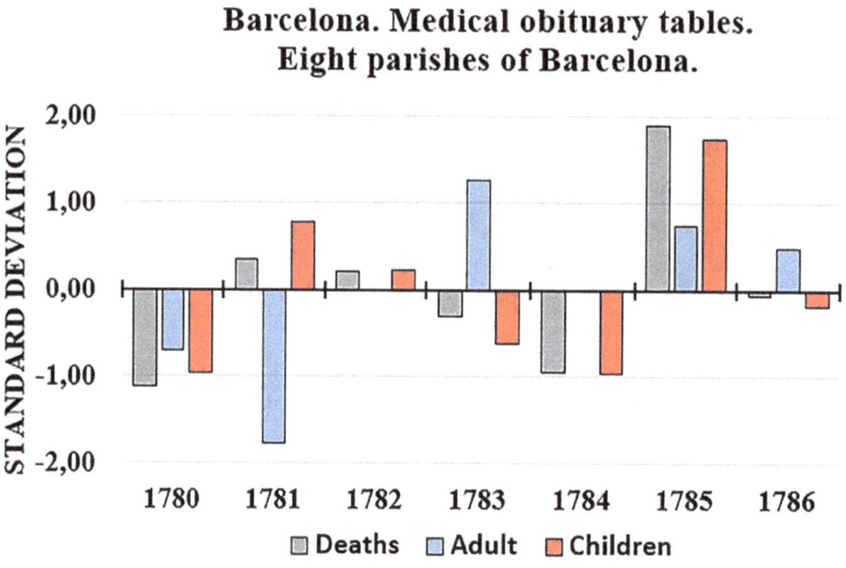

Figure 7. Mortality records of Barcelona in which are reflected the adult and childish mortality from the eight parishes of the city since 1780 until 1786. ARAMC, "Papeles del Dr. D. Francisco Salvà," legajo XII, num 1, "Notas para las tablas necrológicas…," doc. 9. "Muertos en Barcelona, por parroquias, años 1780 a 1786, 1797 a 1800 y primeros meses de 1801, 1802 y 1803."

Childish mortality in 1785 is uniform in all the parishes of the city. However, the most noticeable parishes where mortality wreaked havoc upon the civil population were the Cathedral (160 corpses, 959 children), and the parishes of Santa María del Mar (291 corpses, 528 children), parish of Santa María del Pi (267 adults, 319 children), and Sant Pere de les Puel·les (100 corpses, 222 children). The conjunction of minimal monthly temperatures higher than 22.5°C, a high number of favorable days for sporogony of both analyzed plasmodium, and the critical rain episodes that succeeded since 1782 and 1785 could explain the anomaly in childish population as a consequence of a more favorable environment to the development of malaria. This disease could have been presented in a more prolonged seasonal pattern until the autumn months. In 1785, in the month of July physician Dr. Francisco Salvà noticed a transition based on a more aggressive presence of putrid fevers: *"In the month of July, the constitution was less inflammatory but more putrid than in the previous month (...) tertian fevers were very common this month. Were also detected colic pains and convulsions that were attached by the use of narcotics. In August the epidemical constitution didn't changed, with the exception of some small-poxes, and tertian fevers, there were not more noticeable diseases; but were common diarrheas, dysenteries"* [93].

Finally, a significant high values of child mortality is observed in 1786 in all parishes of Barcelona. In fact, the only exception was Sant Jaume parish (43 adult, 26 children). Children who had the more reduced opportunities to survive due to the combination of malaria along with gastrointestinal diseases *"Those weaning children had the less favorable time. Some of them were affected by a universal weakness after which they died"* [93].

7. Discussion and conclusions

Malaria is a protean disease very sensitive to changes in precipitation, temperature, and wind direction. As shown above, the strong relation between the disease and environment is linked by the principal vector, *Anopheles* female's mosquitoes that give to the disease a high range of territorial affection. Since the progressive disappearance of the plague from European countries, endemic malaria plays a role as a background illness due to the synergic, positive, and negative interactions among other sicknesses such as smallpox, flu, cholera, yellow fever —among others—generating a constant oscillation in mortality peaks. However, historians usually have not paid the merited attention to an illness that was anchored in the quotidian lives, troop movements, the economy, and the landscapes of past Europe since the sixteenth century until the systematic eradication of malaria in the second half of the twentieth century. This illness caused deleterious effects on the health status of peoples of the past, being the children, the newborns were the principal affected collective. This sickness was indirectly fed by those parents who fought for the systematic construction of irrigation trenches to ensure a good alimentation and guarantee a minimum salary for their families.

Malaria is a complex disease with multiple facets and symptoms. In fact, the complexity of the illness resides in the high range of aspects in which it can have an impact on ancient societies. In consequence, the problem to develop historical studies focused on the detection of endemic and epidemic malaria that can only be solved with an interdisciplinary research that will involve a high variety of research fields. One of the most problematic aspects that we usually find in our research was to correctly identify each disease. Due to the above reason, the methodology that we propose is based on to conjunct and compare the most complete range of sources that we can manage. As shown above, from the bibliography we can part a solid basis for the problem to later investigate our corpus of sources. A first step would be the in-depth study of a selection of municipal sources, essentially, municipal chords and municipal proclaims. This step will provide us a rich documentation of quotidian life, hygienic policies, and essential product supplies, all the negative consequences derived from climatic instability and the economic status of the city and the repercussion over the economy as a consequence of the epidemic context. The information extracted from municipal chords can be reinforced with the help of sanitation sources, such as sanitation expedients. The fact to cross and conjunct all the information extracted from municipal sources will provide us an exact chronology of the effects and the perception of epidemics in the past societies.

Public sources such as the documentation extracted from Reial Acadèmia de Medicina de Catalunya show the potential to realize deepest research over medical archives. In fact, from medical records and instrumental meteorological data we detect a high range of interesting sources such as medical topographies, which in their conjunct and confronted to the municipal sources or the information contained in print sources can contribute to an exact description and analysis of the symptomatology detected in epidemics and hygienic measures proposed by the physicians to municipal authorities and state institutions related to epidemics. Instrumental meteorological records open a high range of possible analysis concerning vector or virus diseases. In fact, one of the current problems is to develop precise mathematical models that cannot help historians to better detect the territorial affection of the diseases but also their seasonal behavior. One of our personal interests is to develop the analysis of instrumental meteorological data with the support of mathematics, physics, entomologists, and biologist to further develop the most detailed analysis in our next studies.

Ecclesiastical sources, more importantly baptism records and burial records, deliver to the researcher the possibility to contrast the information with the corpus sources. More important is the possibility to detect mortality peaks that go unusually high and far from their seasonal patterns of mortality. These mortality peaks can also contradict the symptomatology detected by contemporary physicians for a concrete time lapse and can also be put in relation to the resultant analysis of the environmental requisites for vector-borne diseases such as malaria. As an example, unless we cannot say that all childish mortality peaks are clearly caused by malaria, we can undoubtedly detect the presence of the illness associated with gastrointestinal diseases, typhoid fevers or smallpox, among other diseases.

In the late eighteenth century, we found an interesting conjunction of socioeconomic conditions, environmental conditioners, and urban structures that were, in their conjunct, submitted to the historical context derived from the Spanish Succession War. Since the new political order resultant applied the "Real Decreto de Nueva Planta," the pre-existent Catalan sanitation and political institutions were reshuffled to respond to the interest of the Bourbon monarchy. At the end of the eighteenth century, cities such as Barcelona adapted to political changes but were also submitted to the consequences derived from the new political order. In this sense, Barcelona was under a massive income of population that arrived to the city due to the stagnant agricultural patterns of Catalonia in the middle of the eighteenth century. This city offered the possibility to export agricultural surplus due to the important commercial flow and also the opportunity to have a job in the industrial-artisanal areas of the city. The hygienic repercussion of the city with almost 114,100 population fell over the hydric structures that could not be properly adapted.

On the other hand, municipal authorities could not guarantee an appropriate hygienic management of hydric resources due to the drastic reduction of the City budget and the lack of municipal competences. Water that flows through the city carries the miasmas, all the residues of the industrial areas, and the mix of fecal matters with drinking waters. Moreover, the water that came from the Besós River through the channel known as Rec Comtal was the principal cause of contamination due to the traditional presence of legal and illegal cane cultivation rafts.

The relation between stagnant waters and the presence of tertian fevers was well known by physicians and municipal authorities. Barcelona is a good sample that can clearly appreciate through the medical reports presented about the tertian fevers epidemic context that took place between 1783 and 1786. In both medical records, it is clearly detected that the physicians searched the relation with environment and diseases, first inside the city but thereafter doctors refocused their research on the suburban areas of the city and more importantly in both marshlands.

In fact, in the late eighteenth century sanitation institutions were clearly a reminiscence of the pre-existent health structures before the sanitarian institutional reshuffle that took place in 1720. Physicians, in spite of the consequences of the new Bourbonic order, had a considerable impact on the decisions in hygienic policies applied by the municipal authorities. We found a good example which shows that many proclamations detected between 1783 and 1786 focused on the management of marshlands and lagoons that surrounded Barcelona.

However, the dramatic loss of prestige and control over medical studies would be the principal incentive in the constant pursuit of a medical academy in Barcelona. The medical academy since its foundation on 2 July 1770 will rigorously apply and follow the principles of hygienic medicine instigating all the physicians of the medical academy to develop historical medical studies to better understand the causes of illnesses, the relation with environment, the weather, and the sickness.

Acknowledgements

This work is produced within the framework of the Unit of Excellence LabexMed, Social Sciences and Humanities, at the heart of multidisciplinary research for the Mediterranean, under grant number 10-LABX-0090. This work is supported by a state grant administrated by the Agence Nationale de la Recherche for the project Investissements d'Avenir A*MIDEX under grant no. ANR-11-IDEX-0001-02.

Author details

Kevin Pometti

Address all correspondence to: kevin.pometti-benitez@univ-amu.fr

LabexMed, MMSH, CNRS UMR 7303, TELEMME, Aix-Marseille University, Aix-en-Provence, France

References

[1] Mercader J. La ordenación de Cataluña por Felipe V: la Nueva Planta. Hispania: Revista Española de Historia. 1951;43:257–366.

[2] Günzberg Moll J. Instituciones públicas catalanas después del Real Decreto de Nueva Planta. Ivs Fvgit. 2004–2005;13–14:267–295.

[3] Pérez Samper, M. Los regentes de la Real Audiencia de Cataluña (1716–1808). Pedralbes: Revista d'Història Moderna. 1981;1:211–252.

[4] López i Guallar M. L'absolutisme i la dinámica política social. Barcelona. Quaderns d'Història. 2002;7:71–102.

[5] García Espuche A. La Ciutat del Born: economía i vida quotidiana a Barcelona (segles XIV a XVIII). Barcelona: Museu d'Història de Barcelona; 2009. 661 p.

[6] SalvàF. Borrador de una curiosa descripción de la Barcelona de fines del siglo XVIII. Located at: Papeles del Doctor Don Francisco Salvà, Reial Acadèmia de Medicina de Barcelona, Barcelona, RAMB, XIV; no. 8.

[7] Young A. Viatge a Catalunya; traducció i presentació: Ramon Boixareau. Tremp: Garsineu; 1993. 99 pp.

[8] Vilar P. Catalunya dins l'Espanya Moderna: recerques sobre els fonaments econòmics de les estructures nacionals. Barcelona: Curial, Edicions 62; 1988. vol. 1.

[9] Carrera Pujal J. La Barcelona del segle XVIII. Barcelona: Bosch; 1951. vol. 1.

[10] Vilar P. Catalunya dins l'Espanya Moderna: recerques sobre els fonaments econòmics de les estructures nacionals. Barcelona: Curial, Edicions 62; 1988. vol. 2.

[11] En fuerza de la Orden del Real Acuerdo con que se halla el Muy Ilustre Ayuntamiento de esta ciudad, y en atención à que la multitud de Fábricas de Algodón y Lana (...). Located at: Bandos, 1778-1786, Arxiu Històric de la Ciutat de Barcelona, Barcelona, AHCB, Dossier no. 10.

[12] García i Fuertes G. L'Abastament d'aigua a la Barcelona del segle XVIII. Barcelona: Fundació Salvador Vives i Casajuana: Rafael Dalmau; 1990. 206 p.

[13] Salvà F. Letrinas y Albañales. Located at: Papeles del Doctor Don Francisco Salvà, Reial Acadèmia de Medicina de Barcelona, Barcelona, RAMB, XVIII; no. 2.

[14] Alier R. El desplegament de la ciutat manufacturera: 1714–1833. In: Sobrequés i Callicó J, director. Historia de Barcelona. Barcelona: Enciclopèdia Catalana: Ajuntament de Barcelona; 1993. vol. 5.

[15] Martín Corrales E. La contaminación industrial en el litoral catalán durante el siglo XVIII. In: Centemeri L, Daumalin X, directors. Pollutions industrielles et espaces

méditerranéens (XVIIIe-XXIe siècle). Aix-en-Provence: Karthala-MMSH; 2015. pp. 215–238.

[16] Ayala B. Condiciones de trabajo en las fábricas de indianas de Barcelona durante el último tercio del siglo XVIII. Manuscrits: Revista d'Història Moderna. 1987;6:121–134.

[17] Piera Miquel N. Els usos de les indianes a la Barcelona del segle XVIII: decorar la llar o vestir la gent?. Barcelona Quaderns d'Història. 2011;17:67–84.

[18] Bajet M. El mostassaf de Barcelona i les seves funcions en el segle XVI: edició del "Llibre de les Ordinations." Barcelona: Fundació Noguera; 1994. 606 p.

[19] Campos Díez M. El Real Tribunal del Protomedicato Castellano (Siglos XIV-XIX). Cuenca: Servicio de Publicaciones de la Universidad de Castilla-La Mancha; 1999. 424 p.

[20] Zarzoso A. Medicina i il·lustració a Catalunya. Barcelona: Fundació Noguera; 2004. 462 p.

[21] Maestre Maestre J, Pascual Barea J, editors. Humanismo y pervivencia del mundo clásico: homenaje al profesor Antonio Prieto. Madrid: Consejo Superior de Investigaciones Científicas; 2008–2010. vol. 4.

[22] Granjel L S. La Medicina española del siglo XVIII. Salamanca: Ediciones Universidad de Salamanca; 1979. 285 p.

[23] Prats J. La Universitat de Cervera i el reformisme borbònic. Lleida: Pagès; 1993. 436 p.

[24] Peset M, Mancebo P, Peset J. Temores y defensa de España frente a la peste de Marsella de 1720. Asclepio. 1971;23:131–187.

[25] Peset M, Peset J. Muerte en España. Política y sociedad entre la peste y el cólera. Madrid: Seminarios y ediciones; 1972. 258 p.

[26] Perdiguero-Gil E, Zarzoso A. La sanidad marítima en dos ciudades mediterráneas de la Corona de Aragón durante el siglo XVIII: Barcelona y Alicante. In: Perdiguero-Gil E, Vidal Hernández J, editors. La Ciudadela de los fantasmas: lazaretos y protección sanitaria en el mundo moderno. Menorca: Institut Menorquí d'Estudis; 2010. pp. 29–48.

[27] Pardo Tomás J, Martínez Vidal A. Un programa, dues acadèmies: Jaume Bonells i el foment de la medicina i de les ciències naturals a Barcelona (1766–1786). In: Nieto-Galán A, Roca i Rossell A, directors. La Reial Acadèmia de Ciències i Arts de Barcelona als segles XVIII i XIX. Història, ciencia i societat. Barcelona: Acadèmia de Ciències i Arts de Barcelona, Institut d'Estudis Catalans; 2000. pp. 137–164.

[28] Bonells J. Discurso inaugural sobre la utilidad y necesidad de las Academias de Medicina-Practica, leído en la Academia el 10 de octubre de 1779 por el Doctor Don Jayme Bonells... In: RAMB. Memorias de la Real Academia Médico-Práctica de

Barcelona: tomo primero. Madrid: En la Imprenta Real por don Pedro Julian Pereyra; 1798. 656 p.

[29] Barriendos M. Els inicis de la meteorologia instrumental a Catalunya: una història en construcció. Ausa. 2012;25(169):561–595.

[30] Zarzoso A. La pràctica mèdica a la Catalunya del segle XVIII [thesis]. Barcelona: Universitat Pompeu Fabra; 2003.

[31] Salvà, F. Exposición de la enseñanza de medicina Clínica en el Real Estudio erigido por S.M. bajo la dirección de la Real Academia Médico-Práctica de Barcelona. Barcelona: Mateo Barceló; 1801–1802. vol. 3.

[32] Spitzen J, Spoor C, Grieco F, Ter Braak C, Beeuwkes J, et al. A 3D Analysis of flight behavior of anopheles gambiae sensu stricto malaria mosquitoes in response to human odor and heat. PLos ONE. 2013;8(5):e62995. DOI: 10.1371/journal.pone.0062995

[33] WHO. World malaria report 2015. Geneva: World Health Organization Press; 2015. 243 pp.

[34] Cox F E G. History of the discovery of the malaria parasites and their vectors. Parasites & Vectors. 2010;3(1):5. DOI: 10.1186/1756-3305-3-5

[35] Hippocrates. Corpus Hippocratorum. Madrid: Gredos; 1989. 358 p.

[36] Cerdán F. Discursos physico-medicos, político-morales que tratan ser toda calentura hectica o contagiosa, esencia del universal contagio, y medios para precaverlo. Madrid: En la imprenta de Agustín Laborda; 1752. 141 p.

[37] Dobson M. Contours of Death and Disease in Early Modern England. Cambridge: Cambridge University Press; 2003. 672 p.

[38] Don Jacinto Pazuengos y Zurbaran, comendador de museros en la Orden de Santiago... Governador militar y político de la Plaza de Barcelona... que para el dia primero de Septiembre del corriente año, tengan limpias y corrientes las Azequias. Located at: Bandos, 1778-1786, Arxiu Històric de la Ciutat de Barcelona, Barcelona, AHCB, Dossier no. 10.

[39] Terán M. Instrucción y Reglas que por ahora deberán observarse por los Ayuntamientos y Juntas de Propios de los Pueblos de este Principado en las Obras, Reparos, y Conservación de Caminos (...). Segovia; 1784. 22 p.

[40] Terán M. Instrucción y reglas que por ahora deberán observarse en el plantero de arboles que vá à hacerse en los terrenos pertenecientes a S.M. en las inmediaciones del puente de Molins de Rey. Barcelona; 1787. 23 p.

[41] Zamora F. "Diario de los viajes hechos en Cataluña": seguit de la resposta del corregiment de Barcelona al seu qüestionari feta per Josep Albert Navarro-Mas i Marquet. Barcelona: Curial; 1973. 510 p.

[42] Jacquemard N, Faure É. Une association délétère: Les riziéres aux portes des villes. L'exemple de la peste des rizièresà Thiers en 1741 et analyse de la législation. In: Beck C, Franchomme M, Guizard-Duchamp F, Heude J, editors. Zones humides et villes d'hier et d'aujourd'hui: Des premières cités aux fronts d'eau contemporains. Lille: Université Charles-de-Gaulle. Revue Du Nord ; 2011:297–306.

[43] Mateu Tortosa E. Arroz y paludismo: riqueza y conflictos en la sociedad valenciana del siglo XVIII. Valencia: Institució Alfons el Magnànim. Institució Valenciana d'Estudis i Investigació; 1987. 192 p.

[44] Riera Palmero J. Estudios y documentos sobre arroz y paludismo en Valencia (s. XVIII). Valladolid: Universidad de Valladolid. Secretariado de Publicaciones, Seminario de Historia de la Medicina; 1988. 224 p.

[45] Pauly P. Esquisses de climatologie comparée: climats et endèmies. Paris: G. Masson; 1874. 744 p.

[46] Sallarés R. Malaria and Rome. A History of Malaria in Ancient Italy. Oxford: Oxford University Press; 2002. 358 p.

[47] Prieto L, Cortés M, Cabrillo E, González-González A. Malaria y embarazo. Progresos de Obstetricia y Ginecología. 2005:48(1):23–34. DOI: 10.1016/S0304-5013(05)72351-7

[48] Kumar V. Robbins Patología Humana. Barcelona: Elsevier; 2008. 956 p.

[49] Cox F E G. History of human parasitology. Clinical Microbiology Reviews. 2002:15(4): 595–612. DOI: 10.1128/CMR.15.4.595-612.2002

[50] Fernández Astasio B. La erradicación del paludismo en España: aspectos biológicos de la lucha antipalúdica [thesis]. Madrid: Universidad Complutense de Madrid; 2002. 436 p.

[51] Grmek M. Preliminaires d'une étude historique des maladies. Annales, Historie, Sciences Sociales. 1969:6:1473–1483.

[52] Faure É. Malarial pathocoenosis: beneficial and deleterious interactions between malaria and other human diseases. Frontiers in Physiology. 2014;5:441. DOI: 10.3389/fphys.2014.00441

[53] Willem J, Jetten T, Focks D. Sensitivity of malaria, schistosomiasis and dengue to global warming. Climatic Change. 1997;35(2):145–156. DOI: 10.1023/A:1005365413932

[54] Pittaluga G. Enfermedades de los Países Cálidos y Parasitología Tropical. Madrid: Calpe; 1923. 555 p.

[55] Rocaute E, Pichard G, Faure É, Royer-Carenzi M. Analysis of the causes of spawning of large-scale, severe malarial epidemics and their rapid total extinction in western Provence, historically a highly endemic region of France (1745–1850). Malaria Journal. 2014;13:72. DOI: 10.1186/1475-2875-13-72

[56] Markell E, Voge M, John D. Parasitología Médica. 6th ed. Madrid: Interamericana McGraw-Hill; 1994. 395 p.

[57] Rodríguez Ocaña E, et al. La acción médico-social contra el paludismo en la España metropolitana y colonial del siglo XX. Madrid: Consejo Superior de Investigaciones Científicas; 2003. 488 p.

[58] Bueno Marí R, Jiménez Peydró R. Crónicas de arroz, mosquitos y paludismo en España: El caso de la Provincia de Valencia (S. XVIII–XX). Hispania. Revista Española de Historia. 2010:70(236):687–708.

[59] Bueno Marí R. Bioecologia, diversidad e interés epidemiológico de los culícidos mediterráneos (Diptera: Culicidae). Valencia: Universitat de València. Departament de Zoologia. Servei de Publicacions; 2010. 423 p.

[60] Lozano Morales A. El estadio invernante del Anopheles maculipennis atroparvus y su relación con la pausa estacional del paludismo en España. Revista de Sanidad e Higiene Pública. 1953;27:23.

[61] Mordecai E, Paaijmans K, Johnson L, Balzer C, Ben-Horin T, et al. Optimal temperature for malaria transmission is dramatically lower than previously predicted. Ecology Letters. 2013;16(1):22–30. DOI: 10.1111/ele.12015

[62] Ermert V, Fink A, Jones A, Morse A. Development of a new version of the Liverpool Malaria Model. I. Refining the parameter settings and mathematical formulation of basic processes based on a literature review. Malaria Journal. 2011;10:35. DOI: 10.1186/1475-2875-10-35

[63] Desaive J, et al. Médecins, climat et épidémies à la fin du XVIIIe siècle. Paris: La haye, Mouton cop; 1972. 256 p.

[64] Pérez Moreda V. Las Crisis de mortalidad en la España interior, siglos XVI–XIX. Madrid: Siglo XXI; 1980. 526 p.

[65] Giménez-Font P. La epidemia de malaria de 1783–1786: Notas sobre la influencia de anomalías climáticas y cambios de usos del suelo en la salud humana. Investigaciones Geográficas. 2008;46:141–157.

[66] Martín-Vide J, Barriendos M. The use of rogation ceremony records in climatic reconstruction: a case study fom Catalonia (Spain). Climatic Change. 1995;30:201–221. DOI: 10.1007/BF01091842

[67] Villalba J. Epidemiología Española, o historia cronológica de las pestes, contagios, epidemias y epizootias que han acaecido en España desde la venida de los cartagineses hasta el año 1801 [...]. Madrid: Imprenta de D. Fermin Villalpando; 1803, vol. 2.

[68] Cavalli-Sforza L, Moroni A, Zei G. Consanguinity, Inbreeding, and Genetic Drift in Italy (MPB-39). Princeton University Press: Monographs in Population Biology; 2004. 320 p.

[69] Salvà F. Notas para las tablas necrológicas de 25 años, en Barcelona. Años 1786-1824. Located at: Papeles del Doctor Don Francisco Salvà, Reial Acadèmia de Medicina de Barcelona, Barcelona, RAMB, XII; no. 1.

[70] Coll S, Guijarro M. Estadística aplicada a la historia y a las ciencias sociales. Madrid: Ediciones Pirámide; 1998. 544 p.

[71] Floridablanca J. Censo español executado de órden del rey: comunicada por el excelentísimo señor Conde de Floridablanca, primer secretario de estado y del despacho, en el año de 1787. Madrid: Imprenta Real; 1787. 176 p.

[72] Barriendos M, Llasat C. The case of the "Maldà" anomaly in the western Mediterranean basin (AD 1760–1800): An example of a strong climatic variability. Climatic Change. 2003;61:191–216. DOI: 10.1023/A:1026327613698

[73] Salvà F. Tablas Meteorológicas, 1780-1824. Located at: Manuscrits, Reial Acadèmia de Medicina de Barcelona, RAMB, 4 vol.

[74] Prohoms M, Barriendos M, Anfrons E, Ripoll R. Recuperación y análisis de la serie de temperatura diaria de Barcelona, 1780–201. In: Moreno J, director. Cambio climático. Extremos e impactos. Salamanca: Publicaciones de la Asociación Española de Climatología (AEC); 2012. pp. 207–217.

[75] Cram T, et al. The International Surface Pressure Databank version 2. Geoscience Data Journal. 2015;2:31–46. DOI: 10.1002/gdj3.25

[76] García Burunda J. Informe del Real Proto-Medicato: en que se proponen las observaciones médicas para indagar las causas, y método curativo de las tercianas, tomando noticias de los progresos de esta enfermedad en el presente año de 1785, que puedan servir de preservativo en adelante. Madrid: Don Antonio de Sancha; 1785, 22 p.

[77] Tovares J. Descripcion histórico-epidemica ó memoria sobre la epidemia de calenturas intermitentes, observada en España el año de 1786 por el Doctor don Juan Tovares, medico de Puerto-Llano, a la que la Real Academia Medico-Practica de Barcelona adjudicó el accessit en su Junta Pública de 29 de febrero de 1792. In: RAMB. Memorias de la Real Academia Médico-Práctica de Barcelona: tomo primero. Madrid: en la Imprenta Real por don Pedro Julian Pereyra; 1798, 656 p.

[78] Masdevall i Terrades J. Relacion de las epidemias de calenturas pútridas y malignas que en estos últimos años se han padecido en el Principado de Cataluña y principalmente de la que descubrió el año pasado de 1783 en la ciudad de Lérida, Llano de Urgél… con el método… de curar semejantes enfermedades. Madrid: en la Imprenta Real; 1786, 156 p.

[79] Llibre d'Acordats de Sanitat, 1783-1800. Located at: Arxiu Històric de la Ciutat de Barcelona, AHCB, 1L VII-4, f. 19 v. and f. 20 v.

[80] Llibre 1r d'Expedients de Sanitat, 1783-1787. Located at: Arxiu Històric de la Ciutat de Barcelona, AHCB, 1L VIII-1, f. 6 r. and f. 6 v.

[81] Milans B, Balaguer G, Güell P, Steva R, Balmes P, Prats Ll, Pujol B. Informe sobre una epidemia observada en Barcelona en el mes de junio de 1783. Located at: Papeles del Doctor Don Francisco Salvà, Reial Acadèmia de Medicina de Barcelona, Barcelona, RAMB, XIV; no. 17, f. 1 r.

[82] Milans B, Balaguer G, Güell P, Steva R, Balmes P, Prats Ll, Pujol B. Informe sobre una epidemia observada en Barcelona en el mes de junio de 1783. Located at: Papeles del Doctor Don Francisco Salvà, Reial Acadèmia de Medicina de Barcelona, Barcelona, RAMB, XIV: no. 17, f. 4 r.

[83] Milans B, Balaguer G, Güell P, Steva R, Balmes P, Prats Ll, Pujol B. Informe sobre una epidemia observada en Barcelona en el mes de junio de 1783. Located at: Papeles del Doctor Don Francisco Salvà, Reial Acadèmia de Medicina de Barcelona, Barcelona, RAMB, XIV: no. 17, f. 2 r. and f. 2 v.

[84] Milans B, Balaguer G, Güell P, Steva R, Balmes P, Prats Ll, Pujol B.Informe sobre una epidemia observada en Barcelona en el mes de junio de 1783. Located at: Papeles del Doctor Don Francisco Salvà, Reial Acadèmia de Medicina de Barcelona, Barcelona, RAMB, XIV: no. 17, f. 5 v. and f. 6 v.

[85] Balmes P, Prats Ll, Steva R. Informe sobre una epidemia de tercianas. Located at: Papeles del Doctor Don Francisco Salvà, Reial Acadèmia de Medicina de Barcelona, Barcelona, RAMB, XIV: no. 16, f. 1 r.

[86] Balmes P, Prats Ll, Steva R. Informe sobre una epidemia de tercianas. Located at: Papeles del Doctor Don Francisco Salvà, Reial Acadèmia de Medicina de Barcelona, Barcelona, RAMB, XIV: no. 16, f. 1 v.

[87] Balmes P, Prats Ll, Steva R. Informe sobre una epidemia de tercianas. Located at: Papeles del Doctor Don Francisco Salvà, Reial Acadèmia de Medicina de Barcelona, Barcelona, RAMB, XIV: no. 16, f. 1 r. and f. 1 v.

[88] Balmes P, Prats Ll, Steva R. Informe sobre una epidemia de tercianas. Located at: Papeles del Doctor Don Francisco Salvà, Reial Acadèmia de Medicina de Barcelona, Barcelona, RAMB, XIV: no. 16, f. 1 v. and f. 2 r.

[89] Balmes P, Prats Ll, Steva R. Informe sobre una epidemia de tercianas. Located at: Papeles del Doctor Don Francisco Salvà, Reial Acadèmia de Medicina de Barcelona, Barcelona, RAMB, XIV: no. 16, f. 2 r. and f. 2 v.

[90] Balmes P, Prats Ll, Steva R. Informe sobre una epidemia de tercianas. Located at: Papeles del Doctor Don Francisco Salvà, Reial Acadèmia de Medicina de Barcelona, Barcelona, RAMB, XIV: no. 16, f. 4 r.

[91] Balmes P, Prats Ll, Steva R. Informe sobre una epidemia de tercianas. Located at: Papeles del Doctor Don Francisco Salvà, Reial Acadèmia de Medicina de Barcelona, Barcelona, RAMB, XIV: no. 16, f. 4 v. and f. 5 r.

[92] Balmes P, Prats Ll, Steva R. Informe sobre una epidemia de tercianas. Located at: Papeles del Doctor Don Francisco Salvà, Reial Acadèmia de Medicina de Barcelona, Barcelona, RAMB, XIV: no. 16, f. 5 v. and f. 6 v.

[93] Salvà F. Tablas Meteorológicas, 1780-1824. Located at: Manuscrits, Reial Acadèmia de Medicina de Barcelona, RAMB, vol. 4.

Permissions

All chapters in this book were first published in CTM, by InTech Open; hereby published with permission under the Creative Commons Attribution License or equivalent. Every chapter published in this book has been scrutinized by our experts. Their significance has been extensively debated. The topics covered herein carry significant findings which will fuel the growth of the discipline. They may even be implemented as practical applications or may be referred to as a beginning point for another development.

The contributors of this book come from diverse backgrounds, making this book a truly international effort. This book will bring forth new frontiers with its revolutionizing research information and detailed analysis of the nascent developments around the world.

We would like to thank all the contributing authors for lending their expertise to make the book truly unique. They have played a crucial role in the development of this book. Without their invaluable contributions this book wouldn't have been possible. They have made vital efforts to compile up to date information on the varied aspects of this subject to make this book a valuable addition to the collection of many professionals and students.

This book was conceptualized with the vision of imparting up-to-date information and advanced data in this field. To ensure the same, a matchless editorial board was set up. Every individual on the board went through rigorous rounds of assessment to prove their worth. After which they invested a large part of their time researching and compiling the most relevant data for our readers.

The editorial board has been involved in producing this book since its inception. They have spent rigorous hours researching and exploring the diverse topics which have resulted in the successful publishing of this book. They have passed on their knowledge of decades through this book. To expedite this challenging task, the publisher supported the team at every step. A small team of assistant editors was also appointed to further simplify the editing procedure and attain best results for the readers.

Apart from the editorial board, the designing team has also invested a significant amount of their time in understanding the subject and creating the most relevant covers. They scrutinized every image to scout for the most suitable representation of the subject and create an appropriate cover for the book.

The publishing team has been an ardent support to the editorial, designing and production team. Their endless efforts to recruit the best for this project, has resulted in the accomplishment of this book. They are a veteran in the field of academics and their pool of knowledge is as vast as their experience in printing. Their expertise and guidance has proved useful at every step. Their uncompromising quality standards have made this book an exceptional effort. Their encouragement from time to time has been an inspiration for everyone.

The publisher and the editorial board hope that this book will prove to be a valuable piece of knowledge for researchers, students, practitioners and scholars across the globe.

List of Contributors

Wilmer E. Villamil-Gómez
Committee on Zoonoses and Haemorrhagic Fevers, Colombian Association of Infectious Diseases, Bogotá, DC, Colombia
Infectious Diseases and Infection Control Research Group, Sincelejo University Hospital, Sincelejo, Sucre, Colombia
Doctoral Program of Tropical Medicine, SUE - Caribe, University of Atlántico, Barranquilla, Colombia
Biodiversity Research Group of the Colombian Caribbean, Faculty of Basic Sciences, University of Atlántico, Barranquilla, Colombia

Melisa Eyes-Escalante
Doctoral Program of Tropical Medicine, SUE - Caribe, University of Atlántico, Barranquilla, Colombia
Biodiversity Research Group of the Colombian Caribbean, Faculty of Basic Sciences, University of Atlántico, Barranquilla, Colombia

Carlos Franco-Paredes
Children's Hospital of Mexico, Federico Gomez and Infectious Diseases Department and Phoebe Putney Memorial Hospital, Albany, GA, USA

Yaw Asare Afrane
Department of Medical Microbiology, College of Health Sciences, University of Ghana, Accra, Ghana

Mariangela Bonizzoni
Department of Biology and Biotechnology, University of Pavia, Pavia, Italy

Guiyun Yan
Program in Public Health, College of Health Sciences, University of California, Irvine, CA, USA

Tagbo Oguonu and Benedict O. Edelu
Department of Paediatrics, College of Medicine, University of Nigeria, Enugu Campus, Enugu State, Nigeria

Emmanuel Chanda
Department of Biomedical Sciences, School of Medicine, University of Zambia, Lusaka, Zambia

Sunil Dhiman
Defence R&D Establishment (DRDE), Gwalior, Madhya Pradesh, India

Vijay Veer
Defence Research Laboratory, Tezpur, Assam, India

Vas Dev
Senior Scientist (Retired), formerly with the National Institute of Malaria Research, New Delhi, India

Luz García-Longoria, Sergio Magallanes, Manuel González-Blázquez, Yolanda Refollo, Florentino de Lope and Alfonso Marzal
Department of Anatomy, Cellular Biology and Zoology, University of Extremadura, Badajoz, Spain

Amy R. Noe, Vinayaka Kotraiah and Gabriel M. Gutierrez
Leidos Life Sciences, Leidos Inc., Frederick, MD, USA

Che Julius Ngwa, Thiago F. de A. Rosa and Gabriele Pradel
Division of Cellular and Applied Infection Biology, Institute of Zoology, RWTH Aachen University, Aachen, Germany

Josiane Etang
Yaoundé Research Institute, Organisation for the Coordination of Endemic Disease Control in Central Africa, Yaoundé, Cameroon
Faculty of Medicine and Pharmaceutical Sciences, University of Douala, Douala, Cameroon

Betrand Fesuh Nono, Henri Gwet and Eugène Patrice Ndong Nguema
National Advanced School of Engineering, University of Yaoundé I, Yaoundé, Cameroon

Parfait Awono-Ambene and Jean-Claude Toto
Yaoundé Research Institute, Organisation for the Coordination of Endemic Disease Control in Central Africa, Yaoundé, Cameroon

Jude Bigoga
Biotechnology Centre, University of Yaoundé I, Cameroon

Wolfgang Ekoko Eyisap
Yaoundé Research Institute, Organisation for the Coordination of Endemic Disease Control in Central Africa, Yaoundé, Cameroon
Laboratory of Animal Biology and Physiology, University of Douala, Cameroon

Michael Piameu
School of Health Sciences, Catholic University of Central Africa, Yaoundé, Cameroon

Etienne Fondjo
National Malaria Control Programme, Ministry of Public Health, Yaoundé, Cameroon

Abraham Peter Mnzava
Global Malaria Programme, World Health Organization, Geneva, Switzerland

Kevin Pometti
LabexMed, MMSH, CNRS UMR 7303, TELEMME, Aix-Marseille University, Aix-en-Provence, France

Index

R

S

T

U

V

Y

Z

www.ingramcontent.com/pod-product-compliance
Lightning Source LLC
LaVergne TN
LVHW060940220926
848485LV00015B/1146
* 9 7 8 1 6 3 9 8 9 5 3 1 1 *